CONTROVERSIES IN TREATING DIABETES

CONTEMPORARY ENDOCRINOLOGY

P. Michael Conn, SERIES EDITOR

CONTROVERSIES IN TREATING DIABETES

Clinical and Research Aspects

Edited by

DEREK LEROITH, MD, PhD

Division of Endocrinology, Diabetes, and Bone Disease, Department of Medicine, Mount Sinai School of Medicine, New York, NY

AARON I. VINIK, MD, PhD, FCP, FACP

Diabetes Research Institute, Department of Medicine, Eastern Virginia Medical School, The Leonard Strelitz Diabetes Institutes, Norfolk, VA

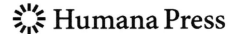 Humana Press

Editors
Derek LeRoith
Division of Endocrinology, Diabetes,
  and Bone Disease
Department of Medicine
Mount Sinai School of Medicine
New York, NY

Aaron I. Vinik
Diabetes Research Institute
Department of Medicine
Eastern Virginia Medical School
The Leonard Strelitz Diabetes Institutes
Norfolk, VA

Series Editor
P. Michael Conn
Oregon Health & Science University
Beaverton, OR

ISBN: 978-1-58829-708-2   e-ISBN: 978-1-59745-572-5

Library of Congress Control Number: 2007933146

PREFACE

Undoubtedly, there is a worldwide epidemic of obesity, the metabolic syndrome and type 2 diabetes, and with these changes comes controversy!

What is the cause of the obesity epidemic? Is the increase in type 2 diabetes caused by obesity alone or are there other factors involved, such as genetics? Is the metabolic syndrome truly a syndrome or merely a grouping of risk factors for cardiovascular disease? How do we effectively prevent and treat the epidemics of obesity, diabetes, and their devastating complications? This book is a compilation of discussions by world experts on these topics. Each chapter was chosen to cover many of the issues that investigators, academics, and healthcare professionals have to deal with in their institutions and private practice.

Stress and dietary excess are presented by Rena Wing, and the explosion of childhood obesity is discussed by Desmond Schatz. On the other hand, treatments for obesity, metabolic syndrome, and hyperlipidemia are discussed separately by Drs. Kaplan, Meigs, and Goldberg, respectively; very practical approaches are presented. The treatment of type 2 diabetes and the anticipation that this would prevent complications are discussed by Vivian Fonseca. Julio Rosenstock presents the case for earlier introduction of insulin in the armamentarium for treating type 2 diabetics. Werner Walthausal presents the pros and cons for a polypill that potentially should improve patient compliance. Incretins are the "new kid on the block" with regard to therapeutic agents and are discussed by Jens Holst. The exciting new concept for hospitalized diabetics (and hyperglycemic nondiabetics) is the use of intensive insulin therapy to manage the hyperglycemia more effectively and reduce mortality and morbidity. This is discussed by Greet van den Berghe, who pioneered the studies.

The underlying mechanisms involved in diabetic complications are summarized by Michael Brownlee and the prevention and treatment of retinopathy and neuropathy is discussed in the chapters by Emily Chew and Aaron Vinik. An important therapeutic area is transplantation. Usually the pancreas is transplanted simultaneously with the kidney once end-stage renal disease requires a kidney transplant. This has generally been shown to help in the control of the diabetes and to protect further complications and damage to vital organs. David Sutherland discusses whether pancreatic transplantation should be performed in the absence of a need for renal transplantation; this is a controversial issue indeed! Another relatively controversial aspect of diabetes management is islet transplantation and David Harlan discusses this important topic in his chapter.

Finally, a critical aspect of patient care is improving quality of life, and for diabetics with such a chronic disorder, this is no less important than all the other aspects discussed in this book! This topic is discussed to Richard Rubin, an expert in this field!

The editors are indebted to the authors who have taken time from their busy schedules to help compile *Controversies in Treating Diabetes: Clinical and Research Aspects* with such important topics. We hope the readers feel likewise.

Derek LeRoith
Aaron I. Vinik

CONTENTS

CONTRIBUTORS

ANDREW J. M. BOULTON, MD, DSC(HONS), FRPC • *Professor of Medicine, Manchester Royal Infirmary, Manchester, United Kingdom*

MICHAEL BROWNLEE, MD • *Professor of Medicine, Albert Einstein College of Medicine, Jack and Pearl Resnick Campus, Morris Park Avenue, Bronx, NY*

EMILY Y. CHEW, MD • *Deputy Director, Division of Epidemiology and Clinical Research, National Eye Institute Health, Bethesda, MD*

CAROLYN F. DEACON, DR. MED SCI • *Associate Professor, University of Copenhagen, Department of Medical Physiology, The Panum Institute, Copenhagen, Denmark*

VIVIAN FONSECA, MD, FRCP • *Professor of Medicine and Pharmacology, Chief of the Section of Endocrinology, Tulane University Health Sciences Center, New Orleans, LA*

RONALD B. GOLDBERG, MD • *Professor of Medicine, Miller School of Medicine, University of Miami, Miami, FL*

ANGELIKA C. GRUESSNER, PhD • *University of Minnesota, Minneapolis, MN*

DAVID M. HARLAN, MD, NIDDK • *Chief, Islet and Autoimmunity Branch, National Institutes of Health, Bethesda, MD*

JENS JUUL HOLST, MD • *Professor of Medical Physiology, Department of Medical Physiology, The Panum Institute, University of Copenhagen, Copenhagen, Denmark*

ALI JAWA, MD • *King Edward Medical College, Mayo Hospital EMW, Lahore, Pakistan*

L. M. KAPLAN, MD • *MGH Weight Center, Massachusetts General Hospital, Boston, MA*

DEREK LEROITH, MD, PhD • *Division of Endocrinology, Diabetes, and Bone Disease, Department of Medicine, Mount Sinai School of Medicine, New York, NY*

ERIC H. LIU, MD • *Diabetes Branch, National Institute of Diabetes and Digestive and Kidney Diseases, Bethesda, MD*

TAKESHI MATSUMURA, MD • *Diabetes Research Center, Albert Einstein College of Medicine, Bronx, NY*

JAMES B. MEIGS, MD, MPH • *Department of Medicine, General Medicine Division, Massachusetts General Hospital, Harvard Medical School, Boston, MA*

ix

HEATHER M. NIEMEIER, PhD • *Brown Medical School, The Miriam Hospital, Providence, RI*

DAVID OWENS, CBE, MD • *Diabetes Research Unit, University of Wales College of Medicine, Llandough Hospital, Cardiff, Wales*

ANGELA MARINILLI PINTO, PhD • *Brown Medical School, The Miriam Hospital, Providence, RI*

JULIO ROSENSTOCK, MD • *Dallas Diabetes and Endocrine Center at Medical City, Dallas, TX*

RICHARD R. RUBIN, MD • *Department of Medicine, John Hopkins University, Monkton, MD*

DESMOND A. SCHATZ, MD • *Associate Chairman of Pediatrics, Medical Director of the Diabetes Center, University of Florida, Gainesville, FL*

MICHAEL S. STALVEY, MD • *Division of Pediatric Endocrinology, Department of Pediatrics, University of Florida, Gainesville, FL*

DAVID E. R. SUTHERLAND, MD, PhD • *Professor, General and Transplant Surgery, Chief, Division of Transplantation Director, Diabetes Institute for Immunology and Transplantation, University of Minnesota, Minneapolis, MN*

GREET VAN DEN BERGHE, MD, PhD • *Department of Intensive Care Medicine, Catholic University of Leuven, Leuven, Belgium*

ILSE VANHOREBEEK, PhD • *Department of Intensive Care Medicine, Catholic University of Leuven, Leuven, Belgium*

AARON I. VINIK, MD, PhD, FCP, FACP • *Director, Diabetes Research Institute, Scientific Director, Department of Medicine, Professor of Medicine, Eastern Virginia Medical School, The Leonard Strelitz Diabetes Institutes, Norfolk, VA*

WERNER WALDHÄUSL, MD • *Professor of Internal Medicine, Department of Medicine III, Division of Endocrinology and Metabolism, Medical University of Vienna, Vienna, Austria*

RENA R. WING, PhD • *Professor, Department of Psychiatry and Human Behavior, Brown Medical School, The Miriam Hospital, Providence, RI*

1

Pancreas Transplantation

Should They be Reserved for Simultaneous Renal Transplants?

David E. R. Sutherland, MD, PhD
and Angelika C. Gruessner, PhD

CONTENTS

SUMMARY

In summary, solitary pancreas transplants (alone in non-uremics—PTA; or after a kidney—PAK) should be done, as well as simultaneous pancreas-kidney (SPK) transplants in uremic diabetics who cannot get a kidney transplant first (to preempt or shorten the time on dialysis). The approach depends on the recipient candidate characteristics and on living or deceased donor availability and suitability. It is regressive to restrict pancreas transplants to just the uremic population, and in this restricted population to just those who cannot get an early kidney transplant to preempt the dialysis that would otherwise be necessary while waiting for both organs from a deceased donor. For the uremic diabetic in centers where there is a long wait time for a deceased donor SPK transplants (because of kidney allocation policies), the best option is a living donor kidney followed by a pancreas transplant; a living donor eliminates waiting for a kidney, and the waiting time for a solitary pancreas at present is relatively short. The patient survival rates are high after either PTA, PAK or SPK transplants, at 3 years 93%, 90% and 91% respectively, with corresponding graft survival (insulin-independence) rates

From: *Contemporary Endocrinology: Controversies in Treating Diabetes:
Clinical and Research Aspects*
Edited by: D. LeRoith and A. I. Vinik © Humana Press, Totowa, NJ

of 60%, 66% and 78%, respectively. Even though pancreas graft survival rates are higher after SPK transplants, the gain in patient survival rates by doing a preemptive kidney transplant more than offsets the lower insulin-independence rates after a PAK. The outcomes justify the continuance of pancreas transplants in all three categories of recipients, with nearly all nephropathic diabetics being PAK or SPK candidates (since immunosuppression will be obligatory for a kidney transplant), and selected non-uremic diabetics, particularly those with hypoglycemic unawareness, being candidates for a PTA.

Key Words: Pancreas, transplant, insulin-independence

PANCREAS TRANSPLANTATION: SHOULD THEY BE RESERVED FOR SIMULTANEOUS RENAL TRANSPLANTS?

The answer is no. Pancreas transplants are currently done in three recipient categories, and that practice should continue:

1. *Pancreas transplants alone (PTA)* in diabetic patients without advanced nephropathy but who have problems that justify the use of immunosuppression to achieve insulin independence, the main one being hypoglycemic unawareness *(1)*.
2. *Pancreas after kidney (PAK) transplants*, done in patients with diabetic nephropathy. The majority receive a living donor (LD) kidney to preempt or remove the need for dialysis *(2)*. Such patients are already obligated to immunosuppression, and it is only the surgical risks that need to be considered. If uremic diabetic patients were not offered the opportunity for a PAK but told they could only get a pancreas as a simultaneous pancreas and kidney (SPK) transplant, it would be a disincentive to perform an LD kidney transplant. Those who opt for a deceased donor (DD) SPK versus an LD kidney transplant alone (KTA) would have to go on a waiting list and accept the increased mortality risk of dialysis versus a preemptive kidney transplant *(3)*.
3. *SPK transplants*, most commonly done with organs from the same DD, in some cases with both from an LD, and in others with the kidney from an LD and the pancreas from a DD *(4)*. Again, the recipient is obligated to immunosuppression in lieu of the kidney, and there is no reason not to add a pancreas other than the additional surgical risk. The main drawback to going on the list for a same DD SPK transplant is the potential long waiting time and the need to go on dialysis versus receiving a preemptive LD kidney transplant. Because the wait time for a DD solitary pancreas transplant is relatively short (as opposed to the wait time for a kidney), an LD kidney followed by a DD pancreas will usually result in insulin-independence being achieved in the nephropathic diabetic sooner than if one waits for an SPK. However, for uremic diabetics without an LD for a kidney graft, an SPK transplant makes sense and in the

USA is associated with higher graft survival rate of the Kidney in SPK Kd than in uremic diabetic recipients of a DD KTA *(5)*. For 1995–2004 DD SPK transplants in the USA, the kidney graft survival rates at 1, 3, and 5 years were 92, 85, and 77%, respectively, versus 89, 77, and 65% for DD KTA diabetic recipients *(5)*. As PAK recipients have a functioning kidney at the time of the pancreas transplant, the kidney graft survival rates are higher in PAK recipients than in SPK recipients, but this is true even when adjustments are made in the calculations to account for the attrition that would occur in PAK candidates *(6,7)*.

Except for the immediate surgical risks, the main drawback of a transplant (allograft) of any kind is the need for immunosuppression and the side effects (both immunosuppressive and non-immunosuppressive) of the antirejection drugs.

Indeed, SPK and PAK recipients get two benefits for the price of immuno-suppression: an insulin-independent, as well as a dialysis-free, state. The benefits are the same whether both organs are transplanted simultaneously or sequentially. The advantages of an SPK over a PAK transplant is placement of both organs with one operation and, when both organs are from the same donor, the ability to use kidney graft function to monitor for rejection episodes that affect both organs, leading to slightly higher graft survival rate of the Pancreas in SPK Px (85% at 1 year for 2000–2004 US cases) than for solitary pancreas transplants (76% for PTA and 78% for PAK) *(2)*, where monitoring for rejection is more difficult *(6)*. However, the advantages of an SPK may be offset by the long waiting time for DD organs when the allocation is primarily by the rules for kidney allocation, and the mortality rate in uremic candidates waiting for an SPK transplant is much higher than in candidates waiting for a PAK transplant who improved their survival probabilities already by having an expeditious LD kidney transplant that preempted the need for or minimized their time on dialysis *(3,5,7)*.

Thus, one must ask the question as to why the question is asked, because the current outcomes (of patient and graft survival rates) in all three categories have to be considered good. Indeed, PTA recipients enjoy the highest patient survival rate following transplantation compared with any other organ allograft recipient groups (not only versus the other categories of pancreas transplants but versus kidney, heart, and liver recipients as well), according to Port et al. *(8)*—91% at 5 years for PTA recipients done between 1998 and 2004, versus 81% for DD KTA and 90% for LD KTA recipients, 85% for PAK and 86% for SPK recipients, and 73% for both liver and heart recipients.

However, there are no randomized trials of pancreas transplantation versus exogenous insulin treatment in any of the categories, and even in the group with simultaneous kidney and pancreas transplants, no randomized comparisons have been done to kidney transplants alone. Thus, even though the graft survival rates are higher for a pancreas with an SPK than the other categories, the impact on patient survival or kidney graft survival of adding the pancreas is technically not known. At least for SPK, it is clear that the relative risk of dying while waiting for a transplant (usually while on dialysis) is higher than that for those who actually receive an SPK transplant. For PAK and PTA recipients, an analysis by Venstrom et al. *(9)* of the United Network for Organ Sharing (UNOS) database suggested that the mortality hazard ratio was slightly higher for PAK and PTA recipients than for those on the waiting list. A subsequent analysis of the same cohort of patients as well as an updated cohort by Gruessner et al. *(10)*, correcting for the counting of patients twice in the Venstrom analysis for those listed at more than one center and for the inappropriate exclusions of patients based on creatinine criteria, showed the hazard ratio for dying was higher for those on the PTA- and PAK-waiting lists than for those who had been transplanted.

The most recent analyses by the International Pancreas Transplant Registry of US cases in all three categories, as reported to the UNOS data base, support the above points *(2,10)*, and the highlights are summarized in detail. First, despite the slightly higher pancreas graft survival rates in the SPK than in the PAK and PTA categories, the number of transplants in the latter categories has increased annually for the past decade, whereas the number of SPK transplants has plateaued (Fig. 1). This change reflects the increased use of LD kidney transplants to treat uremic diabetics who then go on to get a DD pancreas. Over that same interval, the graft survival rates have also improved in all categories but most dramatically in the PAK and PTA recipients (Fig. 2). Patient survival

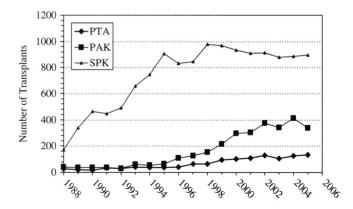

Fig. 1. Annual number of US pancreas transplants by category, 1988–2005.

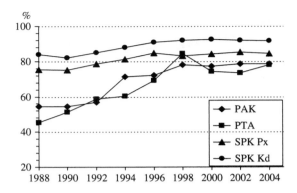

Fig. 2. Pancreas and simultaneous pancreas and kidney (SPK) kidney graft function for 1988–2005 US deceased donor (DD) primary pancreas transplants by recipient category.

rates were high in all categories during the entire decade, ranging from 90 to 98% at 1 year and from 80 to 90% at 5 years for the annual cohorts.

In an analysis of contemporary cases (2000–2005), patient survival rates are shown in Fig. 3 and pancreas graft survival (insulin-independence) rates in Fig. 4. At 3 years, patient survival rates in SPK, PAK, and PTA recipients were 91, 90, and 93%, respectively, and the corresponding 3-year pancreas graft survival rates were 78, 66, and 60%.

In regard to the question of mortality rates while waiting versus after a pancreas transplant, the data from the analysis of the UNOS data base for the period 1995–2003 by Gruessner et al. *(10)* are shown. The survival on the waiting list for each category of patients is shown in Fig. 5. At 1 year, 3% of PTA and PAK candidates died versus 7% of SPK candidates, a relatively

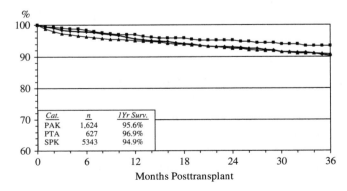

Fig. 3. Patient survival rates in US deceased donor (DD) primary pancreas transplants by recipient category, January 1, 2000 to December 31, 2005.

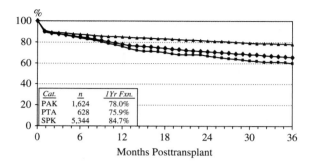

Fig. 4. Pancreas graft functional survival rates in US deceased donor (DD) primary pancreas transplants by recipient category, January 1, 2000 to December 31, 2005.

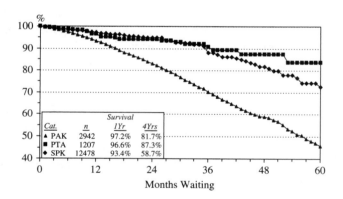

Fig. 5. Patient survival while waiting, all recipient categories, United Network for Organ Sharing (UNOS) pancreas waiting list, January 1, 1995 to May 31, 2003.

small difference, but at 4 years, the mortality rates while waiting were 13, 18, and 41%, respectively, showing the enormous impact remaining uremic has on survival probabilities for diabetic patients. In contrast, recipients of SPK transplants have a dramatically increased probability of survival compared with their counterparts still on the waiting list, with a 45% delta at 4 years (Fig. 6). Although less dramatic, the PTA (Fig. 7) and PAK recipients (Fig. 8) also have higher survival rates at 1 and 4 years than their counterparts on the waiting list, with deltas of 5 and 14% at 4 years. Although of marginal significance, at least we can conclude that solitary pancreas transplants do not increase mortality rates in the recipient population *(10)*. The relative hazard of

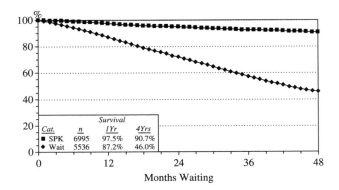

Fig. 6. Simultaneous pancreas and kidney (SPK) patient survival from time of listing, United Network for Organ Sharing (UNOS) pancreas waiting list, January 1, 1995 to May 31, 2003.

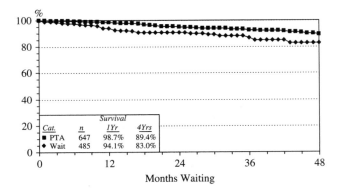

Fig. 7. Pancreas transplants alone (PTA) patient survival from time of listing, United Network for Organ Sharing (UNOS) pancreas waiting list, January 1, 1995 to May 31, 2003.

dying after a pancreas transplant is less by 2 months in SPK, 3 months in PAK, and 8 months in PTA recipients than remaining on the waiting list (Fig. 9).

Retrospective analysis of outcomes done in registries is helpful but does not begin to capture the dilemma facing the patient. For example, if one were to say we should only do a pancreas transplant simultaneous with a kidney transplant from a DD, then one would lose the ability to preempt dialysis with a kidney transplant, as this would then relegate the patient to not being eligible for a pancreas transplant, and they may bypass an LD kidney for an SPK and take the risk of dying while waiting. The apparent advantage of an SPK over PAK is only in one aspect, a 7% higher pancreas graft survival rate at 1 year (9% vs. PTA) *(2)*. However, patient survival rates are much higher in uremic

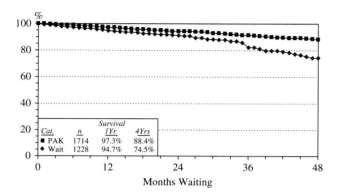

Fig. 8. Pancreas after kidney (PAK) patient survival from time of listing, United Network for Organ Sharing (UNOS) pancreas waiting list, January 1, 1995 to May 31, 2003.

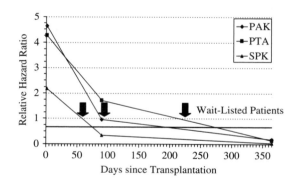

Fig. 9. Relative hazard ratios of patient survival while waiting, all recipient categories, United Network for Organ Sharing (UNOS) pancreas waiting list, January 1, 1995 to May 31, 2003.

patients who receive a preemptive kidney transplant. If allocation favors SPK so it would render moot the advantage of doing an LD kidney to preempt dialysis, then, of course, an SPK is one operation and it has an advantage. Dialysis can always be preempted with LD SPK transplants *(6)*, but again, there are almost for sure not enough living volunteers to donate both a kidney and a pancreas to offset the need. As there are so many non-diabetic uremic patients waiting for kidney transplants, the national allocation program cannot allow all DDs to be used for SPK transplants; so, to utilize all pancreases and not be wasteful, solitary (PAK and PTA) as well as SPK transplants must be offered.

The above arguments for doing solitary (PAK and PTA) than just SPK transplants are also pertinent to the minimally invasive form of beta-cell replacement therapy, islet transplantation *(11)*. What is needed for the liberal application of beta-cell transplants are antirejection protocols in which the non-immunosuppressive as well as immunosuppressive side effects are minimized *(12)*. However, for sure, uremic diabetic patients who undergo kidney transplants should have the option of simultaneous or sequential pancreas transplants to take full advantage of donor availability and suitability, and the use of PTA in selected non-uremic recipients is certainly justified by the current outcomes.

REFERENCES

1. Sutherland DER. Pancreas and islet transplant population. In: Gruessner RWG, Sutherland DER, eds. *Transplantation of the Pancreas*. New York: Springer-Verlag, 2004:91–102.
2. Gruessner AC, Sutherland DE. Pancreas transplant outcomes for United States (US) and non-US cases as reported to the United Network for Organ Sharing (UNOS) and the International Pancreas Transplant Registry (IPTR) as of June 2004. *Clin Transplant* 2005;19:433–455.
3. Schnitzler, MA, et al. The life-years saved by a deceased organ donor. *Am J Transpl* 2005:2289–2296.
4. Farney, AC, et al. Simultaneous cadaver pancreas living donor kidney transplantation (SPLK). *Ann Surg* 2000;232:646–703.
5. Cohen, DJ, et al. Kidney and pancreas transplantation in the United States, 1995–2004. *Am J Transpl* 2006:6(Pt 2):1153–1169.
6. Sutherland, DE, et al. Lessons learned from more than 1,000 pancreas transplants at a single institution. *Ann Surg* 2001;233:463–501.
7. Gruessner, AC, et al. Pancreas after kidney transplants in posturemic patients with type 1 diabetes mellitus. *J Am Soc Nephrol* 2001;12:2490–2499.
8. Port, FK, et al. Recent trends and results for organ donation and transplantation in the United States, 2005. *Am J Transpl* 2006;(pt 2):1095–1100.
9. Venstrom, JM, et al. Survival after pancreas transplantation in patients with diabetes and preserved kidney function. *J Am Med Assoc* 2003;290:2817–2823.
10. Gruessner RWG, Sutherland DER, Gruessner AW. Mortality Assessment in Pancreas Transplants. *Am J Transpl* 2004;4:2018–2026.
11. Feng, S, et al. Developments in clinical islet, liver, thoracic, kidney and pancreas transplantation in the last 5 years. *Am J Transpl* 2006;6:1759–1767.
12. Sutherland, DER. Beta-cell replacement by transplantation in diabetes mellitus: which patients at what risk; which way (when pancreas, when islets), and how to allocate deceased donor pancreases. *Curr Opin Transplant* 2005;10:147–149.

2 Islet Cell Transplantation
How Effective Is It?

Eric H. Liu, MD
and David M. Harlan, MD

CONTENTS

SUMMARY

Islet cell transplantation as a treatment for diabetes has shown great promise, but has significant limitations. Since early animal studies in rats demonstrated its ability to restore euglycemia, islet transplantation has not proven to be a durable or practical therapy for type 1 diabetes. Here we review some of the history, technique, clinical outcomes, and potential alternatives of islet transplantation.

From: *Contemporary Endocrinology: Controversies in Treating Diabetes:
Clinical and Research Aspects*
Edited by: D. LeRoith and A. I. Vinik © Humana Press, Totowa, NJ

Key Words: Islet, transplantation, beta-cell, liberase, immunosuppression, adverse events, encapsulation, progenitors, regeneration, isolation, technique, edmonton protocol, risks, benefits.

Cell-based transplantation has long held great promise as a diabetes treatment alternative. Since islets were first identified in the pancreas by Paul Langerhans in 1869, and after von Mering and Minkowski demonstrated that total pancreatectomy in dogs resulted in diabetes, several attempts have been made to use pancreatic tissue to reverse diabetes (1–4). For instance, in 1894, Williams grafted pancreatic tissue from a slaughtered sheep into the subcutaneous tissue of a 15-year-old boy with diabetes but failed to revive him; the boy died 3 days later (5). Insulin's discovery and first clinical use in 1922 temporarily deflated pressure for transplant approaches. However, with increasing awareness that insulin neither cures diabetes nor absolutely prevents its complications, interest in tissue transplant was revived when Lacy and his colleagues in St. Louis demonstrated in the 1960s and 1970s that isolated pancreatic islets could reverse diabetes in experimental rodent models. That early laboratory animal success was tested in clinical trials, but with minimal success. Another generation passed before enthusiasm was reinfused in clinical islet transplantation with the "Edmonton" Protocol report in 2000. Since then, islet transplantation euphoria again waned when new limitations with the technique were recognized. Thus, although the field has advanced considerably, several barriers must be overcome before cell transplantation as a diabetes treatment can fulfill its long-standing promise.

HISTORY

Since Lacy's early work, a major hurdle was the imperfect technique for isolating viable islets in sufficient numbers and with preserved function (6). Early investigators used a laborious and inefficient microdissection technique but only produced enough tissue to study islet physiology (7,8). A major advance came with the use of collagenase to enzymatically dissociate the pancreas to yield isolated islets (9,10). The techniques were refined, for instance, by injecting the collagenase into the pancreatic duct, and allowed Ballinger and Lacy (11) to transplant syngeneic rat islets intraperitoneally to cure experimental diabetes. The Lacy team further refined the technique by using density gradients to separate islets from pancreatic acinar tissue and implanting the purified islets into the liver by portal vein infusion (12,13). This critical early work, all accomplished in the 1970s, established the basic techniques that while refined since, remain largely unchanged. That is, islet transplantation as currently practiced in both large animal trials and clinical studies isolates islets and infuses them more or less as worked out by those early pioneers. More recent improvements have been to automate, in part, the islet isolation process and to improve the purity and activity of the critical collagenase enzyme (e.g., Liberase® made by Roche).

ISLET ISOLATION

Although the islet isolation technique, using broad brushstrokes, is quite similar to that developed over 20 years ago, a fair amount of variation in technique exists between islet isolation centers (14). We will review the isolation technique in more detail and discuss some of the finer points related to the technique.

The majority of isolated human islets are derived from cadaveric organ donors. As with whole organ procurement, the pancreas is flushed with preservation solution (e.g., University of Wisconsin Solution) and kept on ice. The pancreas is typically procured along with the donor's duodenum and spleen, and special care is given to avoid damaging the pancreatic capsule (15). The organ is then transported to the laboratory on ice in either preservation solution alone or using the more recently developed "two-layer" method that adds the oxygen-carrying solution perfluorocarbon (PFC) (16–18).

Once the organ arrives in the laboratory, isolation proceeds in four general stages. One, the pancreas is isolated from extraneous tissues and "inflated" with collagenase by injecting the enzyme into the pancreatic duct. Two, the collagenase "digests" the pancreas. Three, small pancreatic cell aggregates continuously released by the collagenase digestion are collected and washed to stop continued digestion. Four, islets are isolated from other pancreatic cell aggregates (taking advantage of acinar tissue's greater density) using density gradient separation techniques. All procedures are performed in biological safety cabinets and under otherwise sterile and controlled conditions.

After the organ is cleaned and the pancreatic duct cannulated, cold collagenase (typically Liberase®) solution is injected to "inflate" the pancreas with enzyme. The gland is then often cut into smaller fragments and is transferred into the digestion chamber (named "Ricordi chamber" in honor of Dr. Camillo Ricordi who played an instrumental role improving isolation techniques). The digestion step consists of a closed fluid circuit that includes the Ricordi chamber, a heating coil, a peristaltic pump, a sampling port, and a collection flask (Fig. 1). The inflated pancreas segments and several marbles are placed together into the Ricordi chamber. A screen with 500-μm opening filters the chamber allowing only small pieces of tissue to escape. A pump is started to circulate the fluid, and the chamber is shaken—either by hand or by placing the chamber in a shaker machine. The circulating fluid is warmed to 37°C and then fluid samples are repeatedly taken and examined microscopically to determine when the digestion is complete. The trained islet isolator knows when the islets are sufficiently liberated from the acinar tissue but not "over digested." Over digestion, to be avoided, means that the collagenase has disrupted the islets themselves into smaller cellular fragments thought to be be less viable and functional. Once the digestion is considered complete, the circuit is converted into a linear system design to quickly dilute and inactivate the collagenase, drawing in cold media (inactivating the enzyme with temperature) and adding human albumin to the fluid flowing through the chamber (to chemically inactivate the enzyme). The fluid is collected into multiple chilled conical flasks, pooled, and prepared for the density gradient separation step.

Density gradient separation techniques vary. Most laboratories rely on Ficoll® gradients, but some use non-sucrose-based solutions (e.g., Optiprep®). Either a continuous or a discontinuous gradient can be used as acinar cell aggregates will migrate into the most-dense gradient, whereas islets tend to gravitate to a less-dense layer. After a short centrifugation, the gradient is expelled and collected into chilled tubes to promptly dilute the polysucrose gradient. Each tube is sampled and assessed for islet content and purity. Fractions enriched in pure or relatively pure islets are pooled, samples are taken, and the islets are counted and assessed. The cells are ready now ready for culture or transplantation.

LIMITS OF THE PROCEDURE

Although the islet isolation procedure has been successfully performed in dozens of laboratories around the world, the technique remains imperfect. As many as half the isolation attempts are considered failed because too few islets are isolated, or the isolated islets are overly digested, not sufficiently viable, or unsatisfactorily purified from acinar tissue (19). Several issues may contribute to failed islet isolation efforts, starting with the donor. Lakey and colleagues looked retrospectively at several of their isolation efforts, and using a relatively generous definition of success [150,000 islet equivalents (IEQs)—to be defined later in this section], they reported that increased donor age, higher donor body mass index, and a local procurement team all correlated with a more successful outcome. On the contrary, donor hyperglycemia, cardiac arrest, donor reliances on high dose pressors to maintain blood pressure, and prolonged cold storage had a negative impact (20). Moreover, careful surgical technique and particular attention to keeping the pancreas chilled during the procurement also affected the islet yield (21). While these factors can be used to screen for higher quality donors, recall that all donors are brain dead, and brain death itself has been shown to negatively impact islet yield and function, perhaps through up-regulation of inflammatory cytokine [tumor necrosis factor (TNF)-α, interleukin (IL)-1β, and IL-6] levels (22). To a limited degree, islets have been isolated from living donors (partial pancreatectomy in a single allogeneic donor case report or complete pancreatectomy for autotransplantation), and such efforts appear to generate a higher islet yield and islets with better function (23–27). These data further support the concept that brain death is bad for islet isolation efforts and for ultimate isolated islet function. Unfortunately, until other sources are found, cadaveric pancreas donation will remain the major islet source for clinical transplantation efforts.

Research to refine isolation techniques continues to progress, but the technique remains quite expensive, requires an experienced team, and demands considerable resources. The reagents themselves can be variable—starting with the collagenase enzyme. Many centers use an enzymatic blend (Liberase®) that effectively digests the pancreas, but suffers from some lot-to-lot variability, and many investigators believe the shelf life is relatively short. Furthermore, centers often disagree about which enzyme lots are effective and which are not. And as mentioned above, determining the optimal time to end the pancreas digestion during the isolation procedure requires an experienced islet isolator. This end-of-digestion call remains as much an art as it is a science. Most recently on April 18, 2007, groups around the world using Liberase (R) to isolate islets were informed that the reagent was exposed to cow brain extract during manufacturing. While the risk of transmitting bovine spongiform encephalopathy is quite low, it is not zero. Programs using Liberase (R) have curtailed clinical islet transplantation, thus pointing out the technique's experimental nature.

Investigators have tested many different techniques for quantifying islet quality but none is yet absolutely predictive of clinical function. Even determining the islet yield remains a challenge. As isolated islets vary significantly in size, standard procedure calls for estimating the "IEQs," resulting from the isolation. To assess IEQ number, an aliquot of the digested pancreas is taken, and the number of islets falling within several size ranges is counted (for example, 0–50 μm in diameter, 51–100 μm, 101–150 μm, etc.). Using these counts, the cumulative islet volume is calculated by a mathematical formula to convert that volume into a theoretical IEQ number where all the islets are 150 μm in diameter. Unfortunately, the process is user and sampling dependent, making it a relatively subjective technique (28). Purity has also been a challenging parameter to measure with precision. Currently, islet preparations are stained with dithizone, a dye that takes advantage of β cells' high zinc content by binding to that metal to stain the islets red. The islet isolator then estimates the percentage purity by examining an aliquot of the pancreas digest. This method is even more subjective than islet counting such that different observer's islet purity assessments vary considerably. A variety of islet functional assays also exist including in vitro glucose-stimulated (either using "static" glucose incubations or perifusion assays in which glucose concentrations vary over time) insulin release assays and oxygen consumption assays (29–31). These in vitro assays have the great advantage of generating a result quickly to help decide which islet preparations are of sufficient quality for transplant. The problem is that no assay is yet well validated for its clinical predictive power. That is, some islet preparations measured to be of high quality by in vitro assay results fail to function well in vivo. Many believe that a more laborious and time-consuming in vivo assay for islet function is a better predictor of clinical function. For this in vivo assay, isolated islets are transplanted into diabetic immuno-incompetent mice to see whether the islets restore normal glucose homeostasis to the animal. This type of assay does not provide its information in a timely enough fashion to dictate which islets can be used clinically and is limited by the large number of islets needed. New techniques are being tested in hopes of improving the islet assessment process.

CLINICAL ISLET TRANSPLANTATION

By the late 1980s, improved isolation techniques and breakthroughs in immunosuppression made possible clinical trials to test islet transplantation in patients with type 1 diabetes mellitus (T1DM). Following some not well documented and unsuccessful clinical islet transplantation efforts by others, David Scharp and Paul Lacy of Washington University in St. Louis first reported a clinical islet transplant success when they transplanted islets into the portal vein of a diabetic kidney transplant recipient (32). This patient received nearly 800,000 IEQs (obtained from several donors) and was immuno-suppressed with anti-lymphocyte globulin and cyclosporine. Following the islet infusion, the patient was given intravenous insulin for a few days to maintain tight blood glucose control. Once the insulin infusion was stopped, the patient retained C-peptide production with near-normal fasting blood glucose and significantly improved blood glucose control. All exogenous insulin was stopped 10 days after the islet infusion, and the patient continued to have normal glucose levels until day 25, when insulin therapy was reinstituted because of gradually worsening glycemia control. The St. Louis group expanded their study to include diabetic patients with preserved kidney function, and they tested different immunosuppressive approaches. In most cases, subjects were able to achieve partial graft function with increased C-peptide production. However, only one patient was able to maintain sustained insulin indepen-dence; most patients rejected their grafts. As demonstrated by Scharp and Lacy, patients who only received 6000 IEq/kg body weight were never restored to insulin independence, whereas those who received almost 14,000 IEq/kg were occasionally able to achieve at least temporary insulin independence. With regard to cell quality, all the preparations demonstrated good glucose-stimulated insulin release, reflecting standard assays' inability to predict clinical outcome.

After this initial case series, the procedure was tested at other institutions but with similar mixed results (*33–35*). The International Islet Registry documented several cases of short-term insulin independence but no long-term success (*36*). An overall conclusion of these studies was that in addition to the difficulty of obtaining sufficient numbers and quality of islets for clinical transplantation, perhaps a more significant barrier limiting transplant-based approaches to diabetes was the imperfect efficacy and safety of existing immunosuppressive therapies.

IMMUNOSUPPRESSION

T1DM, at least in theory, represents a most difficult challenge for immuno-suppression because, following the transplant of allogeneic β cells (using either a whole organ transplant or isolated islets) both an alloimmune and an autoimmune response may exist to destroy those islets. That is, T1DM is caused by a T-cell-mediated autoimmune killing of β cells (and data suggest that this autoimmune response never wanes), and in addition to that autoimmune response, transplanting tissues from a cadaveric human donor always generates an alloimmune response. In an effort to control both, combination immuno-suppression was employed (*37–39*). Initial approaches used cyclosporine, one of various anti-lymphocyte antibodies, anti-proliferative agents (e.g., azathio-prine), and corticosteroids. Steroids were appropriately deemed particularly detrimental to the graft, because of the well-known nature of glucocorticoids to raise the blood sugar level. Current data suggest that calcineurin inhibitors (e.g., cyclosporine) probably exacerbated the unfavorable environment for transplanted beta-cell survival and function (*40*).

THE EDMONTON ADVANCE

On the basis of these early studies, the group from Edmonton, Alberta, Canada, developed a protocol to assess whether four modifications to the standard clinical islet transplant approach could improve overall outcome. The "Edmonton" protocol modifications included (i) transplanting more islets from multiple pancreas donors, (ii) using a novel and less diabetogenic immunosup-pressive regimen, (iii) avoiding animal products (i.e., fetal calf serum) during cell processing, and (iv) minimizing cell culture and transplanting the isolated islets as soon as possible after their isolation. In 2000, they reported a series of seven consecutive cadaveric islet transplant recipients all rendered insulin independent for at least 1 year, and with normal blood sugar control (*41*). For the first time, islet transplantation resulted in relatively sustained insulin independence and in a consistent fashion.

Widespread experience since that publication now suggests that of the four modifications made by the Edmonton group, the islet number infused and the immunosuppression employed after the transplant were the most important factors underlying their success. Since "Edmonton," additional technical advances have been reported. The two-layer pancreas preservation method has become more widely used as it appears to reproducibly promote good islet isolation results (17). And centers have resumed culturing islets before transplant. Islets not cultured are comparable with cultured cells for a limited period with regard to function post-transplant, and the culture period allows for more complete testing of the isolated islet "product" and to orchestrate the islet transplant procedure during regular working hours and with a stable and rested transplant team. Moreover, culture time allows unpurified acinar tissue to degrade. A few centers have reasoned that the islet transplant procedure may be feasible wherever a hospital has a trained and equipped interventional radiology suite but that islet isolation may be best performed at centers well versed in that fine art. To that end, a few groups have collaborated by transporting cadaveric pancreata to a specialized center for the isolation procedure, then returning the isolated islets to the original center for transplantation (42–45). Such a strategy would allow the transplant center to focus on patient care and relatively quickly offer a novel therapy, without having to make the significant investment required to build, staff, and equip an islet isolation facility.

ISLET TRANSPLANTATION OUTCOME FOLLOW-UP

The success of the Edmonton Protocol infused the islet transplantation field with tremendous energy. And the excitement was appropriate. The glucocorticoid-free immunosuppressive regimen they employed had enjoyed some limited success in kidney allograft recipients, relying on a monoclonal antibody against the IL-2 receptor (daclizumab) every 2 weeks for five doses as an induction therapy, in conjunction with tacrolimus (FK506) and sirolimus (rapamycin) (46–49). Like cyclosporine, tacrolimus also has significant diabetes-promoting effects, but the Edmonton group used lower doses than typically employed for other organ transplants. In that original series, seven consecutive patients became insulin free after a sufficient number of islets were infused, the patients suffered no significant hypoglycemia, the mean amplitude of glycemic excursion was decreased, and the percentage of glucose values within the normal range markedly improved. There were some complications from the infusion procedure and the immunosuppression, but no patients died from their islet transplants. Islet transplantation had finally succeeded.

Islet transplantation not only offered the reality of insulin independence, it also offered a new model for testing transplant tolerance. Everyone reasoned that if a cell transplant was rejected because an experimental therapy failed, the only risk for the patient was going back on insulin—a much better option compared with dialysis (kidney) or death (liver, heart, lungs). Other centers attempted to replicate Edmonton's historic results. Thanks to significant helpful input from both Edmonton and the University of Miami, our National Institutes of Health (NIH) group quickly replicated the protocol, with results similar to that since reported by centers around the world, including longer follow-up results reported from Edmonton *(50)*. Networks around the world were created to perform more islet transplants. The Immune Tolerance Network (ITN), sponsored by the NIH and the Juvenile Diabetes Research Foundation (JDRF), initiated a multi-center trial to test whether Edmonton's results could be reproduced at other centers, then serve as a model for the testing of novel therapies designed to achieve immunological tolerance *(51)*. Islet Cell Resource centers were created around the USA to provide good quality isolated islets for both research and transplant studies. It was an exciting time.

Gradually however, a more sober view of the field evolved. For the multi-center ITN trial, centers with islet isolation and transplantation experience enjoyed results similar to Edmonton's—but other centers were not so fortunate. Furthermore, follow-up data showed that long-term insulin independence was difficult to maintain. After 1 year, the Edmonton group still had promising data—most patients were insulin free or treated with oral hypoglycemic agents and low-dose insulin *(34)*. But most recently Edmonton reported on 65 islet transplant recipients and reported a 1-year insulin independence rate of 64%, a 3-year insulin independence rate of only 20%, and a 5-year insulin independence rate of <10% (median 15 months) *(35)*. On the contrary, 80% of the patients maintained circulating C-peptide levels suggesting that some of the islets continued to function, and at 5 years, the vast majority enjoyed normal HgA1c values.

Of great concern to many however have been the risks associated with the immunosuppressive therapy and the transplant procedure itself. With longer follow-up, Edmonton protocol immunosuppression with both tacrolimus and sirolimus has been found to produce significant side effects. Common adverse effects of tacrolimus include neurotoxicity (tremor, headache, motor disturbances), gastrointestinal (GI) complaints, hypertension, and hyperkalemia. But the greatest concern is the nephrotoxicity and specific beta-cell toxicity. Patients on sirolimus can exhibit hyperlipidemia, oral ulcers, anemia, leukopenia, thrombocytopenia, hypokalemia or hyperkalemia, fever, gastrointestinal effects, delayed wound healing, and edema. Although not nephrotoxic itself, sirolimus appears to exacerbate the nephrotoxicity of calcineurin inhibitors (cyclosporin and tacrolimus). In the original Edmonton series, 2 of 15 procedures required transfusion secondary to bleeding from the hepatic cannulation, and all patients had at least some minor buccal ulceration from the sirolimus. They reported no changes in lipids and no patients required lipid-lowering therapy, but their follow-up was only 4–15 months. With the more recent report including 5-year follow-up, 15 of 65 subjects had major bleeding from the cannulation requiring intervention (transfusion or laparotomy). Over half of the patients had transient elevations in their liver enzymes that lasted approximately 4 weeks, but 8 of 36 patients who underwent abdominal magnetic resonance imaging were found to have (MRI) developed fatty liver. With regard to the immunosuppression, mouth ulcers were highly prevalent (89%), while also prevalent were diarrhea, acne, edema, ovarian cysts, and anemia. Three patients developed pneumonia and one developed thyroid papillary carcinoma. The use of lipid-lowering medications also increased from 23% of patients pre-transplant to 86% after 5 years. A recent report from Edmonton showed that Islet transplant recipients inexorably lost kidney function over time, from an initial creatinine clearance of 89 ml/min/1.73m^2 at baseline, to 58 ml/min/1.73m^2 four years post transplant (52). The authors attributed the worsening kidney function to the patients underlying chronic diabetes, but recent reports from others call that interpretation into question. For instance, a report from Finland that included nearly every patient diagnosed with T1DM in that country since 1965 found a remarkably low incidence of renal failure (53). On the contrary, myriad studies now suggest that modern immunosuppressive regimens significantly increase the risk of renal insufficiency, suggesting that the declining renal function seen in the islet transplant recipients may have been caused by the immunosuppression given to preserve the allogeneic islets and not the underlying diabetes (54).

Other centers have tried various islet transplantation strategies. At the University of Minnesota, subjects and donor pancreata were carefully selected and eight of eight patients achieved insulin independence, with five of the eight lasting 1 year (55). At the University of Miami, 14 of 16 patients achieved insulin independence, with 11 remaining off insulin for at least 1 year and six off insulin for at least 18 months (56). Other large centers achieved similar results (50,57).

BENEFITS, RISKS, AND LIMITATIONS

The patient with difficult-to-control T1DM facing the option of an islet transplant must ask themselves how much risk is justified in return for short-term relief from insulin injections and longer term improved glycemia control. The patient can reasonably count on fewer to no daily insulin injections (for up to several months), would likely check blood glucose values less frequently, and could expect much less risk of hypoglycemia (58). On the contrary, the patient need recognize the risks associated with: the procedure, the immuno-suppression, and with islets placed within the liver.

Let us then discuss the risk/benefit equation from the most global perspective and based on ever evolving but still incomplete knowledge *(59)*. The benefits of good glucose control to lower both the risk of microvascular complications (retinopathy, nephropathy, and neuropathy), and more recently macrovascular complications (myocardial infarctions, cerebrovascular accidents), have been clearly demonstrated by the diabetes control and complications trial (DCCT) and follow-up studies *(60–62)*. These data, coupled with the improved glycemia control most pancreas or islet transplant recipients achieve, have suggested to some that these transplant therapies may too decrease or reverse micro- and macrovascular complications. Indeed, patients with pancreas allografts functioning for 10 years or more have been reported to display less histological evidence of diabetic nephropathy than was present before their pancreas transplant *(63)*.

The question of transplant-based therapy's effects on long-term diabetes complications is more nuanced however. For instance, the DCCT did not study patients with long-standing, complicated diabetes (i.e., those with advanced microvascular or macrovascular complications) and therefore should be viewed more as a prevention study for those complications. As importantly, no patient in the DCCT was treated with immunosuppressive agents and clearly transplant recipients must be so treated. The question then becomes one of comparing the benefits achieved by transplant-based improved glycemia control weighed against the known toxicities associated with immunosuppression. Indeed, even the report studying patients with long-standing pancreas allografts noted that although the kidney biopsies showed less evidence of diabetic nephropathy, the patient's kidney function was actually worse than that pre-transplant *(63)*. And a previous study by the same group evaluating kidney function in pancreas transplant recipients compared patients with functioning pancreas grafts to those who had no transplant or a transplant but lost it (and therefore discontinued immunosuppression). The group with the failed pancreas allografts that never received a transplant had better kidney function, whereas the transplant patients had declining renal function proportional to cyclosporine levels *(64)*. The point is that the net effect of transplant-based and immunosuppression-requiring treatments on diabetes complication endpoints remains unknown and that we must guard against assuming benefit.

Even with regard to patient survival following transplant-based treatments for diabetes, there is uncertainty. An analysis we performed comparing the survival of pancreas allograft recipients with those listed for but still awaiting their pancreas transplant demonstrated a significantly worse survival in the transplanted group—at least for the T1DM patients with preserved kidney function (i.e., serum creatinine less than 2.0 mg/dl) *(65)*. A similar analysis by the Minnesota group did not find the survival disadvantage we reported, but for that analysis patients with renal insufficiency were not excluded, and everyone agrees that patients with diabetes and renal insufficiency have a poor prognosis *(66)*. Indeed, our original paper and other similar analyses found that patients with diabetes and kidney failure did enjoy a transplantation-associated survival benefit but that most if not all of that benefit was attributable to the transplanted kidney with little or no effect of the simultaneously transplanted pancreas.

Considering the fact that most patients undergo islet transplantation for hypoglycemia unawareness, and that intensive insulin therapy is associated with more hypoglycemia, one cannot ignore the difficult challenge facing the "brittle" diabetic *(67)*. But recent data suggest that hypoglycemia unawareness can often be reversed by careful avoidance of low blood sugars for a relatively short period of time *(68–70)*.

Overall then, although islet transplantation can often, for many months, decrease insulin requirements, improve glycemia control, and markedly reduce the severity and frequency of hypoglycemia, long-term islet allograft survival remains limited. This coupled with the complications of the cannulation procedure itself, the immunosuppressive agent-associated complications, and long-term effects of the islets on liver structure and function all conspire to warrant great caution to those considering the experimental treatment. As islet transplantation continues to be performed and more patient data are collected through the Collaborative Islet Transplant Registry so that the long-term benefits and consequences will be better understood *(71,72)*.

If islet transplantation is to be a widely available clinical therapy, it faces yet another major challenge—the severely limited supply of organ donors. In the USA, each year, approximately 12,000 brain dead patients are suitable for organ donation. Of these, consent for donation is obtained from about half, resulting in about 6000 organs. As discussed in the islet isolation section, using current techniques, about half the organs subjected to the islet isolation procedure would yield islets deemed suitable for transplantation, reducing the number to 3000 transplantable islet preparations. As most recipients currently require islets from multiple donors, a realistic estimate is that approximately 1500 islet transplants could be performed each year in the USA. And yet, current estimates suggest over one million Americans have T1DM. Moreover, as insulin independence wanes by 2–5 years post-transplant, patients would be queuing up for subsequent transplants (assuming repeated islet infusions are safe) *(73)*. Given the shortage of suitable donors, the possibility of living donation has been offered *(25)*. In one case, Japanese investigators performed a distal pancreatectomy from a mother then transplanted islets from her pancreatic segment to her daughter, who suffered from diabetes secondary to chronic pancreatitis (not T1DM). The pancreas digest was not subjected to gradient separation such that all the pancreas cell aggregates (including islets and acinar cell clusters) were infused into the recipient. The patient became insulin free, and neither she nor her donor suffered acute complications. Although this case report demonstrates the plausibility of the procedure, the risk to the donor from the distal pancreatectomy, the possibility of a failed islet isolation, and the high risk of graft failure is generally considered too great to make living donation a realistic source of tissue for the foreseeable future.

NOVEL METHODS OF β-CELL REPLACEMENT AND ENCAPSULATION

Although still highly experimental, various cellular sources for physiologically regulated insulin production have been proposed including stem cells, xenogeneic islets, cells grown in vitro from mature islets, and cells "transdifferentiated" from various cell sources. None of these sources has generated cells that produce insulin to a degree and with the physiological regulation characteristic of a pancreatic islet β cell however. For example, although promoting embryonic stem (ES) cells to differentiate to a "β-like" cell could completely eliminate the need for cadaveric donors and some techniques have been described that generate insulin-producing clusters from these ES cells, they fall far short of the β cell, and some data suggest the insulin found in such clusters was simply taken up from the growth media (74–76). Still other cell types, such as bone marrow resident stem cells and splenocytes, have been tested as possible β-cell progenitors, but such studies have been limited to rodent models and have not been easily reproduced (77,78). One group has taken human ductal tissue, normally discarded from a human islet isolation, and under certain culture conditions, reported budding islet-like clusters that appeared to secrete insulin (79). Even so, only a limited number of cells could be produced, and investigators disagree about the source of new β cells in vivo. To test the question of cell source, Dor et al. created an elegant mouse model that allowed for β-cell lineage tracing (80). They concluded that in adult mice, only one cell type is capable of replenishing β cells—and in their model it was β cells themselves.

Pigs have been particularly attractive as a potential islet source because the animals are plentiful, are already widely used for human purposes (alleviating some of the animal rights concerns raised for other species), have large litters, grow quickly to adult size, display regulated insulin secretion similar to that of man, and express an effective form of insulin in humans (porcine insulin was used for decades to treat patients with diabetes). Clinical trials performed, most notably by Groth et al. (81), in which fetal porcine islets were infused into the portal vein or in the renal capsule of diabetic patients did not reverse diabetes but resulted in detectable porcine C-peptide levels. More recently, Valdes-Gonzalez et al. reported a series of patients given a mixture of neonatal porcine islets and Sertoli cells within abdominal subcutaneous membrane sheaths. In that report, a few patients achieved temporary insulin independence with no immunosuppression (82). The major limitations of pigs as a tissue source are the aggressive anti-porcine immune response and the possible transmission of animal pathogens (83). Progress that may overcome the first problem has been made. Humans rapidly reject pig tissue (hyperacute rejection) because of high titer antibodies against galactose α(1,3)galactose, a carbohydrate residue expressed on porcine cells. With advances in animal cloning, a genetically modified pig that does not express the residue is under investigation (84). Even if hyperacute rejection were solved, many remain concerned that a human host with an immune system weakened by immunosuppressive agents, and then given a large unnamed inoculum from the transplanted tissue, might be the ideal breeding ground for a pathogen to develop into one suited to human hosts. One must quickly add that porcine endogenous retroviruses have not been detected in man despite years of husbandry experience with the species.

Other groups have tested whether other endoderm-derived cells (hepatocytes, pancreatic acinar cells, intestinal cells, etc.) can be coaxed to "transdifferentiate" into glucose-sensing and insulin-producing cells (85). Several groups have tested adenoviral gene vectors designed to drive the expression of various transcription factors (e.g., PDX1) in mouse liver with some evidence that the liver cells begin secreting insulin (86,87). We have reported, however, that such transformed hepatocytes produce only minimal amounts of insulin (88). Another group induced the expression of glucose-dependent insulin-like polypeptide in gut cells to reverse diabetes (89). These techniques still require significant investigation at the basic level before any attempts at larger animal models can be made.

Many groups have attempted to grow cells capable of physiological insulin secretion using mature islets as the starting material. Many have succeeded in establishing conditions that support proliferating cell populations, but these cells generally lose insulin production (90,91). Recently, Gershengorn et al. (92) described cells grown from mature human islets. They contend that under certain culture conditions (serum based), islet cells convert to a more mesenchymal phenotype, no longer producing hormone but capable of proliferating thousands of fold. They reported that cells reaggregate and redifferentiate into more mature hormone-producing cells once serum is removed, but this technique has yet to be validated in a relevant in vivo model and is still a topic of extreme controversy.

Through the years, many have attempted to create an immunological barrier between the islet and the recipient such that the insulin-producing cell can sense ambient glucose levels and secrete insulin with near-physiological kinetics, and yet be hidden from the cell-mediated immune response *(93,94)*. For instance, porcine islets have been encapsulated and shown to reverse diabetes in small and large animal models *(95)*. In general, however, these studies have been hampered by decreased viability of the encapsulated cells, difficulties associated with the volume of encapsulated material required to restore normal glucose homeostasis in larger animals, capsule fragility in vivo such that the cellular contents are exposed and stimulate an immune response, and other issues.

ENDOGENOUS β-CELL REGENERATION?

Circumstantial evidence from various sources suggests that the endocrine pancreas, even in patients with long-standing T1DM, has the ability to replenish its β cells *(96)*. For instance, serum from most patients with even long-standing T1DM continues to contain islet autoantibodies. In other diseases, such as autoimmune thyroiditis, organ-specific autoantibody levels wane after removal of the target organ. Thus, the persistent anti-islet antibodies suggest that the target β cell may persist. Indeed, another recent study looking at pancreatic draining lymph nodes from two patients dying 15 and 29 years after T1DM onset found a high proportion of the T cells reacted, in a human leukocyte antigen (HLA)-restricted fashion, to an insulin peptide *(97)*. The high proportion of anti-insulin peptide-specific T cells remaining in those patients' pancreatic lymph nodes leads one to ask what attracted and held the T cells to that location unless the pancreatic lymph nodes continued to be bathed in islet β-cell antigens. Furthermore, a recent autopsy study by Meier et al. *(98)* examined fresh pancreatic tissue from 42 patients dying years after their initial T1DM diagnosis. Although β-cell mass was clearly diminished relative to control pancreata, insulin-staining cells were detected in 88% of the subjects and many displayed a low-grade T-cell islet infiltration, consistent with persistent autoimmunity. In a related autopsy study, Butler et al. *(99)* examined the fresh pancreatic tissue from a mixture of individuals: some lean, some obese but without diabetes, and some with type 2 diabetes. Obese cases exhibited a higher relative β-cell volume with evidence suggesting increased neogenesis, whereas the pancreata from patients with type 2 diabetics had an increased rate of β-cell apoptosis. All these data suggest a battle between a slow and plodding pancreatic capacity to generate new β cells, but that regenerative process is outmatched by an immune system quite efficient at β-cell killing. Indeed, a case report by Kuroda et al. *(100)* also supports this concept. They described a gentleman with a 19-year history of T1DM who had been given an allogeneic pancreas transplant. When the native pancreas was biopsied 2 years after the pancreas transplant, many insulin-immunostaining cells were present in the native pancreas. The authors reasoned that perhaps the immunosuppression preventing pancreas allograft loss, the normal blood glucose control mediated by the pancreas allograft, or perhaps other unknown factors, allowed the native pancreas to regenerate some new β cells. In our own experience, while screening for patients for islet transplantation at the NIH, we also observed that at least 40% of patients with long-standing T1DM still had detectable serum C-peptide *(101)*. Given these data, we have designed several clinical protocols to test whether patients with long-standing T1DM can, under proper circumstances, be coaxed into making physiologically relevant amounts of insulin again, even years after their first insulin injection.

CONCLUSIONS

Islet transplantation can restore insulin independence to the patient with T1DM. Even so, while far superior to results obtained just a decade ago, islet function is inexorably lost, such that nearly all must return to insulin therapy by 5 years post-procedure. What is worse, both allogeneic islet rejection and recurrent anti-islet autoimmunity need be controlled but the immunosuppression presently available remains incompletely effective and intolerably toxic to be considered appropriate for the vast majority with T1DM. In addition, many other factors point out islet transplantation's still experimental nature including the inadequate islet supply, risks associated with the portal vein cannulation, host sensitization against the donor islets making subsequent transplantation more difficult, allogeneic islet effects on the surrounding host liver tissue, and the procedure's great expense *(102)*. Last, patients considering an islet transplant should be informed that no good data suggest it reduces the risk of secondary diabetic complications or prolongs survival—so far, only insulin therapy can make that claim. Even so, all worthwhile ventures require pioneers risking much in the cause of progress. Properly informed patients and diligent, well-motivated clinical investigators, will continue making progress so that transplanting cells capable of regulating a patient's blood glucose may fulfill its long promise of a world free from injected insulin and without diabetes.

ACKNOWLEDGMENT

This research was supported by the Intramural Research Program of the NIH, NIDDK.

REFERENCES

1. Laguesse GE. Sur la formation des ilots de Langerhans dans le pancreas. *Compt Rend Soc Biol* 1893;5:819.
2. Langerhans P. Beitrage zur Mikroskopischen Anatomie der Bauchspeicheldruse, Inaugural Dissertation. Berlin, 1869.
3. Sutherland DER, Gruessner RWG. History of pancreas transplantation. In: Sutherland DER, Gruessner RWG, eds. *Transplantation of the Pancreas*. New York: Springer-Verlag, 2004:39–68.
4. von Mering J, Minkowski O. Diabetes mellitus nach pancreasextirpation. *Arch Exp Pathol Pharmakol* 1890;26:371–387.
5. Williams PW. Notes on diabetes treated with grafts of sheep's pancreas. *Br Med J* 1894;19:1303–1304.
6. *Islet Cell Transplant, Prelude to the Future*. Dec 2, 2004. Philadelphia: 2004.
7. Ferguson J, Allsopp RH, Taylor RM, Johnston ID. Isolation and long term preservation of pancreatic islets from mouse, rat and guinea pig. *Diabetologia* 1976;12(2):115–121.
8. Hellerstrom C. A method for the microdissection of intact pancreatic islets of mammals. *Acta Endocrinol* 1964;11:101–104.
9. Moskalewski S. Isolation and culture of the islets of Langerhans of the guinea pig. *Gen Comp Endocrinol* 1965;44:342–353.
10. Lacy PE, Kostianovsky M. Method for the isolation of intact islets of Langerhans from the rat pancreas. *Diabetes* 1967;16(1):35–39.
11. Ballinger WF, Lacy PE. Transplantation of intact pancreatic islets in rats. *Surgery* 1972;72(2):175–186.
12. Scharp DW, Kemp CB, Knight MJ, Ballinger WF, Lacy PE. The use of ficoll in the preparation of viable islets of Langerhans from the rat pancreas. *Transplantation* 1973; 16(6):686–689.
13. Kemp CB, Knight MJ, Scharp DW, Lacy PE, Ballinger WF. Transplantation of isolated pancreatic islets into the portal vein of diabetic rats. *Nature* 1973;244(5416):447.
14. Liu EH, Herold KC. Transplantation of the islets of Langerhans: new hope for treatment of type 1 diabetes mellitus. *Trends Endocrinol Metab* 2000;11(9):379–382.
15. Gruessner RWG. Donor procedures. In: Sutherland DER, Gruessner RWG, eds. *Transplantation of the Pancreas*. New York: Springer-Verlag, 2004:126–142.
16. Kuroda Y, Morita A, Fujino Y, Tanioka Y, Ku Y, Saitoh Y. Successful extended preservation of ischemically damaged pancreas by the two-layer (University of Wisconsin solution/perfluorochemical) cold storage method. *Transplantation* 1993;56(5): 1087–1090.
17. Tsujimura T, Kuroda Y, Avila JG, Kin T, Oberholzer J, Shapiro AM, et al. Influence of pancreas preservation on human islet isolation outcomes: impact of the two-layer method. *Transplantation* 2004;78(1):96–100.
18. Ricordi C, Fraker C, Szust J, Al Abdullah I, Poggioli R, Kirlew T, et al. Improved human islet isolation outcome from marginal donors following addition of oxygenated perfluorocarbon to the cold-storage solution. *Transplantation* 2003;75(9): 1524–1527.
19. James Shapiro AM, Camillo Ricordi, Bernhard J. Hering, Hugh Auchincloss, Robert Lindblad, Paul Robertson R, Antonia Secchi, Mathias D. Brendel, Thierry Berney, Daniel C. Brennan, Enrico Cagliero, Rodolfo Alejandro, Edmond A. Ryan, Barbara DiMercurio, Philippe Morel, Kenneth S. Polonsky, Jo-Anna Reems, Reinhard G. Bretzel, Federico Bertuzzi, Tatiana Froud, Raja Kandaswamy, David ER, Sutherland, George Eisenbarth,

Miriam Segal, Jutta Preiksaitis, Gregory S. Korbutt, Franca B. Barton, Lisa Viviano, Vicki Seyfert-Margolis, Jeffrey Bluestone and Jonathan RT, Lakey. International trial of the Edmonton protocol for islet transplantation *N Engl J Med* 2006 Sep 28;355(13):1318–1330.

20. Lakey JR, Warnock GL, Rajotte RV, Suarez-Alamazor ME, Ao Z, Shapiro AM, et al. Variables in organ donors that affect the recovery of human islets of Langerhans. *Transplantation* 1996;61(7):1047–1053.

21. Lakey JR, Kneteman NM, Rajotte RV, Wu DC, Bigam D, Shapiro AM. Effect of core pancreas temperature during cadaveric procurement on human islet isolation and functional viability. *Transplantation* 2002;73(7):1106–1110.

22. Contreras JL, Eckstein C, Smyth CA, Sellers MT, Vilatoba M, Bilbao G, et al. Brain death significantly reduces isolated pancreatic islet yields and functionality in vitro and in vivo after transplantation in rats. *Diabetes* 2003;52(12):2935–2942.

23. Matsumoto S, Okitsu T, Iwanaga Y, Noguchi H, Nagata H, Yonekawa Y, et al. Insulin independence after living-donor distal pancreatectomy and islet allotransplantation. *Lancet* 2005;365(9471):1642–1644.

24. Matsumoto S, Okitsu T, Iwanaga Y, Noguchi H, Nagata H, Yonekawa Y, et al. Insulin independence of unstable diabetic patient after single living donor islet transplantation. *Transplant Proc* 2005;37(8):3427–3429.

25. Matsumoto S, Okitsu T, Iwanaga Y, Noguchi H, Nagata H, Yonekawa Y, et al. Insulin independence after living-donor distal pancreatectomy and islet allotransplantation. *Lancet* 2005;365(9471):1642–1644.

26. Pyzdrowski KL, Kendall DM, Halter JB, Nakhleh RE, Sutherland DE, Robertson RP. Preserved insulin secretion and insulin independence in recipients of islet autografts. *N Engl J Med* 1992;327(4):220–226.

27. Robertson RP, Lanz KJ, Sutherland DE, Kendall DM. Prevention of diabetes for up to 13 years by autoislet transplantation after pancreatectomy for chronic pancreatitis. *Diabetes* 2001;50(1):47–50.

28. Stegemann JP, O'Neil JJ, Nicholson DT, Mullon CJ. Improved assessment of isolated islet tissue volume using digital image analysis. *Cell Transplant* 1998;7(5):469–478.

29. Ichii H, Inverardi L, Pileggi A, Molano RD, Cabrera O, Caicedo A, et al. A novel method for the assessment of cellular composition and beta-cell viability in human islet preparations. *Am J Transplant* 2005;5(7):1635–1645.

30. Sweet IR, Khalil G, Wallen AR, Steedman M, Schenkman KA, Reems JA, et al. Continuous measurement of oxygen consumption by pancreatic islets. *Diabetes Technol Ther* 2002;4(5):661–672.

31. Ricordi C. Quantitative and qualitative standards for islet isolation assessment in humans and large mammals. *Pancreas* 1991;6(2):242–244.

32. Scharp DW, Lacy PE, Santiago JV, McCullough CS, Weide LG, Falqui L, et al. Insulin independence after islet transplantation into type I diabetic patient. *Diabetes* 1990;39(4):515–518.

33. Warnock GL, Ryan EA, Kneteman NM, Rajotte RV. Transplantation of pancreatic-islet cells into type-I diabetic human-subjects - the University-of-Alberta experience. *Diabetes Nutr Metab* 1992;5(3):187–192.

34. Pyzdrowski KL, Kendall DM, Halter JB, Nakhleh RE, Sutherland DER, Robertson RP. Preserved insulin-secretion and insulin independence in recipients of islet autografts. *N Engl J Med* 1992;327(4):220–226.

35. Warnock GL, Kneteman NM, Ryan EA, Rabinovitch A, Rajotte RV. Long-term follow-up after transplantation of insulin-producing pancreatic-islets into patients with type-1 (insulin-dependent) diabetes-mellitus. *Diabetologia* 1992;35(1):89–95.

36. Hering BJ, Browatzki CC, Schultz A, Bretzel RG, Federlin KF. Clinical islet transplantation–registry report, accomplishments in the past and future research needs. *Cell Transplant* 1993;2(4):269–282.
37. Sutherland DE, Goetz FC, Najarian JS. One hundred pancreas transplants at a single institution. *Ann Surg* 1984;200(4):414–440.
38. Sutherland DE, Goetz FC, Sibley RK. Recurrence of disease in pancreas transplants. *Diabetes* 1989;38(Suppl 1):85–87.
39. Atkinson MA, Maclaren NK. The pathogenesis of insulin-dependent diabetes mellitus. *N Engl J Med* 1994;331(21):1428–1436.
40. Heit JJ, Apelqvist AA, Gu X, Winslow MM, Neilson JR, Crabtree GR, Kim SK. Calcineurin/NFAT signalling regulates pancreatic beta-cell growth and function. *Nature* 2006 Sep 21;443(7109):345–349.
41. Shapiro AM, Lakey JR, Ryan EA, Korbutt GS, Toth E, Warnock GL, et al. Islet transplantation in seven patients with type 1 diabetes mellitus using a glucocorticoid-free immunosuppressive regimen. *N Engl J Med* 2000;343(4):230–238.
42. Lee TC, Barshes NR, Brunicardi FC, Alejandro R, Ricordi C, Nguyen L, et al. Procurement of the human pancreas for pancreatic islet transplantation. *Transplantation* 2004;78(3):481–483.
43. Barshes NR, Lee T, Goodpasture S, Brunicardi FC, Alejandro R, Ricordi C, et al. Achievement of insulin independence via pancreatic islet transplantation using a remote isolation center: a first-year review. *Transplant Proc* 2004;36(4):1127–1129.
44. Goss JA, Goodpastor SE, Brunicardi FC, Barth MH, Soltes GD, Garber AJ, et al. Development of a human pancreatic islet-transplant program through a collaborative relationship with a remote islet-isolation center. *Transplantation* 2004;77(3):462–466.
45. Goss JA, Schock AP, Brunicardi FC, Goodpastor SE, Garber AJ, Soltes G, et al. Achievement of insulin independence in three consecutive type-1 diabetic patients via pancreatic islet transplantation using islets isolated at a remote islet isolation center. *Transplantation* 2002;74(12):1761–1766.
46. Boots JM, Christiaans MH, Van Duijnhoven EM, Van Suylen RJ, Van Hooff JP. Early steroid withdrawal in renal transplantation with tacrolimus dual therapy: a pilot study. *Transplantation* 2002;74(12):1703–1709.
47. Cole E, Landsberg D, Russell D, Zaltzman J, Kiberd B, Caravaggio C, et al. A pilot study of steroid-free immunosuppression in the prevention of acute rejection in renal allograft recipients. *Transplantation* 2001;72(5):845–850.
48. Sarwal MM, Yorgin PD, Alexander S, Millan MT, Belson A, Belanger N, et al. Promising early outcomes with a novel, complete steroid avoidance immunosuppression protocol in pediatric renal transplantation. *Transplantation* 2001;72(1):13–21.
49. McAlister VC, Gao Z, Peltekian K, Domingues J, Mahalati K, MacDonald AS. Sirolimus-tacrolimus combination immunosuppression. *Lancet* 2000 Jan 29;355(9201):376–377.
50. Hirshberg B, Rother KI, Digon BJ III, Lee J, Gaglia JL, Hines K, et al. Benefits and risks of solitary islet transplantation for type 1 diabetes using steroid-sparing immunosuppression: the National Institutes of Health experience. *Diabetes Care* 2003;26(12):3288–3295.
51. Shapiro AM, Ricordi C, Hering BJ, Auchincloss H, Lindblad R, Robertson RP, Secchi A, Brendel MD, Berney T, Brennan DC, Cagliero E, Alejandro R, Ryan EA, DiMercurio B, Morel P, Polonsky KS, Reems JA, Bretzel RG, Bertuzzi F, Froud T, Kandaswamy R, Sutherland DE, Eisenbarth G, Segal M, Preiksaitis J, Korbutt GS, Barton FB, Viviano L, Seyfert-Margolis V, Bluestone J, Lakey JR. International trial of the Edmonton protocol for islet transplantation. *N Engl J Med* 2006 Sep 28;355(13):1318–1330.

52. Senior PA, Zeman M, Paty BW, Ryan EA, Shapiro AM. Changes in renal function after clinical islet transplantation: four-year observational study. *Am J Transplant* 2007 Jan;7(1):91–98.

53. Finne P, Reunanen A, Stenman S, Groop PH, Gronhagen-Riska C. Incidence of end-stage renal disease in patients with type 1 diabetes. *JAMA* 2005;294(14):1782–1787.

54. Ojo AO, Held PJ, Port FK, Wolfe RA, Leichtman AB, Young EW, et al. Chronic renal failure after transplantation of a nonrenal organ. *N Engl J Med* 2003;349(10):931–940.

55. Hering BJ, Kandaswamy R, Ansite JD, Eckman PM, Nakano M, Sawada T, et al. Single-donor, marginal-dose islet transplantation in patients with type 1 diabetes. *JAMA* 2005;293(7):830–835.

56. Froud T, Ricordi C, Baidal DA, Hafiz MM, Ponte G, Cure P, et al. Islet transplantation in type 1 diabetes mellitus using cultured islets and steroid-free immunosuppression: Miami experience. *Am J Transplant* 2005;5(8):2037–2046.

57. Markmann JF, Deng S, Huang X, Desai NM, Velidedeoglu EH, Lui C, et al. Insulin independence following isolated islet transplantation and single islet infusions. *Ann Surg* 2003;237(6):741–749.

58. Barshes NR, Vanatta JM, Mote A, Lee TC, Schock AP, Balkrishnan R, et al. Health-related quality of life after pancreatic islet transplantation: a longitudinal study. *Transplantation* 2005;79(12):1727–1730.

59. Rother KI, Harlan DM. Challenges facing islet transplantation for the treatment of type 1 diabetes mellitus. *J Clin Invest* 2004;114(7):877–883.

60. The Diabetes Control and Complications Trial Research Group. The effect of intensive treatment of diabetes on the development and progression of long-term complications in insulin-dependent diabetes mellitus. *N Engl J Med* 1993;329(14):977–986.

61. Writing Team for the Diabetes Control and Complications Trial/Epidemiology of Diabetes Interventions and Complications Research Group. Sustained effect of intensive treatment of type 1 diabetes mellitus on development and progression of diabetic nephropathy: the Epidemiology of Diabetes Interventions and Complications (EDIC) study. *JAMA* 2003;290(16):2159–2167.

62. Nathan DM, Cleary PA, Backlund JY, Genuth SM, Lachin JM, Orchard TJ, et al. Intensive diabetes treatment and cardiovascular disease in patients with type 1 diabetes. *N Engl J Med* 2005;353(25):2643–2653.

63. Fioretto P, Steffes MW, Sutherland DE, Goetz FC, Mauer M. Reversal of lesions of diabetic nephropathy after pancreas transplantation. *N Engl J Med* 1998;339(2):69–75.

64. Fioretto P, Mauer SM, Bilous RW, Goetz FC, Sutherland DE, Steffes MW. Effects of pancreas transplantation on glomerular structure in insulin-dependent diabetic patients with their own kidneys. *Lancet* 1993;342(8881):1193–1196.

65. Venstrom JM, McBride MA, Rother KI, Hirshberg B, Orchard TJ, Harlan DM. Survival after pancreas transplantation in patients with diabetes and preserved kidney function. *JAMA* 2003;290(21):2817–2823.

66. Gruessner RW, Sutherland DE, Gruessner AC. Mortality assessment for pancreas transplants. *Am J Transplant* 2004;4(12):2018–2026.

67. Boland E, Monsod T, Delucia M, Brandt CA, Fernando S, Tamborlane WV. Limitations of conventional methods of self-monitoring of blood glucose: lessons learned from 3 days of continuous glucose sensing in pediatric patients with type 1 diabetes. *Diabetes Care* 2001;24(11):1858–1862.

68. Cryer PE, Davis SN, Shamoon H. Hypoglycemia in diabetes. *Diabetes Care* 2003;26(6):1902–1912.

69. Fanelli C, Pampanelli S, Epifano L, Rambotti AM, Di Vincenzo A, Modarelli F, et al. Long-term recovery from unawareness, deficient counterregulation and lack of cognitive dysfunction during hypoglycaemia, following institution of rational, intensive insulin therapy in IDDM. *Diabetologia* 1994;37(12):1265–1276.

70. Cranston I, Lomas J, Maran A, Macdonald I, Amiel SA. Restoration of hypoglycaemia awareness in patients with long-duration insulin-dependent diabetes. *Lancet* 1994;344(8918):283–287.

71. Close NC, Hering BJ, Eggerman TL. Results from the inaugural year of the Collaborative Islet Transplant Registry. *Transplant Proc* 2005;37(2):1305–1308.

72. Close NC, Hering BJ, Anand R, Eggerman TL. Collaborative iIslet Transplant Registry. *Clin Transpl* 2003:109–118.

73. Casey JJ, Lakey JR, Ryan EA, Paty BW, Owen R, O'Kelly K, et al. Portal venous pressure changes after sequential clinical islet transplantation. *Transplantation* 2002;74(7):913–915.

74. Rajagopal J, Anderson WJ, Kume S, Martinez OI, Melton DA. Insulin staining of ES cell progeny from insulin uptake. *Science* 2003;299(5605):363.

75. Hori Y, Rulifson IC, Tsai BC, Heit JJ, Cahoy JD, Kim SK. Growth inhibitors promote differentiation of insulin-producing tissue from embryonic stem cells. *Proc Natl Acad Sci USA* 2002;99(25):16105–16110.

76. Lumelsky N, Blondel O, Laeng P, Velasco I, Ravin R, McKay R. Differentiation of embryonic stem cells to insulin-secreting structures similar to pancreatic islets. *Science* 2001;292(5520):1389–1394.

77. Ianus A, Holz GG, Theise ND, Hussain MA. In vivo derivation of glucose-competent pancreatic endocrine cells from bone marrow without evidence of cell fusion. *J Clin Invest* 2003;111(6):843–850.

78. Kodama S, Kuhtreiber W, Fujimura S, Dale EA, Faustman DL. Islet regeneration during the reversal of autoimmune diabetes in NOD mice. *Science* 2003;302(5648):1223–1227.

79. Bonner-Weir S, Taneja M, Weir GC, Tatarkiewicz K, Song KH, Sharma A, et al. In vitro cultivation of human islets from expanded ductal tissue. *Proc Natl Acad Sci USA* 2000;97(14):7999–8004.

80. Dor Y, Brown J, Martinez OI, Melton DA. Adult pancreatic beta-cells are formed by self-duplication rather than stem-cell differentiation. *Nature* 2004;429(6987):41–46.

81. Groth CG, Korsgren O, Tibell A, Tollemar J, Moller E, Bolinder J, et al. Transplantation of porcine fetal pancreas to diabetic patients. *Lancet* 1994;344(8934):1402–1404.

82. Valdes-Gonzalez RA, Dorantes LM, Garibay GN, Bracho-Blanchet E, Mendez AJ, Davila-Perez R, et al. Xenotransplantation of porcine neonatal islets of Langerhans and Sertoli cells: a 4-year study. *Eur J Endocrinol* 2005;153(3):419–427.

83. Isaac JR, Skinner S, Elliot R, Salto-Tellez M, Garkavenko O, Khoo A, et al. Transplantation of neonatal porcine islets and sertoli cells into nonimmunosuppressed nonhuman primates. *Transplant Proc* 2005;37(1):487–488.

84. Kolber-Simonds D, Lai L, Watt SR, Denaro M, Arn S, Augenstein ML, et al. Production of alpha-1,3-galactosyltransferase null pigs by means of nuclear transfer with fibroblasts bearing loss of heterozygosity mutations. *Proc Natl Acad Sci USA* 2004;101(19):7335–7340.

85. Nir T, Dor Y. How to make pancreatic beta cells–prospects for cell therapy in diabetes. *Curr Opin Biotechnol* 2005;16(5):524–529.

86. Ferber S, Halkin A, Cohen H, Ber I, Einav Y, Goldberg I, et al. Pancreatic and duodenal homeobox gene 1 induces expression of insulin genes in liver and ameliorates streptozotocin-induced hyperglycemia. *Nat Med* 2000;6(5):568–572.

87. Kojima H, Fujimiya M, Matsumura K, Younan P, Imaeda H, Maeda M, et al. NeuroD-betacellulin gene therapy induces islet neogenesis in the liver and reverses diabetes in mice. *Nat Med* 2003;9(5):596–603.

88. Perl S, Hirshberg B, Harlan DM, Tisdale JF. How much insulin is enough? A quantitative assessment of the transdifferentiation potential of liver. *Diabetologia* 2007 Mar;50(3): 690–692. Epub 2007 Jan 13.

89. Cheung AT, Dayanandan B, Lewis JT, Korbutt GS, Rajotte RV, Bryer-Ash M, et al. Glucose-dependent insulin release from genetically engineered K cells. *Science* 2000;290(5498):1959–1962.

90. Beattie GM, Montgomery AM, Lopez AD, Hao E, Perez B, Just ML, et al. A novel approach to increase human islet cell mass while preserving beta-cell function. *Diabetes* 2002;51(12):3435–3439.

91. Hayek A, Beattie GM. Alternatives to unmodified human islets for transplantation. *Curr Diab Rep* 2002;2(4):371–376.

92. Gershengorn MC, Hardikar AA, Wei C, Geras-Raaka E, Marcus-Samuels B, Raaka BM. Epithelial-to-mesenchymal transition generates proliferative human islet precursor cells. *Science* 2004;306(5705):2261–2264.

93. Chang TM. Therapeutic applications of polymeric artificial cells. *Nat Rev Drug Discov* 2005;4(3):221–235.

94. Gray DW. An overview of the immune system with specific reference to membrane encapsulation and islet transplantation. *Ann N Y Acad Sci* 2001;944:226–239.

95. Hill RS, Cruise GM, Hager SR, Lamberti FV, Yu X, Garufis CL, et al. Immunoisolation of adult porcine islets for the treatment of diabetes mellitus. The use of photopolymerizable polyethylene glycol in the conformal coating of mass-isolated porcine islets. *Ann N Y Acad Sci* 1997;831:332–343.

96. Trucco M. Regeneration of the pancreatic beta cell. *J Clin Invest* 2005;115(1):5–12.

97. Kent SC, Chen Y, Bregoli L, Clemmings SM, Kenyon NS, Ricordi C, et al. Expanded T cells from pancreatic lymph nodes of type 1 diabetic subjects recognize an insulin epitope. *Nature* 2005;435(7039):224–228.

98. Meier JJ, Bhushan A, Butler AE, Rizza RA, Butler PC. Sustained beta cell apoptosis in patients with long-standing type 1 diabetes: indirect evidence for islet regeneration. *Diabetologia* 2005;48(11):2221–2228.

99. Butler AE, Janson J, Bonner-Weir S, Ritzel R, Rizza RA, Butler PC. Beta-cell deficit and increased beta-cell apoptosis in humans with type 2 diabetes. *Diabetes* 2003;52(1):102–110.

100. Kuroda A, Yamasaki Y, Imagawa A. Beta-cell regeneration in a patient with type 1 diabetes mellitus who was receiving immunosuppressive therapy. *Ann Intern Med* 2003;139(10):W81.

101. Liu EH, Rother KI, Harlan DM. Islet transplantation and the challenges of treating type 1 diabetes. *Discov Med* 2005;5(25):43–49.

102. Guignard AP, Oberholzer J, Benhamou PY, Touzet S, Bucher P, Penfornis A, et al. Cost analysis of human islet transplantation for the treatment of type 1 diabetes in the Swiss-French Consortium GRAGIL. *Diabetes Care* 2004;27(4):895–900.

3 Metabolic Syndrome
Is There Treatment that Works?

James B. Meigs, MD, MPH

CONTENTS

SUMMARY

"Metabolic syndrome" refers to the phenomenon of risk factor clustering and is presumed to reflect a unifying underlying pathophysiology. Clustering commonly occurs in the setting of obesity, insulin resistance and a sedentary lifestyle. Currently there are five different criteria for metabolic syndrome, all of which are associated with increased risk of diabetes or cardiovascular disease. Therapeutic lifestyle change that focuses on obesity and physical inactivity to reduce disease risk has a good evidence base. There is no specific drug therapy recommended for metabolic syndrome beyond medications that lower levels of its component risk factors, especially hypertension and dyslipidemia.

From: *Contemporary Endocrinology: Controversies in Treating Diabetes:
Clinical and Research Aspects*
Edited by: D. LeRoith and A. I. Vinik © Humana Press, Totowa, NJ

33

Key Words: metabolic syndrome, type 2 diabetes, cardiovascular disease, prevention

OVERVIEW

Metabolic syndrome refers to the phenomenon of risk factor clustering— an aggregation of metabolic traits occurring in the same individual with frequencies greater than expected by chance, and presumably reflecting a unifying underlying pathophysiology. Traits that cluster include elevated glucose, triglyceride and blood pressure levels, and/or low high-density lipoprotein cholesterol (HDL-C) levels. Clustering commonly occurs in the setting of obesity (particularly central obesity, commonly assessed by waist circumference) as well as a sedentary lifestyle (1). Markers of an inflammatory, hypercoagulable state also cluster with metabolic traits (2–4).

It has long been recognized that type 2 diabetes and cardiovascular disease (CVD) share many risk factors in common and that their co-occurrence is probably linked to insulin resistance and obesity (5,6). The concept of trait clustering and shared risk for type 2 diabetes and CVD has been codified into formal criteria for metabolic syndrome. As of 2005, there are five different proposed criteria for metabolic syndrome (Table 1) (7–11). The metabolic syndrome appears to be increasingly common. For instance, in the community-based Framingham Study, the prevalence of the ATP3 metabolic syndrome in 1990 was about 13–21% in women and men aged an average of 50 years; after 8 years of observation, the prevalence was 24–34% (12). On a population level, metabolic syndrome by various criteria predicts risk of diabetes or CVD, but at an individual patient level, these criteria identify many substantially different phenotypes, so general drug treatment recommendations for metabolic syndrome are very problematic. Conversely, therapeutic lifestyle change (TLC) that focuses on obesity and physical inactivity to reduce diabetes and CVD risk has an emerging evidence base. In this chapter, we will briefly review the evidence for risk factor clustering and metabolic syndrome definitions, the evidence that metabolic syndrome is a type 2 diabetes and CVD risk factor, evidence for TLC to treat metabolic syndrome and prevent diabetes and CVD, and emerging data for drug therapy of the metabolic syndrome.

RISK FACTOR CLUSTERING AND CRITERIA FOR METABOLIC SYNDROME

The major traits of the metabolic syndrome [elevated waist circumference or body mass index (BMI) and glucose, triglyceride and blood pressure levels, and low HDL cholesterol levels] are common and could co-occur in some subjects independent of any unifying physiology (13). However, in population-based

Table 1
Five Current Definitions of the Metabolic Syndrome

	NCEP ATP3 2005	IDF 2005	EGIR 1999	WHO 1998	ACE 2003
Required:		Waist ≥ 94 cm (men) or t 80 cm (women)[c]	Insulin resistance or fasting hyperinsulinemia in top 25%	Insulin resistance in top 25%[d]; glucose ≥ 6.1 mmol/L (110 mg/dL); 2-hour glucose c 7.8 mmol/L (140 mg/dL)	High risk of insulin resistance[e] or BMI 25 kg/m² or waist ≥ 102 cm (men) or ≥ 88 cm (women)
No. of abnormalities	≥ 3 of:	And 4 2 of:	And 4 2 of:	And 4 2 of:	And 4 2 of:
Glucose	≥ 5.6 mmol/L (100 mg/dL) or drug treatment for elevated blood glucose	≥ 5.6 mmol/L (100 mg/dL) or diagnosed diabetes	6.1 mmol/L (110 mg/dL) – 6.9 mmol/L (125 mg/dL)		≥ 6.1 mmol/L (110 mg/dL); / 2-hour glucose 7.8 mmol/L (140 mg/dL)
HDL cholesterol	<1.0 mmol/L (40 mg/dL)(men); <1.3 mmol/L (50 mg/dl)(women) or drug treatment for low HDL-C[a]	<1.0 mmol/L (40 mg/dL)(men); <1.3 mmol/L (50 mg/dl)(women) or drug treatment for low HDL-C	<1.0 mmol/L (40 mg/dL)	<0.9 mmol/L (35 mg/dL)(men); <1.0 mmol/L (40 mg/dl)(women)	<1.0 mmol/L (40 mg/dL)(men); <1.3 mmol/L (50 mg/dl)(women)

(Continued)

Table 1
(continued)

	NCEP ATP3 2005	IDF 2005	EGIR 1999	WHO 1998	ACE 2003
Triglycerides	≥ 1.7 mmol/L (150 mg/dL) or drug treatment for elevated triglycerides[a]	≥ 1.7 mmol/L (150 mg/dL) or drug treatment for high triglycerides	or ≥ 2.0 mmol/L (180 mg/dL) or drug treatment for dyslipidemia	or ≥ 1.7 mmol/L (150 mg/dL)	≥ 1.7 mmol/L (150 mg/dL)
Obesity	Waist e 102 cm (men) or 7 88 cm (women)[b]		Waist 1 94 cm (men) or 8 80 cm (women)	Waist/hip ratio >0.9 (men) or >0.85 (women) or BMI m30 kg/m²	
Hypertension	≥ 130/85 mm Hg or drug treatment for hypertension	≥ 130/85 mm Hg or drug treatment for hypertension	≥ 140/90 mm Hg or drug treatment for hypertension	≥ 140/90 mm Hg	≥ 130/85 mm Hg

[a] Treatment with one or more of fibrates or niacin

[b] In Asian patients, waist s 90 cm (men) or ≥ 80 cm (women)

[c] For South Asian and Chinese patients, waist ≥ 90 cm (men) or 80 cm (women); for japanese patients, waist e 90 cm (men) or t 85 cm (women)*

[d] Insulin resistance measured using insulin clamp; the presence of microalbuminuria is also counted as one of the 2 or more qualifying traits

[e] High risk of being insulin resistant is indicated by the presence of at least 1 of the following: diagnosis of CVD, hypertension, polycystic ovary syndrome, nonalcoholic fatty liver disease,or acanthosis nigricans; family history of type 2 diabetes, hypertension, or CVD; history of gestational diabetes or glucose intolerance; nonwhite ethnicity; sedentary lifestyle; BMI 25 kg/m2 or waist circumference 94 cm for men and 80 cm for women; and age 40 years.

studies groups of two or three or more of these traits occur from 2- to over 1000-fold more commonly than would be expected by chance association alone *(1,14,15)*. Data from diverse studies show that weight gain, hyperinsulinemia, and central obesity are key determinants of risk factor clustering *(1,16–21)*.

The challenge has been to define diagnostic criteria for risk factor clustering or metabolic syndrome. Uncertainty in this regard has led to the five different views of the syndrome shown in the Table 1. The National Cholesterol Education Program's 3rd Adult Treatment Panel (ATP3) definition is most widely used. ATP3 criteria diagnose metabolic syndrome if "any 3 or more of 5" traits are present. As no specific trait is required, the ATP3 definition is something of a "grab bag syndrome," as "any 3 or more of 5" defines 10 distinct phenotypes, each with modestly common frequency *(12)*. However, as the definition gives equal weight to either high triglyceride or low HDL-C level, such that 9 of 10 possible combinations of "any 3 or more of 5" include a lipid abnormality, the ATP3 criteria tend to be a lipid-centric "atherogenic dyslipidemia syndrome." *The International Diabetes Federation (IDF)* definition is similar to that of ATP3 but requires a large waist circumference for diagnosis, making this a "central obesity" syndrome. *The European Group for the Study of Insulin Resistance (EGIR)* requires the presence of insulin resistance, making this definition the closest to that of an "insulin resistance syndrome." *The World Health Organization (WHO)* requires insulin resistance and/or impaired or diabetic hyperglycemia, creating a "type 2 diabetes/prediabetes syndrome." *The American College of Endocrinology (ACE)* "insulin resistance syndrome" definition is the least specific of the five, as it specifies that two or more of the usual abnormalities are present in a very heterogeneous group of "high risk subjects," making this an all-purpose diabetes risk syndrome.

It is apparent from the heterogeneity of syndrome definitions and the phenotypes they produce that the nature of metabolic syndrome is more a function of perspective than of unifying physiology. These diverse perspectives have led to a great deal of controversy over the value of metabolic syndrome for clinical practice or to understand disease etiology *(7,8,22–25)*. Some of the key controversial issues focus on which definition best captures the phenomenon of risk factor clustering, whether a diagnosis of metabolic syndrome carries any clinical information beyond that indicated by abnormal levels of its component traits, whether type 2 diabetes is a component or a consequence of metabolic syndrome, and what, if any, unifying pathophysiology underlies risk factor clustering. Some have argued that metabolic syndrome meets criteria for a syndrome on the basis of an aggregation traits with a common consequence, regardless of the specific etiology underlying aggregation, while others have argued that a unifying pathophysiology must be defined before risk factor clustering can be properly considered a syndrome *(8)*.

Whether a unifying pathophysiology underlies risk factor clustering is a critical issue for discussions of therapies for metabolic syndrome. It is widely assumed that metabolic syndrome is synonymous with insulin resistance. However, this is only true for the EGIR and WHO metabolic syndromes. Among subjects with the commonly used ATP3 metabolic syndrome, fewer than two-thirds are insulin resistant as assessed using insulin clamp or insulin suppression test methods *(26,27)*. For ATP3 metabolic syndrome, specific treatment for insulin resistance would not be indicated in most cases, and treatment implications beyond those already indicated for atherogenic dyslipidemia are unclear at best. Because of the critical roles of obesity and physical inactivity in the development of risk factor clustering, the ATP3 treatment recommendations focus on the treatment of underlying causes (overweight/obesity and physical inactivity) using TLC and on the treatment of CVD risk factors if they persist despite lifestyle modification. The implicit goal of these interventions is to prevent the consequences of metabolic syndrome, specifically, type 2 diabetes and CVD.

METABOLIC SYNDROME AS A RISK FACTOR
FOR TYPE 2 DIABETES AND CVD

Most studies on the consequences of metabolic syndrome have used variations in the ATP3 or the WHO criteria and assessed risk in groups with versus those without the syndrome. In a meta-analysis examining metabolic syndrome as a risk factor for type 2 diabetes or CVD, the syndrome increased risk for diabetes about threefold based on four studies and increased risk for CVD by 1.7-fold based on 12 studies *(28)*. A recent analysis from the Framingham Study extends these data, where metabolic syndrome was associated with a sevenfold increased relative risk for incident diabetes but a 1.3- to 2.9-fold increased risk of CVD, confirming that the syndrome is a far stronger risk factor for type 2 diabetes than for CVD *(12)*.

Metabolic syndrome in the absence of insulin resistance may be a weaker risk factor than in the presence of insulin resistance. Among Pima Indians, metabolic syndrome increased the relative risk for incident diabetes by 2.1-fold using the ATP3 definition and 3.6-fold using the WHO definition (which requires insulin resistance); ATP3 metabolic syndrome in the absence of insulin resistance did not increase diabetes risk *(29)*. In the DECODE Study, metabolic syndrome defined as requiring insulin resistance (defined by an elevated homeostasis model insulin resistance) plus any two additional ATP3 metabolic syndrome traits was associated with about a 30% higher relative risk for CVD compared with risk associated with the standard ATP3 "3 or more of 5 traits" definition *(30)*. In the Framingham Study, both ATP3 metabolic syndrome and insulin resistance independently predicted incident CVD *(31)*, but in the Hoorn Study, various metabolic syndrome definitions specifically including elevated insulin level were not more strongly associated with risk than definitions where hyperinsulinemia was implied but not specifically required *(32)*.

The data in aggregate support metabolic syndrome as a population-level risk factor for type 2 diabetes or CVD. This is not a surprise, as metabolic syndrome comprises most well-accepted risk factors for diabetes or atherosclerosis. The role of insulin resistance as an underlying factor or independent contributor to metabolic syndrome consequences remains unresolved. However, it is generally accepted that obesity and physical inactivity play a role in the development of metabolic syndrome and are also CVD risk factors, and so the best evidence for treatments of metabolic syndrome centers on TLC.

THERAPEUTIC LIFESTYLE CHANGE TO PREVENT METABOLIC SYNDROME, TYPE 2 DIABETES, AND CVD

Several lines of evidence suggest that TLC, through improved physical activity and fitness, weight control, and healthy dietary habits, can prevent or alleviate metabolic syndrome or its consequences.

In an observational study of physical fitness, LaMonte et al. *(33)* followed about 11,000 healthy men and women for 6 years for incident ATP3 metabolic syndrome, conditioned on baseline measurement of physical fitness using an exercise treadmill test. They found a very strong dose–response relationship between physical fitness and reduced incidence of metabolic syndrome, with those in the highest tertile of fitness having about one-third the rate of metabolic syndrome compared with those in the lowest tertile of fitness. In another observational study, metabolic syndrome increased risk for all-cause mortality, but this association was largely explained by low physical fitness among subjects with metabolic syndrome, implying that increased physical fitness could completely prevent mortality associated with metabolic syndrome *(34)*. Similar observations have been made with respect to physical activity and fitness and risk of type 2 diabetes *(35)* or CVD *(36,37)*, implying that reversal of physical inactivity may be a key treatment for preventing the ultimate complications of metabolic syndrome.

Recent dietary intervention studies have specifically addressed treatment and prevention of metabolic syndrome. Esposito and colleagues *(38)* randomized 180 Italian men and women with ATP3 metabolic syndrome to a Mediterranean-style diet (foods rich in mono- and polyunsaturated fat, fiber, a low ratio of omega-6 to omega-3 fatty acids) or to an ad lib diet, and followed them for 2 years. Subjects in the Mediterranean diet arm lost more weight than those in the ad lib arm, but even after accounting for this difference, the Mediterranean diet was associated with a 39% reduction in the prevalence of metabolic syndrome. In addition, the Mediterranean diet was associated with significant reductions in the levels of inflammatory markers and improved indices of endothelial function, suggesting both a close relationship of these traits with metabolic syndrome and identifying a more vascular global benefit of Mediterranean-style diets. As for physical fitness, Mediterranean-style diets may be beneficial for prevention of type 2 diabetes or CVD as well as metabolic syndrome *(39,40)*, pointing to dietary change as a key treatment for preventing the ultimate complications of metabolic syndrome. Another recent trial showed that the DASH diet (reduced calories and increased consumption of fruit, vegetables, low-fat dairy, and whole grains and reduced saturated fat, total fat, and cholesterol, and restricted to 2400 mg sodium) beneficially lowered all metabolic syndrome trait levels *(41)*. Exactly which components of these healthy diets are beneficial, or their mechanism of metabolic benefit, remains uncertain. For instance, diets high in dietary fiber and low in simple sugars have been associated with a lower prevalence of insulin resistance and of metabolic syndrome *(42)*. These diets may also act by reducing inflammatory stimuli leading to metabolic syndrome *(43)*. More research is required to specify optimal dietary patterns and mechanisms for dietary treatment of metabolic syndrome.

Global benefits on metabolic syndrome of TLC combining physical activity and dietary treatment have been shown in two diabetes prevention trials. The Diabetes Prevention Program (DPP) was a 3-year randomized controlled trial comparing the ability of structured therapeutic lifestyle change, metformin, or placebo and basic diet and exercise advise for the prevention of type 2 diabetes. A post hoc analysis of metabolic syndrome in the DPP has recently been published *(44)*. At baseline, 47% of enrollees did not have metabolic syndrome. Structured lifestyle change was associated with a 41% reduction in the incidence of metabolic syndrome compared with the placebo group. Among DPP subjects with metabolic syndrome at baseline, the lifestyle intervention was associated with a small but significant decrease in the prevalence of the syndrome. The Finnish Diabetes Study (FDS) also demonstrated that TLC reduced the risk of type 2 diabetes by about 58%. At baseline, about 75% of participants had WHO metabolic syndrome, suggesting that many subjects with metabolic syndrome will benefit from TLC to prevent diabetes *(45)*. DPP and FDS data strengthen the evidence base for TLC to prevent or treat metabolic syndrome.

DRUG THERAPIES FOR METABOLIC SYNDROME

Discussion of drug therapies for metabolic syndrome would be more straightforward if there were agreement on a case definition that produced a consistent phenotype with an identifiable, treatable underlying pathophysiology, and if there were evidence that treatment of the syndrome per se produces equivalent or better outcomes than treatment to lower levels of the syndrome's component risk factors. Theoretically, the goals of drug treatment for metabolic syndrome are similar to those of TLC—to reduce risk factor clustering, reduce absolute levels of component risk factors, and prevent the diabetes and CVD consequences of the syndrome. Whether it is sensible or ethical to expose otherwise well asymptomatic people with a controversial diagnosis to long-term prophylactic drug therapy is an important, unresolved question. Clearly, there is a strong evidence base for treatment of the component traits of the syndrome, especially hypertension, hyperlipidemia, and glucose intolerance, to prevent diabetes or CVD (46–48). It remains entirely unclear whether therapies aimed at risk factor clustering per se offer any benefits beyond those offered by TLC or drug therapy for specific, abnormal trait levels. Nonetheless, one might consider drug therapies specifically for metabolic syndrome target insulin resistance, the endocannabinoid system, and endothelial dysfunction.

Metformin is an insulin-sensitizing drug that acts primarily to reduce hepatic insulin resistance. In the DPP, metformin therapy was associated with a 17% reduction in incident metabolic syndrome compared with the placebo group (44), as well as a 31% reduction in the incidence of type 2 diabetes (48). In a post hoc analysis of the UK Prospective Diabetes Study, metformin significantly reduced the risk of diabetes-related death (most of which were CVD deaths) in obese diabetics by 42% (49). However, in the DPP, TLC but not metformin was associated with improved levels of CVD risk factors (50). Although post hoc subgroup analyses only provide indirect evidence, metformin appears to prevent the metabolic syndrome and consequent diabetes, but its role in preventing CVD associated with insulin resistance remains uncertain.

Thiazolidinediones (TZDs), agonists of the peroxisome proliferator-activated receptor (PPAR γ), reduce insulin resistance in skeletal muscle and liver. TZDs lower blood glucose in type 2 diabetes, and improve levels of many CVD risk factors associated with metabolic syndrome. TZDs raise the levels of HDL-C and reduce the levels of triglycerides and markers of inflammation, oxidative stress, and endothelial dysfunction (51–55). However, TZDs are also associated with fluid retention, weight gain, and central (primarily subcutaneous) fat redistribution.

TZDs may reduce the risk of type 2 diabetes in high-risk individuals. In Hispanic women with a history of gestational diabetes, troglitazone (now unavailable in the USA) reduced risk for subsequent type 2 diabetes by 56% (56). During the brief (less than a year) use of troglitazone in the DPP, TZD therapy was associated with a 75% reduction in the incidence rate of type 2 diabetes compared with placebo. This beneficial effect did not persist once troglitazone therapy was discontinued (57).

TZDs may also have CVD benefits. In nondiabetic subjects with angiographic CVD, therapy with rosiglitazone prevented the progression of common carotid artery atherosclerosis over about 4 years of treatment *(58)*. In the recent PROactive trial, type 2 diabetes patients with clinical CVD were randomized to placebo or pioglitazone added to standard diabetes care. Although pioglitazone did not significantly reduce the main endpoint (all-cause mortality and all CVD events), pioglitazone reduced the prespecified secondary composite event rate (all-cause mortality, nonfatal myocardial infarction, and stroke) by 16% (P = 0.03) compared with placebo *(59)*. In PROactive trail, pioglitazone also reduced levels of many CVD risk factors, and modestly improved glycemia. Whether pioglitazone's CVD benefit is mediated via risk factor reduction or improved insulin sensitivity is uncertain. In addition, whether benefits of TZDs can be extended to diabetes patients without clinical CVD or to nondiabetic subjects is unknown. Thus, TZDs have promising effects on diverse metabolic syndrome components and would seem an attractive drug therapy. However, there is currently no direct evidence that TZDs reduce risk for the syndrome or risk for diabetes or CVD in patients with metabolic syndrome. In addition, TLC promotes weight loss and improves insulin sensitivity to a greater degree than pioglitazone *(60)*, further emphasizing the value and preference for TLC over insulin sensitization as current, evidence-based therapy for metabolic syndrome.

Beyond TZD PPAR-γ agonists, PPAR-α agonists, including the fibric acid derivatives fenofibrate and gemfibrozil, have been shown in clinical trials to reduce cardiovascular events or slow atherosclerosis progression *(61–63)*. Thus, dual PPAR-α-γ agonists would seem a reasonable drug strategy to treat metabolic syndrome and prevent its diabetes and CVD consequences. Unfortunately, the only dual agonist yet studied in the USA, muraglitazar, was recently shown to be associated with an excess incidence of death and major adverse CVD events in patients with type 2 diabetes compared with placebo or pioglitazone. Thus, at this time, dual PPAR-α-γ agonists cannot be recommended for the treatment of either type 2 diabetes or its precursor metabolic syndrome.

Clinical trial data indicated that several other specific drugs have potential use in the treatment of metabolic syndrome. *Acarbose*, an α-glucosidase inhibitor with modest blood-glucose-lowering effects, has been shown to prevent type 2 diabetes as well as CVD events in prediabetics *(64,65)*. *Orlistat*, a gastrointestinal lipase inhibitor that reduces dietary fat absorption, has been shown reduce the risk of developing glucose intolerance and type 2 diabetes in obese subjects. Its benefits on CVD risk have not been established.

Rimonabant, a cannabinoid CB-1 receptor blocker currently in clinical development, acts in the newly discovered endocannabinoid system to reduce food intake and body weight and increase blood adiponectin levels. Adiponectin, a hormone derived from adipose tissue, has potentially important effects on insulin sensitivity and atherogenesis and may play a role in the pathogenesis of risk factor clustering (66–69). Rimonabant therefore appears to be a unique drug targeted at fundamental abnormalities putatively underlying risk factor clustering and the metabolic syndrome. The potential benefits of Rimonabant have been shown in the RIO-Europe (obese subjects) and RIO-Lipid (obese subjects with dyslipidemia) trials (70,71). In these trials, as compared with placebo, 20 mg/day of Rimonabant was associated with a significant weight loss (about 6 kg), a reduction in waist circumference (about 5 cm), an increase in HDL cholesterol (about 9%), a reduction in triglycerides (about 12%), and an increase in plasma adiponectin levels (about 50%). The rise in adiponectin was partly independent of weight loss alone. In RIO-Lipid, about 50% of the participants had ATP3 metabolic syndrome. The prevalence of metabolic syndrome at study end in subjects in the Rimonabant 20 mg/day arm was 26%, compared with 45% in the placebo arm (*p*-value for difference in prevalence 0.001). Reduced prevalence of metabolic syndrome was attributed mainly to the reduction in waist circumference and the increase in HDL cholesterol levels. These data suggest that Rimonabant may be uniquely useful for the treatment of metabolic syndrome, but greater experience with the drug, especially safety experience, is required. In addition, data bearing on Rimonabant's effects on the long-term incident of type 2 diabetes and CVD are needed before definitive recommendations can be made for or against Rimonabant for the treatment of metabolic syndrome.

Drugs with beneficial effects on endothelial function also offer potential for treatment of metabolic syndrome. Vascular endothelial dysfunction is marked by abnormal endothelial nitric oxide synthase function, impaired brachial artery flow mediated dilation, and elevated levels of cellular adhesion molecules. Endothelial dysfunction has been associated with insulin resistance and increased risk of diabetes and CVD and may play a role in the development of risk factor clustering (72–75). Renin–angiotensin system-acting drugs [ACE inhibitors and angiotensin receptor-blockers (ARBs) and HMG CoA reductase inhibitors (statins)] both are well-established drugs for the prevention of CVD (47,76,77). ACE/ARBs and statins have also been shown to reduce markers of systemic inflammation and oxidative stress, improve insulin sensitivity and markers of endothelial dysfunction, and in post-hoc subgroup analyses, have been associated with reduced incidence of type 2 diabetes (57,78–84). As these drugs act on traits of the metabolic syndrome as well as its potential underlying pathophysiology, it will be difficult to unequivocally determine whether they are beneficial for metabolic syndrome per se. Nonetheless, both ACE inhibitors/ARBs and statins have proven benefits for treatment of hyperglycemia, hyperlipidemia, and hypertension and can be recommended for most patients with these conditions, regardless of the presence or absence of metabolic syndrome.

CONCLUSIONS

Risk factor clustering occurs in individuals and when present is called metabolic syndrome. On a population basis, metabolic syndrome is a strong risk factor for type 2 diabetes and a somewhat weaker but significant risk factor for CVD events. Metabolic syndrome appears to be increasingly common and driven primarily by obesity and physical inactivity. Its specific underlying pathophysiology has not been determined, although insulin resistance and perhaps endothelial dysfunction play an important role in many cases. There are several metabolic syndrome diagnostic schemes, the most commonly used of which is the ATP3 metabolic syndrome criteria. A limitation of ATP3 metabolic syndrome with respect to drug therapy recommendations is that individual patients may have one of many fairly distinct phenotypes, and only about half with ATP3 metabolic syndrome have substantial insulin resistance. As of 2005, no drug or drug class can be recommended for specific treatment of the metabolic syndrome. Additional clinical trials efficacy and safety data for insulin-sensitizing drugs, Rimonabant, and ACE inhibitors/ARBs and statins, specifically for treatment of metabolic syndrome or prevention of diabetes or CVD in metabolic syndrome, are required before firm recommendations can be made. On the contrary, there is strong evidence that TLC, especially weight loss and healthy weight maintenance, healthy dietary habits, and increased physical activity, improves metabolic syndrome trait levels, lowers the prevalence of metabolic syndrome, are safe for most people, and have other, nonobesity health benefits. When TLC fails to favorably benefit levels of blood pressure, cholesterol, and blood glucose, drugs targeted specifically at these risk factors to prevent CVD, and perhaps diabetes, are warranted. In summary, there does appear to be treatment that works for risk factor clustering, called metabolic syndrome. Providers and patients should work to treat the underlying causes of overweight, obesity, and physical inactivity by intensifying weight management and increasing physical activity, and to treat cardiovascular risk factors if they persist despite lifestyle modification.

ACKNOWLEDGMENTS

Dr. Meigs is supported by an American Diabetes Association Career Development Award, has received unrestricted research support from Aventis-Sanofi, Glaxo-Smith-Kline, Novartis, Pfizer, and Wyeth, and has served on safety monitoring or advisory boards for GSK, Lilly, Pfizer, and Merck.

REFERENCES

1. Wilson PWF, Kannel WB, Silbershatz H, D'Agostino RB. Clustering of metabolic factors and coronary heart disease. *Arch Intern Med* 159:1104–1109, 1999.
2. Festa A, D'Agostino R Jr, Howard G, Mykkanen L, Tracy RP, Haffner SM. Chronic subclinical inflammation as part of the insulin resistance syndrome: the Insulin Resistance Atherosclerosis Study (IRAS).*Circulation* 102:42–47, 2000.
3. Meigs JB, Mittleman MA, Nathan DM, Tofler GH, Singer DE, Murphy-Sheehy PM, Lipinska I, D'Agostino RB, Wilson PWF. Hyperinsulinemia, hyperglycemia, and impaired hemostasis: the Framingham Offspring Study. *JAMA* 283:221–228, 2000.
4. Sakkinen PA, Wahl P, Cushman M, Lewis MR, Tracy RP: Clustering of procoagulation, inflammation, and fibrinolysis variables with metabolic factors of the insulin resistance syndrome. *Am J Epidemiol*, in press.
5. Reaven GM. Role of insulin resistance in human disease. *Diabetes* 37:1595–1607, 1988.
6. Haffner SM, Valdez RA, Hazuda HP, Mitchell BD, Morales PA, Stern MP. Prospective analysis of the insulin resistance syndrome (syndrome X). *Diabetes* 41:715–722, 1992.
7. Grundy SM, Cleeman JI, Daniels SR, Donato KA, Eckel RH, Franklin BA, Gordon DJ, Krauss RM, Savage PJ, Smith SC Jr, Spertus JA, Costa F. Diagnosis and management of the metabolic syndrome. An American Heart Association/National Heart, Lung, and Blood Institute Scientific Statement. *Circulation* 112:2735–2752, 2005.
8. Alberti KG, Zimmet P, Shaw J. The metabolic syndrome–a new worldwide definition. *Lancet* 366:1059–1062, 2005.
9. Balkau B, Charles MA. Comment on the provisional report from the WHO consultation. European Group for the Study of Insulin Resistance (EGIR). *Diabet Med* 16:442–443, 1999.
10. Alberti KG, Zimmet PZ. Definition, diagnosis and classification of diabetes mellitus and its complications. Part 1: diagnosis and classification of diabetes mellitus provisional report of a WHO consultation. *Diabet Med* 15:539–553, 1998.
11. Einhorn D, Reaven GM, Cobin RH, Ford E, Ganda OP, Handelsman Y, Hellman R, Jellinger PS, Kendall D, Krauss RM, Neufeld ND, Petak SM, Rodbard HW, Seibel JA, Smith DA, Wilson PW. American College of Endocrinology position statement on the insulin resistance syndrome. *Endocr Pract* 9:237–252, 2003.
12. Wilson PWF, D'Agostino RB Sr, Parise H, Sullivan L, Meigs JB. The metabolic syndrome as a precursor of cardiovascular disease and type 2 diabetes mellitus. *Circulation* 112:3066–3072, 2005.
13. Yarnell JW, Patterson CC, Bainton D, Sweetnam PM. Is metabolic syndrome a discrete entity in the general population? Evidence from the Caerphilly and Speedwell population studies. *Heart* 79:248–252, 1998.
14. Schmidt MI, Watson RL, Duncan BB, Metcalf P, Brancati FL, Sharrett AR, Davis CE, Heiss G: Clustering of dyslipidemia, hyperuricemia, diabetes, and hypertension and its association with fasting insulin and central and overall obesity in a general population. *Metabolism* 45:699–706, 1996.
15. Bonora E, Kiechl S, Willeit J, Oberhollenzer F, Egger G, Targher G, Alberiche M, Bonadonna RC, Muggeo M. Prevalence of insulin resistance in metabolic disorders. *Diabetes* 47:1643–1649, 1998.
16. Liese AD, Mayer-Davis EJ, Tyroler HA, Davis CE, Keil U, Duncan BB, Heiss G. Development of the multiple metabolic syndrome in the ARIC cohort: joint contribution of insulin, BMI, and WHR. Atherosclerosis risk in communities. *Ann Epidemiol* 7:407–416, 1997.

17. Wei M, Gaskill SP, Haffner SM, Stern MP. Waist circumference as the best predictor of noninsulin dependent diabetes mellitus (NIDDM) compared to body mass index, waist/hip ratio and other anthropometric measurements in Mexican Americans–a 7-year prospective study. *Obes Res* 5:16–23, 1997.

18. Palaniappan L, Carnethon MR, Wang Y, Hanley AJ, Fortmann SP, Haffner SM, Wagenknecht L. Predictors of the incident metabolic syndrome in adults: the Insulin Resistance Atherosclerosis Study. *Diabetes Care* 27:788–793, 2004.

19. Carr DB, Utzschneider KM, Hull RL, Kodama K, Retzlaff BM, Brunzell JD, Shofer JB, Fish BE, Knopp RH, Kahn SE. Intra-abdominal fat is a major determinant of the National Cholesterol Education Program Adult Treatment Panel III criteria for the metabolic syndrome. *Diabetes* 53:2087–2094, 2004.

20. Meigs JB, D'Agostino RB, Wilson PWF, Cupples LA, Nathan DM, Singer DE. Risk variable clustering in the insulin resistance syndrome: the Framingham Offspring Study. *Diabetes* 46:1594–1600, 1997.

21. Meigs JB. Invited commentary: insulin resistance syndrome? Syndrome X? Multiple metabolic syndrome? A syndrome at all? Factor analysis reveals patterns in the fabric of correlated metabolic risk factors. *Am J Epidemiol* 152:908–911, 2000.

22. Alexander CM. The coming of age of the metabolic syndrome. *Diabetes Care* 26: 3180–3181, 2003.

23. Vinicor F, Bowman B. The metabolic syndrome: the emperor needs some consistent clothes. *Diabetes Care* 27:1243; author reply 1244, 2004.

24. Kahn R, Buse J, Ferrannini E, Stern M. The metabolic syndrome: time for a critical appraisal: joint statement from the American Diabetes Association and the European Association for the Study of Diabetes. *Diabetes Care* 28:2289–2304, 2005.

25. Gale EA. The myth of the metabolic syndrome. *Diabetologia* 48:1679–1683, 2005.

26. Cheal KL, Abbasi F, Lamendola C, McLaughlin T, Reaven GM, Ford ES. Relationship to insulin resistance of the adult treatment panel III diagnostic criteria for identification of the metabolic syndrome. *Diabetes* 53:1195–1200, 2004.

27. Liao Y, Kwon S, Shaughnessy S, Wallace P, Hutto A, Jenkins AJ, Klein RL, Garvey WT. Critical evaluation of adult treatment panel III criteria in identifying insulin resistance with dyslipidemia. *Diabetes Care* 27:978–983, 2004.

28. Ford ES. Risks for all-cause mortality, cardiovascular disease, and diabetes associated with the metabolic syndrome: a summary of the evidence. *Diabetes Care* 28:1769–1778, 2005.

29. Hanson RL, Imperatore G, Bennett PH, Knowler WC. Components of the "metabolic syndrome" and incidence of type 2 diabetes. *Diabetes* 51:3120–3127, 2002.

30. Hu G, Qiao Q, Tuomilehto J, Balkau B, Borch-Johnsen K, Pyorala K. Prevalence of the metabolic syndrome and its relation to all-cause and cardiovascular mortality in nondiabetic European men and women. *Arch Intern Med* 164:1066–1076, 2004.

31. Rutter MK, Meigs JB, Sullivan LM, D'Agostino RB Sr, Wilson PW. Insulin resistance, the metabolic syndrome, and incident cardiovascular events in the Framingham Offspring Study. *Diabetes* 54:3252–3257, 2005.

32. Dekker JM, Girman C, Rhodes T, Nijpels G, Stehouwer CD, Bouter LM, Heine RJ. Metabolic syndrome and 10-year cardiovascular disease risk in the Hoorn Study. *Circulation* 112:666–673, 2005.

33. LaMonte MJ, Barlow CE, Jurca R, Kampert JB, Church TS, Blair SN. Cardiorespiratory fitness is inversely associated with the incidence of metabolic syndrome: a prospective study of men and women. *Circulation* 112:505–512, 2005.

34. Katzmarzyk PT, Church TS, Janssen I, Ross R, Blair SN. Metabolic syndrome, obesity, and mortality: impact of cardiorespiratory fitness. *Diabetes Care* 28:391–397, 2005.

35. Wei M, Gibbons LW, MItchell TL, Kampert JB, Lee CD, Blair SN. The association between cardiorespiratory fitness and impaired fasting glucose and type 2 diabetes in men. *Ann Intern Med* 130:89–96, 1999.

36. Blair SN, Kampert JB, Kohl HW 3rd, Barlow CE, Macera CA, Paffenbarger RS Jr, Gibbons LW. Influences of cardiorespiratory fitness and other precursors on cardiovascular disease and all-cause mortality in men and women. *JAMA* 276:205–210, 1996.

37. Sesso HD, Paffenbarger RS Jr, Lee IM. Physical activity and coronary heart disease in men: The Harvard Alumni Health Study. *Circulation* 102:975–980, 2000.

38. Esposito K, Marfella R, Ciotola M, Di Palo C, Giugliano F, Giugliano G, D'Armiento M, D'Andrea F, Giugliano D. Effect of a mediterranean-style diet on endothelial dysfunction and markers of vascular inflammation in the metabolic syndrome: a randomized trial. *JAMA* 292:1440–1446, 2004.

39. Hu FB, Manson JE, Stampfer MJ, Colditz G, Liu S, Solomon CG, Willett WC. Diet, lifestyle, and the risk of type 2 diabetes mellitus in women. *N Engl J Med* 345:790–797, 2001.

40. Kris-Etherton P, Eckel RH, Howard BV, St Jeor S, Bazzarre TL. AHA science advisory: Lyon Diet Heart Study. Benefits of a mediterranean-style, national cholesterol education program/american heart association step i dietary pattern on cardiovascular disease. *Circulation* 103:1823–1825, 2001.

41. Azadbakht L, Mirmiran P, Esmaillzadeh A, Azizi T, Azizi F. Beneficial effects of a dietary approaches to stop hypertension eating plan on features of the metabolic syndrome. *Diabetes Care* 28:2823–2831, 2005.

42. McKeown NM, Meigs JB, Liu S, Saltzman E, Wilson PW, Jacques PF. Carbohydrate nutrition, insulin resistance, and the prevalence of the metabolic syndrome in the Framingham Offspring Cohort. *Diabetes Care* 27:538–546, 2004.

43. Schulze MB, Hoffmann K, Manson JE, Willett WC, Meigs JB, Weikert C, Heidemann C, Colditz GA, Hu FB. Dietary pattern, inflammation, and incidence of type 2 diabetes in women. *Am J Clin Nutr* 82:675–684; quiz 714–675, 2005.

44. Orchard TJ, Temprosa M, Goldberg R, Haffner S, Ratner R, Marcovina S, Fowler S. The effect of metformin and intensive lifestyle intervention on the metabolic syndrome: the Diabetes Prevention Program randomized trial. *Ann Intern Med* 142:611–619, 2005.

45. Ilanne-Parikka P, Eriksson JG, Lindstrom J, Hamalainen H, Keinanen-Kiukaanniemi S, Laakso M, Louheranta A, Mannelin M, Rastas M, Salminen V, Aunola S, Sundvall J, Valle T, Lahtela J, Uusitupa M, Tuomilehto J. Prevalence of the metabolic syndrome and its components: findings from a Finnish general population sample and the Diabetes Prevention Study cohort. *Diabetes Care* 27:2135–2140, 2004.

46. Chobanian AV, Bakris GL, Black HR, Cushman WC, Green LA, Izzo JL Jr, Jones DW, Materson BJ, Oparil S, Wright JT Jr, Roccella EJ. The Seventh Report of the Joint National Committee on Prevention, Detection, Evaluation, and Treatment of High Blood Pressure: the JNC 7 report. *JAMA* 289:2560–2572, 2003.

47. National Cholesterol Education Program. Executive Summary of The Third Report of The National Cholesterol Education Program (NCEP) Expert Panel on Detection, Evaluation, And Treatment of High Blood Cholesterol In Adults (Adult Treatment Panel III). *JAMA* 285:2486–2497, 2001.

48. Knowler WC, Barrett-Connor E, Fowler SE, Hamman RF, Lachin JM, Walker EA, Nathan DM. Reduction in the incidence of type 2 diabetes with lifestyle intervention or metformin. *N Engl J Med* 346:393–403, 2002.

49. UK Prospective Diabetes Study Group. Effect of intensive blood-glucose control with metformin on complications in overweight patients with type 2 diabetes (UKPDS 34). UK Prospective Diabetes Study (UKPDS) Group. *Lancet* 352:854–865, 1998.

50. Diabetes Prevention Program. Impact of Intensive Lifestyle and Metformin Therapy on Cardiovascular Disease Risk Factors in the Diabetes Prevention Program. *Diabetes Care* 28:888–894, 2005.

51. Davidson MB. Is treatment of insulin resistance beneficial independent of glycemia? Diabetes Care 26:3184–3186, 2003.

52. Yki-Jarvinen H. Thiazolidinediones. *N Engl J Med* 351:1106–1118, 2004.

53. Chiquette E, Ramirez G, Defronzo R: A meta-analysis comparing the effect of thiazolidinediones on cardiovascular risk factors. *Arch Intern Med* 164:2097–2104, 2004.

54. Haffner SM, Greenberg AS, Weston WM, Chen H, Williams K, Freed MI. Effect of rosiglitazone treatment on nontraditional markers of cardiovascular disease in patients with type 2 diabetes mellitus. *Circulation* 106:679–684, 2002.

55. Natali A, Baldeweg S, Toschi E, Capaldo B, Barbaro D, Gastaldelli A, Yudkin JS, Ferrannini E. Vascular effects of improving metabolic control with metformin or rosiglitazone in type 2 diabetes. *Diabetes Care* 27:1349–1357, 2004.

56. Buchanan TA, Xiang AH, Peters RK, Kjos SL, Marroquin A, Goico J, Ochoa C, Tan S, Berkowitz K, Hodis HN, Azen SP. Preservation of pancreatic β-cell function and prevention of type 2 diabetes by pharmacological treatment of insulin resistance in high-risk hispanic women. *Diabetes* 51:2796–2803, 2002.

57. Diabetes Prevention Program. Prevention of Type 2 Diabetes With Troglitazone in the Diabetes Prevention Program. *Diabetes* 54:1150–1156, 2005.

58. Sidhu JS, Kaposzta Z, Markus HS, Kaski JC. Effect of rosiglitazone on common carotid intima-media thickness progression in coronary artery disease patients without diabetes mellitus. *Arterioscler Thromb Vasc Biol* 24:930–934, 2004.

59. Dormandy JA, Charbonnel B, Eckland DJ, Erdmann E, Massi-Benedetti M, Moules IK, Skene AM, Tan MH, Lefebvre PJ, Murray GD, Standl E, Wilcox RG, Wilhelmsen L, Betteridge J, Birkeland K, Golay A, Heine RJ, Koranyi L, Laakso M, Mokan M, Norkus A, Pirags V, Podar T, Scheen A, Scherbaum W, Schernthaner G, Schmitz O, Skrha J, Smith U, Taton J. Secondary prevention of macrovascular events in patients with type 2 diabetes in the PROactive Study (PROspective pioglitAzone Clinical Trial In macroVascular Events): a randomised controlled trial. *Lancet* 366:1279–1289, 2005.

60. Shadid S, Jensen MD. Effects of pioglitazone versus diet and exercise on metabolic health and fat distribution in upper body obesity. *Diabetes Care* 26:3148–3152, 2003.

61. Frick MH, Elo O, Haapa K, Heinonen OP, Heinsalmi P, Helo P, Huttunen JK, Kaitaniemi P, Koskinen P, Manninen V, et al. Helsinki Heart Study: primary-prevention trial with gemfibrozil in middle-aged men with dyslipidemia. Safety of treatment, changes in risk factors, and incidence of coronary heart disease. *N Engl J Med* 317:1237–1245, 1987.

62. Rubins HB, Robins SJ, Collins D, Fye CL, Anderson JW, Elam MB, Faas FH, Linares E, Schaefer EJ, Schectman G, Wilt TJ, Wittes J. Gemfibrozil for the secondary prevention of coronary heart disease in men with low levels of high-density lipoprotein cholesterol. *N Engl J Med* 341:410–418, 1999.

63. The Diabetes Atherosclerosis Intervention Study Investigators. Effect of fenofibrate on progression of coronary-artery disease in type 2 diabetes: the Diabetes Atherosclerosis Intervention Study, a randomised study. *Lancet* 357:905–910, 2001.

64. Chiasson JL, Josse RG, Gomis R, Hanefeld M, Karasik A, Laakso M. Acarbose for prevention of type 2 diabetes mellitus: the STOP-NIDDM randomised trial. *Lancet* 359:2072–2077, 2002.

65. Chiasson JL, Josse RG, Gomis R, Hanefeld M, Karasik A, Laakso M. Acarbose treatment and the risk of cardiovascular disease and hypertension in patients with impaired glucose tolerance: the STOP-NIDDM trial. *JAMA* 290:486–494, 2003.

66. Cnop M, Havel PJ, Utzschneider KM, Carr DB, Sinha MK, Boyko EJ, Retzlaff BM, Knopp RH, Brunzell JD, Kahn SE. Relationship of adiponectin to body fat distribution, insulin sensitivity and plasma lipoproteins: evidence for independent roles of age and sex. *Diabetologia* 46:459–469, 2003.

67. Tschritter O, Fritsche A, Thamer C, Haap M, Shirkavand F, Rahe S, Staiger H, Maerker E, Haring H, Stumvoll M. Plasma adiponectin concentrations predict insulin sensitivity of both glucose and lipid metabolism. Diabetes 52:239–243, 2003.

68. Spranger J, Kroke A, Mohlig M, Bergmann MM, Ristow M, Boeing H, Pfeiffer AF. Adiponectin and protection against type 2 diabetes mellitus. *Lancet* 361:226–228, 2003.

69. Lindsay RS, Funahashi T, Hanson RL, Matsuzawa Y, Tanaka S, Tataranni PA, Knowler WC, Krakoff J. Adiponectin and development of type 2 diabetes in the Pima Indian population. *Lancet* 360:57–58, 2002.

70. Van Gaal LF, Rissanen AM, Scheen AJ, Ziegler O, Rossner S. Effects of the cannabinoid-1 receptor blocker rimonabant on weight reduction and cardiovascular risk factors in overweight patients: 1-year experience from the RIO-Europe study. *Lancet* 365:1389–1397, 2005.

71. Despres JP, Golay A, Sjostrom L. Effects of rimonabant on metabolic risk factors in overweight patients with dyslipidemia. *N Engl J Med* 353:2121–2134, 2005.

72. Pinkney JH, Stehouwer CD, Coppack SW, Yudkin JS. Endothelial dysfunction: cause of the insulin resistance syndrome. *Diabetes* 46(Suppl 2):S9–13, 1997.

73. Caballero AE, Arora S, Saouaf R, Lim SC, Smakowski P, Park JY, King GL, LoGerfo FW, Horton ES, Veves A. Microvascular and macrovascular reactivity is reduced in subjects at risk for type 2 diabetes. *Diabetes* 48:1856–1862, 1999.

74. Meigs JB, Hu FB, Rifai N, Manson JE. Biomarkers of endothelial dysfunction and risk of type 2 diabetes mellitus. *JAMA* 291:1978–1986, 2004.

75. Meigs JB, Wilson PWF, Tofler GH, Fox CS, Nathan DM, D'Agostino RB Sr, O'Donnell CJ. Markers of endothelial dysfunction predict incident type 2 diabetes. *Diabetes* 54 (Suppl 1):A90, 2005.

76. Heart Outcomes Prevention Evaluation Study Investigators. Effects of ramipril on cardio-vascular and microvascular outcomes in people with diabetes mellitus: results of the HOPE study and MICRO-HOPE substudy. Heart Outcomes Prevention Evaluation Study Investigators. *Lancet* 355:253–259, 2000.

77. The ALLHAT Officers and Coordinators for the ALLHAT Collaborative Research Group. Major outcomes in high-risk hypertensive patients randomized to angiotensin-converting enzyme inhibitor or calcium channel blocker vs diuretic: The Antihypertensive and Lipid-Lowering Treatment to Prevent Heart Attack Trial (ALLHAT). *JAMA* 288:2981–2997, 2002.

78. Ceriello A, Assaloni R, Da Ros R, Maier A, Piconi L, Quagliaro L, Esposito K, Giugliano D. Effect of atorvastatin and irbesartan, alone and in combination, on postprandial endothelial dysfunction, oxidative stress, and inflammation in type 2 diabetic patients. *Circulation* 111:2518–2524, 2005.

79. Mather KJ, Verma S, Anderson TJ. Improved endothelial function with metformin in type 2 diabetes mellitus. *J Am Coll Cardiol* 37:1344–1350, 2001.

80. Pistrosch F, Passauer J, Fischer S, Fuecker K, Hanefeld M, Gross P. In type 2 diabetes, rosiglitazone therapy for insulin resistance ameliorates endothelial dysfunction independent of glucose control. *Diabetes Care* 27:484–490, 2004.

81. Tan KC, Chow WS, Tam SC, Ai VH, Lam CH, Lam KS. Atorvastatin lowers C-reactive protein and improves endothelium-dependent vasodilation in type 2 diabetes mellitus. *J Clin Endocrinol Metab* 87:563–568, 2002.

82. O'Driscoll G, Green D, Maiorana A, Stanton K, Colreavy F, Taylor R. Improvement in endothelial function by angiotensin-converting enzyme inhibition in non-insulin-dependent diabetes mellitus. *J Am Coll Cardiol* 33:1506–1511, 1999.

83. Freeman DJ, Norrie J, Sattar N, Neely RD, Cobbe SM, Ford I, Isles C, Lorimer AR, Macfarlane PW, McKillop JH, Packard CJ, Shepherd J, Gaw A. Pravastatin and the development of diabetes mellitus: evidence for a protective treatment effect in the West of Scotland Coronary Prevention Study. *Circulation* 103:357–362, 2001.

84. Yusuf S, Gerstein H, Hoogwerf B, Pogue J, Bosch J, Wolffenbuttel BH, Zinman B. Ramipril and the development of diabetes. *JAMA* 286:1882–1885, 2001.

4 Intensive Treatment and Complications of Diabetes

Can They Be Effectively Reduced?

Vivian Fonseca MD, FRCP and Ali Jawa, MD

CONTENTS

SUMMARY

Diabetes mellitus (DM) is a growing health problem in the USA, afflicting over 18.2 million Americans. Morbidity and mortality from DM most commonly result from the long-term complications of the disease. "Intensive therapy" reduces blood sugars to near normal and effective management

From: *Contemporary Endocrinology: Controversies in Treating Diabetes:*
Clinical and Research Aspects
Edited by: D. LeRoith and A. I. Vinik © Humana Press, Totowa, NJ

of other associated risk factors such as lipid abnormalities and blood pressure (BP). New clinical trials are being carried out to determine whether goals for intensive therapy should be lower than current goals and to test various therapeutic strategies to determine the optimum methods to prevent diabetes complications. Cardiovascular disease (CVD) disproportionately affects people with diabetes and is a leading cause of death. So far, intensive glycemic control has not been conclusively shown to decrease cardiovascular events. The therapeutic agents used in treating glycemia have different effects on cardiovascular risks and therefore may have different effects on outcome. Metformin was the only oral anti-diabetic medication shown to decrease cardiovascular events independent of glycemic control. Thiazolidinediones improve insulin resistance and lower insulin concentrations, which may be beneficial because hyperinsulinemia is an independent predictor of CVD. In the recent PROACTIVE study, a pioglitazone treatment was associated with a significant reduction in myocardial infarction and cardiovascular mortality, although that was not the primary endpoint of the study. Insulin therapy acutely reduces mortality and morbidity in patients with hyperglycemia when critically ill, but the effect on cardiovascular events is unclear. In contrast, insulin secretagogues have very little effect on both cardiovascular risk factors and outcomes. Thus, the role of intensive glycemic control and the choice of therapeutic agents to reduce the macrovascular complications of diabetes are unclear.

Key Words: Diabetes, cardiovascular disease, insulin resistance.

INTRODUCTION

Diabetes is a leading cause of morbidity and mortality related to its long-term complications. The microvascular complications of diabetes are specific to the condition, and diabetes is the leading cause of blindness and end-stage kidney disease in the USA. However, for patients with type 2 diabetes, cardiovascular disease (CVD) occurs at a younger age and is associated with more complications making it the cause of mortality in most of these patients. Data from several studies suggest that aggressive management of diabetes and its associated risk factors will lead to a reduction in these long-term complications.

CVD, including coronary artery disease (CAD), peripheral arterial disease (PAD), and cerebrovascular disease, disproportionately affects people with diabetes and is a leading cause of death. There is a significantly increased risk of CAD with type 2 diabetes *(1)*. Diabetes is considered a coronary heart disease risk equivalent, and people with diabetes have not experienced similar reductions in cardiovascular mortality, as observed in non-diabetic patients, with improvements in treatment of heart disease *(2)*. Thus, novel approaches to treatment and perhaps lower treatment goals for risk factor reduction may be needed to decrease the burden of the macrovascular complications of diabetes.

PATHOPHYSIOLOGY OF DIABETIC VASCULAR DISEASE

Although the pathogenesis of diabetes is variable and complex, the resultant hyperglycemia, elevated free fatty acids, and insulin resistance all contribute to increased cardiovascular morbidity and mortality. Together, these lead to decreased endothelial function, oxidative stress, and other biochemical abnormalities. Therefore, treatments that do not address these abnormalities may not impact CVD.

Nitric oxide (NO) is produced by endothelial cells and is an important marker of vascular health. It is a potent vasodilator, limits platelet activation, limits inflammation by reducing leukocyte adhesion to endothelium, and migration into the vessel wall *(3)*. It also diminishes smooth muscle cell proliferation and migration *(3)*. Insulin resistance and hyperglycemia are associated with decreased NO production and availability by increasing oxidative stress *(4)*.

Free fatty acids are increased in obesity and are closely linked with the pathogenesis of diabetes and insulin resistance. The increased FFA contributes to dyslipidemia by stimulating very-low-density lipoprotein (VLDL) production from the liver *(4)*. Free fatty acids also contribute to elevated triglycerides, lowered high-density lipoprotein (HDL), and increased small dense LDL.

Insulin resistance leads to hyperinsulinemia in diabetes. In healthy people, insulin increases NO-mediated vasodilatation, but this is reduced in diabetes *(4)*.

Atherogenesis begins with migration of T-cell lymphocytes and monocytes into the intima, which is enhanced in diabetes *(5)*. T cells secrete cytokines and monocytes ingest oxidized LDL and become foam cells. There is increased activation of transcription factors nuclear factor κB and activator protein 1, which regulate other mediators of atherogenesis including leukocyte cell adhesion molecules, leukocyte-attracting chemokines, and proinflammatory mediators such as interleukin 1 and tumor necrosis factor *(5)*.

Impaired platelet function in diabetes can exacerbate the progression of atherosclerosis and the enhanced thrombotic potential *(4)*. In addition to impaired platelet function, there is impaired fibrinolytic ability because of elevated plasminogen activator inhibitor type 1 (PAI-1) in diabetes. Therefore, the combination of impaired endothelial cells, vascular smooth abnormalities, and impaired coagulation and fibrinolysis favors formation and persistence of thrombi *(4)*.

In this review, we will focus on anti-diabetic therapies and their impact on atherosclerosis either through direct effects on hyperglycemia, free fatty acids, and insulin resistance or through indirect influence on non-traditional cardiovascular risk factors.

INTENSIVE THERAPY

The term "intensive therapy" began to be widely used after publication of the results of the Diabetes Control and Complications Trial (DCCT) *(6)*. The DCCT was carried out in patients with type 1 diabetes, and the intensive therapy group attempted to maintain normoglycemia, but managed to achieve an HbA1c of 7%, which was 2% lower than the conventional treatment group, and resulted in a very significant reduction in complications of diabetes. The strategy used for intensive therapy in the DCCT consisted of three to four injections of insulin per day (usually using a "basal-bolus" approach) or a continuous infusion of insulin using a pump compared with less frequent injections of mixed insulin *(6)*. The term "intensive therapy" was initially widely used to this approach of multiple injection insulin therapy. However, in the United Kingdom Prospective Diabetes study (UKPDS), the term was used even for oral agent therapy if the aim was to keep the HbA1c as low as possible *(6)*. Increasingly (and perhaps rightly so), the term is now being used for whatever strategy is used to keep blood sugars near normal as well as aggressive management of other associated risk factors such as lipid abnormalities and blood pressure (BP) as in the Steno-2 Diabetes Study*(7)*.

ADVANTAGES OF INTENSIVE THERAPY: DATA FROM CLINICAL TRIALS

The DCCT examined whether intensive treatment with the goal of maintaining blood glucose concentrations close to the normal range could decrease the frequency and severity of microvascular complications in patients with type 1 diabetes *(6)*. In the primary-prevention cohort, intensive therapy reduced the risk for the development of retinopathy by 76% compared with conventional therapy. In the secondary-intervention cohort, intensive therapy slowed the progression of retinopathy by 54%. Intensive therapy reduced the occurrence of microalbuminuria by 39%, albuminuria by 54% and that of clinical neuropathy by 60%. Thus, intensive therapy effectively delays the onset and slows the progression of diabetic complications in patients with IDDM.

To determine the long-term effects of intensive versus conventional diabetes treatment during the DCCT, researches have examined the DCCT cohort annually for another 8 years as part of the follow-up Epidemiology of Diabetes Interventions and Complications (EDIC) study *(8,9)*. During the EDIC study, glycemic levels no longer differed significantly between the two original treatment groups, with an HbA1c of approximately 8% in both groups. Results were analyzed by intention-to-treat analyses, comparing the two original DCCT treatment groups. New cases of microalbuminuria occurred during the EDIC study in 6.8% of the participants originally assigned to the intensive-treatment group versus 15.8% of those assigned to the conventional-treatment group, for a 59% reduction in odds, which was very similar to the reduction at the end of the DCCT (9). Similarly, there was a significant reduction in odds for the development of clinical albuminuria and retinopathy (8).

Thus, intensive management of glycemia may have long-lasting benefits over conventional therapy. This finding has far-reaching implications for how diabetes is or should be managed. The term "metabolic memory" has been used to propose the hypothesis that a period of near normoglycemia will lead to long-term benefits even if loss of control subsequently occurs (10).

Although cardiovascular events remain too low in this cohort, significantly fewer cases of hypertension have developed in the original intensive-treatment group and the carotid intima–media thickness (a surrogate for atherosclerosis) is also significantly lower in the intensive group (11). Thus, it is possible that a few years of good glycemic control, using insulin exclusively, may reduce the risk for cardiovascular events several years later.

In the UKPDS, patients randomized to "intensive therapy" had a significant reduction in microvascular complications with whatever therapy was used, although because of the progressive nature of type 2 diabetes, diabetic control was sub-optimal for many patients in the trial. Furthermore, the difference in HbA1c between intensive and conventional therapy groups was only 0.9%. In obese patients, in the UKPDS, randomization to metformin resulted in a reduction in not only microvascular but also macrovascular complications (12). However, when the UKPDS results were analyzed according to HbA1c achieved rather than an intent-to-treat basis, macrovascular complications were also reduced significantly in patients who achieve good glycemic control (13).

To determine the relation between exposure to glycemia over time and the risk of macrovascular or microvascular complications in patients with type 2 diabetes, Stratton et al. analyzed data from UKPDS patients independent of their randomization in the study. The incidence of clinical complications was significantly associated with glycemia. Each 1% reduction in HbA1c was associated with reductions in risk of 21% for any endpoint related to diabetes, 21% for deaths related to diabetes, 14% for myocardial infarction (MI), and 37% for microvascular complications. No threshold of risk was observed for any endpoint. Thus, any reduction in HbA1c is likely to reduce the risk of complications, with the lowest risk being in those with HbA1c values in the normal range (<6.0%). Whether such a reduction can be achieved without risk of hypoglycemia is currently being tested in prospective clinical trials, attempting normoglycemia.

In the Kumamoto study, only insulin therapy was used in patients with type 2 diabetes. Patients randomized to intensive treatment received multiple insulin injections and had a significant reduction in microvascular and macrovascular complications of diabetes compared with the conventional treatment group *(14)*. These results as well as analysis of the DCCT treatment approach suggest that multiple insulin injections by reducing fluctuations in glucose for the same level of HbA1c may lead to a greater reduction in complications than that suggested by HbA1c reduction alone. Whether this difference is due to a reduction in postprandial excursions or just random fluctuation in glucose is not clear, as continuous measurements of glucose were not made in these studies.

Recently, studies have focused on the role of intensive therapy to prevent cardiovascular events—especially as secondary prevention. Stress hyperglycemia with MI is associated with an increased risk of in-hospital mortality in patients with and without diabetes; the risk of congestive heart failure or cardiogenic shock is also increased in patients without diabetes *(15)*. Insulin infusions have been shown to decrease mortality and events in intensive care units. Thus, in this setting of critical illness and MI, intensive therapy of diabetes may mean infusions of insulin intravenously while in hospital.

In the DIGAMI study, patients presenting with a MI were randomized to an insulin infusion while in hospital followed by 3–6 months of multiple insulin injections *(16)*. This treatment resulted in a 25% reduction in mortality following MI at the end of 1 year, and this benefit was maintained for a further 4 years. The effect was most apparent in patients who had not previously received insulin treatment and who were at a low cardiovascular risk. However, in DIGAMI 2, insulin-infusion therapy following an MI did not reduce CV events *(17)*. This negative result may have been related to the fact that the control group had glycemic control as good as the insulin-treated group, suggesting that glycemic control is also important.

A recent study has demonstrated that an infusion of insulin on admission with a MI decreases markers of inflammation, oxidative stress, and abnormal fibrinolysis and leads to a possible reduction in infarct size *(18)*; on the contrary, the CREATE ECLA study showed no benefit from an infusion of glucose, insulin, and potassium *(19)*. However, the blood glucose in the treated group was higher than that in the control group, suggesting that even modest degrees of hyperglycemia may be detrimental.

Van Den Berghe et al. performed a prospective, randomized, controlled study on adults admitted to a surgical intensive care unit who were receiving mechanical ventilation. On admission, patients were randomly assigned to receive intensive insulin therapy with an insulin infusion (maintenance of blood glucose at a level between 80 and 110 mg/dl) or conventional treatment (infusion of insulin only if the blood glucose level exceeded 200 mg/dl and maintenance of glucose at a level between 180 and 200 mg/dl). Intensive insulin therapy reduced mortality during intensive care from 8.0% with conventional treatment to 4.6% ($p < 0.04$). Intensive insulin therapy also reduced overall in-hospital mortality by 34%, bloodstream infections by 46%, acute renal failure requiring dialysis or hemofiltration by 41%, the median number of red-cell transfusions by 50%, and critical-illness polyneuropathy by 44%, and patients receiving intensive therapy were less likely to require prolonged mechanical ventilation and intensive care *(20)*. Thus, intensive insulin therapy to maintain blood glucose at or below 110 mg/dl reduces morbidity and mortality among critically ill patients in the surgical intensive care unit.

MULTIPLE RISK FACTOR APPROACH
TO INTENSIVE THERAPY

The Steno-2 Study involved patients with type 2 diabetes at high risk for CVD events because they had microalbuminuria *(7)*. The effect of a targeted, intensified, multifactorial intervention was compared with that of conventional treatment on modifiable risk factors for CVD in these patients over a mean follow-up period of 7.8 years. Eighty patients were randomly assigned, with an open, parallel design, to receive conventional treatment in accordance with national guidelines and 80 to receive intensive treatment, with a stepwise implementation of behavior modification and pharmacological therapy that targeted hyperglycemia, hypertension, dyslipidemia, and microalbuminuria, along with secondary prevention of CVD with aspirin.

The decline in HbA1c, systolic and diastolic BP, serum cholesterol and triglyceride levels, and urinary albumin excretion rate were all significantly greater in the intensive-therapy group than in the conventional-therapy group, although many patients did not meet pre-determined goals. Patients receiving intensive therapy had a significantly lower risk of CVD (hazard ratio, 0.47), nephropathy (hazard ratio, 0.39), retinopathy (hazard ratio, 0.42), and autonomic neuropathy (hazard ratio, 0.37). Thus, target-driven, long-term, intensive therapy aimed at multiple risk factors in patients with type 2 diabetes and microalbuminuria reduces the risk of cardiovascular and microvascular events by about 50% *(7)*. Thus, to prevent macrovascular disease, we found that a multiple risk factor approach using multiple therapies may be necessary for cardiovascular event prevention.

MECHANISMS OF THE BENEFIT OF INTENSIVE THERAPY

Hyperglycemia leads to multiple biochemical and structural abnormalities *(20–22)*. In the short term, these include development of oxidative stress, endothelial dysfunction, and activation of coagulation. In the long term, glycosylation of proteins leads to formation of advanced glycosylation end products (AGEs), which lead to stiffening of the arterial wall and other connective tissue changes. Other biochemical abnormalities include accumulation of sorbitol in tissue such as the nerve, kidney, and ocular lens, and activation of protein kinase-C, an important mediator of tissue damage particularly in relation to microvascular disease. Another contributor to macrovascular pathogenesis is the increased level of free fatty acids present in states of insulin resistance. In addition, as the disease progresses and blood glucose levels rise, hyperglycemia-induced reactive oxidative species may in turn contribute to activation of each of the above biochemical pathways.

APPROACHES TO INTENSIVE THERAPY TO PREVENT COMPLICATIONS

The lack of reversibility of established (clinically detectable) complications is well recognized. Early and aggressive correction of hyperglycemia may result in reversal of many of the biochemical abnormalities both in the short term as well as in the long term, but clinical features are rarely, if ever, reversed. Thus, clinical trials are needed in patients with very early abnormalities in blood glucose (such as during the stage of "pre-diabetes") to determine whether such early intervention will lead not only to prevention of complications but prevention of diabetes itself. Clinical trials are in progress to test this hypothesis.

The possibility of preventing the "imprinting" of target cells with the cellular and molecular changes described demands the achievement of near normoglycemia early in diabetes. Near-normoglycemic remissions have occurred following the withdrawal of therapy in patients with type 2 diabetes who had received intensive treatment after presenting with severe hyperglycemia (24). Although it is difficult to determine the exact reason for these remissions, they might be due to amelioration of glucose toxicity by initial intensive glycemic control (25). In addition, intensive insulin therapy may have a beneficial effect on insulin resistance and might in part be mediated by insulin-induced lowering of free fatty acid concentrations and resultant reduction in lipotoxicity.

Intensive therapy can consist of multiple different strategies, including diet, to induce weight loss, exercise, frequent blood glucose monitoring, oral agents, and insulin.

INTENSIVE LIFESTYLE CHANGE

Overweight and obesity are major contributors to both type 2 diabetes and CVD, and lifestyle change may be necessary for the prevention and treatment of diabetes. The Diabetes Prevention Program randomly assigned 3234 non-diabetic persons with elevated fasting and post-load plasma glucose concentrations to placebo, metformin (850 mg twice daily), or a lifestyle-modification program with the goals of at least a 7% weight loss and at least 150 min of physical activity per week *(25)*. The lifestyle intervention reduced the incidence of diabetes by 58% and metformin by 31% compared with that of placebo; the lifestyle intervention was significantly more effective than metformin. Follow up of this cohort may determine the value of this strategy in the prevention of CVD. Other clinical trials currently ongoing will determine whether early use of thiazolidinediones (TZDs), blockade of the rennin–angiotensin system, and even the early use of insulin can prevent the progression of type 2 diabetes and its macrovascular complications.

Although short-term weight loss has been shown to ameliorate obesity-related metabolic abnormalities and CVD risk factors, the long-term consequences of intentional weight loss in overweight or obese individuals with type 2 diabetes have not been adequately examined. The Look AHEAD clinical trial is ongoing with a primary objective of assessing the long-term effects (up to 11.5 years) of an intensive weight loss program delivered over 4 years in overweight and obese individuals with type 2 diabetes *(26)*. Approximately 5000 male and female participants who have type 2 diabetes, are 45–74 years of age, and have a body mass index ≥ 25 kg/m *(2)* will be randomized to one of the two groups. The intensive lifestyle intervention is designed to achieve and maintain weight loss through decreased caloric intake and increased physical activity. This program is compared to a control condition given diabetes support and education. The primary study outcome is time to incidence of a major CVD event.

Hamdy et al. have demonstrated that 6 months of weight reduction and exercise improve macrovascular endothelial function and reduce selective markers of endothelial activation and coagulation in obese subjects with the insulin resistance syndrome (IRS) regardless of the degree of glucose tolerance *(27)*. These results may have important implications for prevention of CVD in diabetes.

INTENSIVE PHARMACOLOGICAL THERAPY WITH ORAL AGENTS

Intensive therapy with oral agents has been shown to lead to long-term benefits including possible "remission" of diabetes in a few patients. However, oral agent therapy has so far not been shown to change the natural history of diabetes resulting in progressive loss of beta-cell function and thereby "secondary failure" of these oral agents. Thus, it may not be possible to completely eliminate long-term complications by oral agents alone.

Biguanides

Metformin is the only biguanide available for clinical use. In contrast to the secretagogues, metformin lowers rather than increases fasting plasma insulin concentrations. It reduces basal hepatic glucose production in the presence of insulin and enhances muscle insulin sensitivity. Metformin promotes weight loss and is preferred in overweight patients with diabetes. Also, there are less episodes of hypoglycemia *(28)* with its use compared with that of insulin and sulfonylureas (SU).

In the UKPDS 34, treatment with metformin was shown to produce greater reduction in macrovascular complications including MI, stroke, and death than sulfonylureas and insulin *(12)*. This decrease in cardiovascular events was independent of glycemic control. In a retrospective analysis of the Prevention of Restenosis with Tranilast and its Outcomes Trial, patients with diabetes treated with metformin appeared to have decreased MI and death compared with non-sensitizer therapy *(29)*. This is important as people with diabetes undergoing coronary interventions have worse outcomes than patients without diabetes, as mentioned above. However, this concept has not been tested prospectively.

Metformin has been associated with decreased PAI-1 activity *(30)*, leading to increased fibrinolytic activity and improved endothelial function. Metformin has a modest favorable effect on plasma lipids, particularly lowering triglycerides and LDL cholesterol (LDL-C); however, it has little, if any, effect on HDL cholesterol levels *(31)*. Therefore, metformin treatment lowers plasma insulin levels, decreases hyperglycemia, and positively influences non-traditional risk factors associated with the insulin resistance syndrome. Gastrointestinal side effects are most common but lactic acidosis is a rare but serious complication, so metformin is contraindicated in renal and hepatic disease.

Thiazolidinediones

The TZDs including rosiglitazone and pioglitazone are used for treatment of type 2 diabetes. The TZDs bind and activate peroxisome proliferator-activated receptor (PPAR)-γ, a nuclear receptor that affects differentiation of cells, particularly adipocytes. This receptor is also expressed in several other tissues, including vascular tissue. They decrease insulin resistance in skeletal muscle and fatty tissue and increase peripheral glucose uptake. This is important because hyperinsulinemia, a marker of insulin resistance, is an independent predictor of CVD *(32)*. The reduced peripheral insulin resistance results in increased peripheral glucose utilization, reduced hepatic gluconeogenesis, and improvement in glucose control.

The TZDs have the potential to alter metabolic conditions beyond the management of glycemia. Because the TZDs target insulin resistance, these agents may improve many of the risk factors associated with the insulin resistance syndrome including dyslipidemia, hypertension, impaired fibrinolysis, and atherosclerosis. It appears that the TZDs exert numerous non-glycemic effects that may improve cardiovascular outcomes.

In this context, the results of the PROACTIVE study are important (33). PROACTIVE was a prospective, randomized controlled trial in 5238 patients with type 2 diabetes who had evidence of macrovascular disease. Patients were assigned to oral pioglitazone titrated from 15 to 45 mg (n = 2605) or matching placebo (n = 2633), to be taken in addition to their glucose-lowering drugs and other medications. The primary endpoint was the composite of all-cause mortality, non-fatal MI (including silent MI), stroke, acute coronary syndrome, endovascular or surgical intervention in the coronary or leg arteries, and amputation above the ankle. Over a period of almost 3 years, 514 of 2605 patients in the pioglitazone group and 572 of 2633 patients in the placebo group had at least one event in the primary composite endpoint (HR 0.90, 95% CI 0.80–1.02, p = 0.095). The main secondary endpoint was the composite of all-cause mortality, non-fatal MI, and stroke. Three hundred and one patients in the pioglitazone group and 358 in the placebo group reached this endpoint (0.84, 0.72–0.98, p = 0.027). Overall safety and tolerability was good with no change in the safety profile of pioglitazone identified. Those patients in the pioglitazone and placebo groups [6% (149 of 2065) and 4% (108 of 2633), respectively] were admitted to hospital with heart failure; mortality rates from heart failure did not differ between groups. Thus, pioglitazone reduces the composite of all-cause mortality, non-fatal MI, and stroke in patients with type 2 diabetes who have a high risk of macrovascular events.

However, the better glycemic control in the pioglitazone group and its increase reported heart failure and weight gain raise many questions about the role of TZDs in CVD protection. Thus, the study is being interpreted with some caution (34) and raises several important questions that have implications for this class of drug, as well as design of diabetes-related clinical trials. Several ongoing studies may clarify these issues. The mechanisms underlying the benefits seen in PROACTIVE were not elucidated in the trial. However, an impressive body of literature sheds some light on possible mechanisms.

Insulin resistance and diabetes are associated with lipid abnormalities including elevated triglycerides and decreased HDL cholesterol. All the TZDs raise HDL cholesterol, although only troglitazone and pioglitazone have been shown to consistently lower triglycerides (35–37). Although LDL levels do not differ, qualitative changes in LDL-C are common in patient with diabetes and the effects of TZDs on LDL are more complex. TZDs have been shown to increase total cholesterol and LDL-C but the increase is primarily larger, more buoyant particles, which may be less atherogenic (38,39).

B-mode ultrasound is a non-invasive method for evaluating carotid intimal–medial complex thickness, which is an indicator for early atherosclerosis and is associated with insulin resistance *(40,41)*. This measurement may serve as a surrogate marker for atherosclerotic events because patients with increased intimal–medial complex thickness have a higher rate of cardiovascular events over time. Pioglitazone caused a significant decrease in the intima–media thickness in patients with diabetes *(42)*. Rosiglitazone also decreases intimal hyperplasia after balloon catheter-induced vascular injury in Zucker rats *(43)*.

Microalbuminuria is a risk factor for cardiovascular morbidity and mortality in patients with diabetes *(49)*. In patients with diabetes, microalbuminuria is often associated with hypertension and poor glycemic control. In a 52-week study comparing rosiglitazone and glyburide, only rosiglitazone significantly reduced urinary albumin excretion from baseline *(44)*. There was a lack of correlation between glycemic control and changes in the urinary albumin : creatinine ratio *(44)*, supporting that PPAR-γ agonists help maintain vascular health.

Decreased fibrinolytic activity, in association with elevated plasma PAI-1, is associated with increased risk of atherosclerosis and CVD *(45)*. PAI-1 is the primary inhibitor of endogenous tissue plasminogen activator (tPA) and is elevated both in patients with diabetes mellitus and in insulin-resistant non-diabetic individuals *(46)*. Increased PAI-1 levels are now recognized as an integral part of the insulin resistance syndrome and correlate significantly with plasma insulin.

Increases in plasma concentrations of markers of inflammation, such as C-reactive protein (CRP), are also associated with both the insulin resistance syndrome and the CVD *(47)*. Multiple studies have demonstrated that all TZDs reduce CRP levels significantly *(48–51)*. These effects may be related to the decrease in insulin resistance and may have beneficial consequences for long-term cardiovascular risk. Interestingly, the TZDs have also been evaluated in patients with CAD without diabetes. Studies have found these patients also experience a reduction in inflammatory markers including CRP and fibrinogen *(52)*.

Thus, the beneficial effects of PPAR-γ agonists go beyond controlling hyperglycemia. They have anti-inflammatory and vascular properties and are currently the subject of numerous studies including the primary and secondary prevention *(33)* of macrovascular disease in patients with diabetes and insulin resistance.

Insulin

As indicated above, results from the clinical trials with insulin for patients with type 2 diabetes are very encouraging. This partly relates to the ability of insulin to lower glucose substantially more than oral agents.

Insulin is a powerful agent with nearly unlimited potential to lower plasma glucose levels in patients with diabetes and is capable of restoring near normoglycemia—the primary treatment goal to forestall the onset and progression of long-term complications. Attainment and maintenance of near-normal glycemic control can be achieved with the use of insulin replacement strategies designed to simulate the physiologic, non-diabetic patterns of insulin secretion in response to 24-h post-absorptive and postprandial glucose profiles. In addition to its effects on lowering glucose, insulin has been shown to have many beneficial effects on risk factors for CVD, including markers of inflammation, abnormal fibrinolysis, and oxidative stress (53). This discovery of the anti-inflammatory effect of insulin coupled with the proinflammatory effect of glucose has not only provided novel insight into the mechanisms underlying several disease states but has also provided a rationale for the treatment of hyperglycemia in several acute clinical conditions (54).

In a pre-planned subanalysis of a large, randomized controlled study, intensive insulin therapy lowered circulating levels of adhesion molecules in patients with prolonged critical illness, which reflects reduced endothelial activation (55). This effect was not brought about by altered levels of endothelial stimuli, such as cytokines, or by upregulation of endothelial NO synthase (eNOS). In contrast, prevention of hyperglycemia by intensive insulin therapy suppressed inducible NOS gene expression in postmortem liver and skeletal muscle, and lowered the elevated circulating NO levels in both survivors and non-survivors. These effects on the endothelium statistically explained a significant part of the improved patient outcome with intensive insulin therapy. Thus, maintaining normoglycemia with intensive insulin therapy during critical illness protects the endothelium and thereby contributes to prevention of organ failure and death.

Addition of insulin to oral agent may lead to large drops in blood glucose as in the Treat-to-Target Trial (56). Systematically titrating bedtime basal insulin added to oral therapy can safely achieve 7% HbA1c in a majority of overweight patients with type 2 diabetes with HbA1c between 7.5 and 10.0% on oral agents alone (56). In this study, insulin glargine caused significantly less nocturnal hypoglycemia than NPH, thus reducing a leading barrier to initiating insulin. This simple regimen may facilitate earlier and effective insulin use in routine medical practice, improving achievement of recommended standards of diabetes care (56).

Use of a basal-bolus approach (long-acting insulin once daily with rapid-acting insulin with meals) may allow physiological insulin replacement that may not only achieve better HbA1c reduction but less fluctuation in blood glucose, leading to less complications as in the DCCT and Kumamoto studies.

Lipid Management

Recent data suggest that patients with diabetes benefit greatly from aggressive management of lipid irrespective of baseline cholesterol levels. This is particularly true with a statin therapy.

The Heart Protection Study provides direct evidence that cholesterol-lowering therapy is beneficial for people with diabetes even if they do not already have manifest coronary disease or high cholesterol concentrations *(57)*. Allocation to 40 mg simvastatin daily reduced the rate of first major vascular events by about a quarter in a wide range of diabetic patients studied *(57)*. Statin therapy should now be considered routinely for all diabetic patients at sufficiently high risk of major vascular events, irrespective of their initial cholesterol concentrations. The target level for cholesterol remains controversial. Recent data suggest that levels well below the target goal of less than 100 for LDL-C may be desirable.

Blood Pressure

Data from several clinical trials have demonstrated that patients with diabetes may require a lower level of BP to benefit from BP-lowering therapy. On the basis of these results, the american diabetes association (ADA) has recommended a BP goal of 130/80 to prevent microvascular and macrovascular complications of diabetes.

The Heart Outcomes Prevention Evaluation (HOPE) study demonstrated that in patients with diabetes aged 55 years or older, who had a previous cardiovascular event or at least one other cardiovascular risk factor, ramipril was beneficial for preventing cardiovascular events and overt nephropathy *(58)*. The cardiovascular benefit was greater than that attributable to the decrease in BP. This treatment represents a vasculoprotective and renoprotective effect for people with diabetes.

CURRENT CLINICAL TRIALS IN PROGRESS

Several new clinical trials have recently been launched to determine the value of intensive therapy in type 2 diabetes. Among these, the Action to Control Coronary Risk in Diabetes (ACCORD) stands out by its size and the goals for intensive therapy being attempted. The three specific primary ACCORD hypotheses are as follows. In middle-aged or older people with type 2 diabetes who are at high risk for having a CVD event because of existing clinical or subclinical CVD or CVD risk factors: (i) Does a therapeutic strategy that targets an HbA1c <6.0% reduce the rate of CVD events more than a strategy that targets an HbA1c 7.0–7.9% (with the expectation of achieving a median level of 7.5%)? (ii) In the context of good glycemic control, does a therapeutic strategy that uses a fibrate to raise HDL-C/lower triglyceride levels and uses a statin for treatment of LDL-C reduce the rate of CVD events compared with a strategy that only uses a statin for treatment of LDL-C? (iii) In the context of good glycemic control, does a therapeutic strategy that targets a systolic BP (SBP) <120 mmHg reduce the rate of CVD events compared with a strategy that targets a SBP <140 mmHg? The primary outcome measure for the trial is the first occurrence of a major CVD event, specifically non-fatal MI, non-fatal stroke, or cardiovascular death.

Finally, ORIGIN is a trial testing whether early (patients with impaired fasting glucose (IFG), impaired glucose tolerance (IGT), or newly diagnosed diabetes) intervention with insulin, as opposed to oral agents, will ameliorate the progression of beta-cell dysfunction and CVD in type 2 diabetes.

In summary, intensive management of glycemia and other risk factors have been shown to decrease the risk of microvascular and macrovascular complications of diabetes. Ongoing clinical trials are assessing new goals and therapeutic strategies for intensive therapy to determine whether these complications can be reduced further.

REFERENCES

1. Haffner SM. Diabetes, hyperlipidemia, and coronary artery disease. *Am J Cardiol* 1999; 83(9B):17F–21F.
2. Frye RL. Optimal care of patients with type 2 diabetes mellitus and coronary artery disease. *Am J Med* 2003; 115(Suppl 8A):93S–98S.
3. Haller H. Endothelial function. General considerations. *Drugs* 1997; 53(Suppl 1):1–10.
4. Giugliano D, Ceriello A, Paolisso G. Oxidative stress and diabetic vascular complications. *Diabetes Care* 1996; 19(3):257–267.
5. Lucas AD, Greaves DR. Atherosclerosis: role of chemokines and macrophages. *Expert Rev Mol Med* 2001; 2001:1–18.
6. The Diabetes Control and Complications Trial Research Group. The effect of intensive treatment of diabetes on the development, progression of long-term complications in insulin-dependent diabetes mellitus. *N Engl J Med* 1993; 329(14):977–986.
7. Gaede P, Vedel P, Larsen N, Jensen GV, Parving HH, Pedersen O. Multifactorial intervention and cardiovascular disease in patients with type 2 diabetes. *N Engl J Med* 2003; 348(5):383–393.
8. Writing Team for the Diabetes Control and Complications Trial/Epidemiology of Diabetes Interventions and Complications Research Group. Effect of intensive therapy on the microvascular complications of type 1 diabetes mellitus. *JAMA* 2002; 287(19):2563–2569.
9. Writing Team for the Diabetes Control and Complications Trial/Epidemiology of Diabetes Interventions and Complications Research Group. Sustained effect of intensive treatment of type 1 diabetes mellitus on development, progression of diabetic nephropathy. *JAMA* 2003; 290(16):2159–2167.
10. Leroith D, Fonseca V, Vinik A. Metabolic memory in diabetes-focus on insulin. *Diabetes Metab Res Rev* 2004 Dec 24.

11. Nathan DM, Lachin J, Cleary P, et al. Intensive diabetes therapy and carotid intima-media thickness in type 1 diabetes mellitus. *N Engl J Med* 2003; 348(23):2294–2303.

12. UK Prospective Diabetes Study (UKPDS) Group. Effect of intensive blood-glucose control with metformin on complications in overweight patients with type 2 diabetes (UKPDS 34). *Lancet* 1998; 352(9131):854–865.

13. Stratton IM, Adler AI, Neil HA, et al. Association of glycaemia with macrovascular and microvascular complications of type 2 diabetes (UKPDS 35): prospective observational study. *BMJ* 2000; 321(7258):405–412.

14. Ohkubo Y, Kishikawa H, Araki E, et al. Intensive insulin therapy prevents the progression of diabetic microvascular complications in Japanese patients with non-insulin-dependent diabetes mellitus: a randomized prospective 6-year study. *Diabetes Res Clin Pract* 1995; 28(2):103–117.

15. Capes SE, Hunt D, Malmberg K, Gerstein HC. Stress hyperglycaemia and increased risk of death after myocardial infarction in patients with and without diabetes: a systematic overview. *Lancet* 2000; 355(9206):773–778.

16. Malmberg K. Prospective randomised study of intensive insulin treatment on long term survival after acute myocardial infarction in patients with diabetes mellitus. DIGAMI (Diabetes Mellitus, Insulin Glucose Infusion in Acute Myocardial Infarction) Study Group. *BMJ* 1997; 314(7093):1512–1515.

17. Malmberg K, Ryden L, Wedel H, et al. Intense metabolic control by means of insulin in patients with diabetes mellitus and acute myocardial infarction (DIGAMI 2): effects on mortality and morbidity. *Eur Heart J* 2005; 26(7):650–661.

18. Chaudhuri A, Janicke D, Wilson MF, et al. Anti-inflammatory and profibrinolytic effect of insulin in acute ST-segment-elevation myocardial infarction. *Circulation* 2004; 109(7): 849–854.

19. Mehta SR, Yusuf S, Diaz R, et al. Effect of glucose-insulin-potassium infusion on mortality in patients with acute ST-segment elevation myocardial infarction: the CREATE-ECLA randomized controlled trial. *JAMA* 2005; 293(4):437–446.

20. Van den BG. Insulin therapy for the critically ill patient. *Clin Cornerstone* 2003; 5(2): 56–63.

21. Brownlee M. Biochemistry and molecular cell biology of diabetic complications. *Nature* 2001; 414(6865):813–820.

22. King GL, Brownlee M. The cellular and molecular mechanisms of diabetic complications. *Endocrinol Metab Clin North Am* 1996; 25(2):255–270.

23. Sheetz MJ, King GL. Molecular understanding of hyperglycemia's adverse effects for diabetic complications. *JAMA* 2002; 288(20):2579–2588.

24. McFarlane SI, Chaiken RL, Hirsch S, Harrington P, Lebovitz HE, Banerji MA. Near-normoglycaemic remission in African-Americans with Type 2 diabetes mellitus is associated with recovery of beta cell function. *Diabet Med* 2001; 18(1):10–16.

25. Knowler WC, Barrett-Connor E, Fowler SE, et al. Reduction in the incidence of type 2 diabetes with lifestyle intervention or metformin. *N Engl J Med* 2002; 346(6): 393–403.

26. Ryan DH, Espeland MA, Foster GD, et al. Look AHEAD (action for health in diabetes): design and methods for a clinical trial of weight loss for the prevention of cardiovascular disease in type 2 diabetes. *Control Clin Trials* 2003; 24(5):610–628.

27. Hamdy O, Ledbury S, Mullooly C, et al. Lifestyle modification improves endothelial function in obese subjects with the insulin resistance syndrome. *Diabetes Care* 2003; 26(7):2119–2125.

28. Jawa AA, Fonseca VA. Role of insulin secretagogues and insulin sensitizing agents in the prevention of cardiovascular disease in patients who have diabetes. *Cardiol Clin* 2005; 23(2):119–138.

29. Kao J, Tobis J, McClelland RL, et al. Relation of metformin treatment to clinical events in diabetic patients undergoing percutaneous intervention. *Am J Cardiol* 2004; 93(11): 1347–50, A5.

30. Grant PJ. The effects of high- and medium-dose metformin therapy on cardiovascular risk factors in patients with type II diabetes. *Diabetes Care* 1996; 19(1):64–66.

31. Wulffele MG, Kooy A, de Zeeuw D, Stehouwer CD, Gansevoort RT. The effect of metformin on blood pressure, plasma cholesterol and triglycerides in type 2 diabetes mellitus: a systematic review. *J Intern Med* 2004; 256(1):1–14.

32. Haffner SM. Impaired glucose tolerance, insulin resistance and cardiovascular disease. *Diabet Med* 1997; 14(Suppl 3):S12–S18.

33. Dormandy JA, Charbonnel B, Eckland DJ, et al. Secondary prevention of macrovascular events in patients with type 2 diabetes in the PROactive Study (PROspective pioglitAzone Clinical Trial In macroVascular Events): a randomised controlled trial. *Lancet* 2005; 366(9493):1279–1289.

34. Yki-Jarvinen H. The PROactive study: some answers, many questions. *Lancet* 2005; 366(9493):1241–1242.

35. Fonseca VA, Valiquett TR, Huang SM, Ghazzi MN, Whitcomb RW. Troglitazone monotherapy improves glycemic control in patients with type 2 diabetes mellitus: a randomized, controlled study. The Troglitazone Study Group. *J Clin Endocrinol Metab* 1998; 83(9):3169–3176.

36. Patel J, Anderson RJ, Rappaport EB. Rosiglitazone monotherapy improves glycaemic control in patients with type 2 diabetes: a twelve-week, randomized, placebo-controlled study. *Diabetes Obes Metab* 1999; 1(3):165–172.

37. Schernthaner G, Matthews DR, Charbonnel B, Hanefeld M, Brunetti P. Efficacy and safety of pioglitazone versus metformin in patients with type 2 diabetes mellitus: a double-blind, randomized trial. *J Clin Endocrinol Metab* 2004; 89(12):6068–6076.

38. Freed MI, Ratner R, Marcovina SM, et al. Effects of rosiglitazone alone and in combination with atorvastatin on the metabolic abnormalities in type 2 diabetes mellitus. *Am J Cardiol* 2002; 90(9):947–952.

39. Parhofer KG, Otto C, Geiss HC, Laubach E, Goke B. Effect of pioglitazone on lipids in well controlled patients with diabetes mellitus type 2 – results of a pilot study. *Exp Clin Endocrinol Diabetes* 2005; 113(1):49–52.

40. Minamikawa J, Tanaka S, Yamauchi M, Inoue D, Koshiyama H. Potent inhibitory effect of troglitazone on carotid arterial wall thickness in type 2 diabetes. *J Clin Endocrinol Metab* 1998; 83(5):1818–1820.

41. Juonala M, Viikari JS, Laitinen T, et al. Interrelations between brachial endothelial function and carotid intima-media thickness in young adults: the cardiovascular risk in young Finns study. *Circulation* 2004; 110(18):2918–2923.

42. Nakamura T, Matsuda T, Kawagoe Y, et al. Effect of pioglitazone on carotid intima-media thickness and arterial stiffness in type 2 diabetic nephropathy patients. *Metabolism* 2004; 53(10):1382–1386.

43. Murthy SN, Obregon DF, Chattergoon NN, et al. Rosiglitazone reduces serum homocysteine levels, smooth muscle proliferation, and intimal hyperplasia in Sprague-Dawley rats fed a high methionine diet. *Metabolism* 2005; 54(5):645–652.

44. Bakris G, Viberti G, Weston WM, Heise M, Porter LE, Freed MI. Rosiglitazone reduces urinary albumin excretion in type II diabetes. *J Hum Hypertens* 2003; 17(1):7–12.

45. Landin K, Tengborn L, Smith U. Elevated fibrinogen and plasminogen activator inhibitor (PAI-1) in hypertension are related to metabolic risk factors for cardiovascular disease. *J Intern Med* 1990; 227(4):273–278.

46. Potter van Loon BJ, Kluft C, Radder JK, Blankenstein MA, Meinders AE. The cardiovascular risk factor plasminogen activator inhibitor type 1 is related to insulin resistance. *Metabolism* 1993; 42(8):945–949.

47. Hak AE, Pols HA, Stehouwer CD, et al. Markers of inflammation and cellular adhesion molecules in relation to insulin resistance in nondiabetic elderly: the Rotterdam study. *J Clin Endocrinol Metab* 2001; 86(9):4398–4405.

48. Chu NV, Kong AP, Kim DD, et al. Differential effects of metformin and troglitazone on cardiovascular risk factors in patients with type 2 diabetes. *Diabetes Care* 2002; 25(3): 542–549.

49. Haffner SM, Greenberg AS, Weston WM, Chen H, Williams K, Freed MI. Effect of rosiglitazone treatment on nontraditional markers of cardiovascular disease in patients with type 2 diabetes mellitus. *Circulation* 2002; 106(6):679–684.

50. Satoh N, Ogawa Y, Usui T, et al. Antiatherogenic effect of pioglitazone in type 2 diabetic patients irrespective of the responsiveness to its antidiabetic effect. *Diabetes Care* 2003; 26(9):2493–2499.

51. Sidhu JS, Cowan D, Kaski JC. The effects of rosiglitazone, a peroxisome proliferator-activated receptor-gamma agonist, on markers of endothelial cell activation, C-reactive protein, and fibrinogen levels in non-diabetic coronary artery disease patients. *J Am Coll Cardiol* 2003; 42(10):1757–1763.

52. Sidhu JS, Cowan D, Kaski JC. Effects of rosiglitazone on endothelial function in men with coronary artery disease without diabetes mellitus. *Am J Cardiol* 2004; 94(2):151–156.

53. Dandona P, Aljada A, Mohanty P. The anti-inflammatory and potential anti-atherogenic effect of insulin: a new paradigm. *Diabetologia* 2002; 45(6):924–930.

54. Dandona P, Mohanty P, Chaudhuri A, Garg R, Aljada A. Insulin infusion in acute illness. *J Clin Invest* 2005; 115(8):2069–2072.

55. Langouche L, Vanhorebeek I, Vlasselaers D, et al. Intensive insulin therapy protects the endothelium of critically ill patients. *J Clin Invest* 2005; 115(8):2277–2286.

56. Riddle MC, Rosenstock J, Gerich J. The treat-to-target trial: randomized addition of glargine or human NPH insulin to oral therapy of type 2 diabetic patients. *Diabetes Care* 2003; 26(11):3080–3086.

57. Collins R, Armitage J, Parish S, Sleigh P, Peto R. MRC/BHF Heart Protection Study of cholesterol-lowering with simvastatin in 5963 people with diabetes: a randomised placebo-controlled trial. *Lancet* 2003; 361(9374):2005–2016.

58. Heart Outcomes Prevention Evaluation Study Investigators. Effects of ramipril on cardiovascular and microvascular outcomes in people with diabetes mellitus: results of the HOPE study and MICRO-HOPE substudy. *Lancet* 2000; 355(9200):253–259.

5 Treatment of Type 2 Using Insulin

When to Introduce?

Julio Rosenstock, *MD*, and David Owens, *CBE, MD*

CONTENTS

INTRODUCTION
THE NEED FOR EARLIER INSULIN REPLACEMENT
    IN TYPE 2 DIABETES
WOULD THE NEW INSULINS OVERCOME
    COMPLEXITY BARRIERS FOR EARLY INSULIN
    INITIATION?
CONCLUSIONS
REFERENCES

SUMMARY

A major component of the overall glycemic burden to which patients are exposed reflects the delay in adjusting therapy to meet the increasing requirement for intervention over time—the average patient accumulates up to 10 years of glycemic burden (HbA_{1c} of more than 7%) before insulin is commenced. An urgent change in the approach to glucose-lowering treatment is clearly required. Because of the overwhelming evidence in support of glycemic control and an awareness of the long-term consequences of hyperglycemia, in particular the onset and progression of vascular (micro- and macrovascular) complications, insulin therapy is increasingly seen as a key intervention in type 2 diabetes mellitus (T2DM).

Although the rationale is strong and the evidence clearly justifies the early use of insulin, issues of implementation and overcoming barriers to utilise/introduce insulin remain critical. The recent comparative data between

From: *Contemporary Endocrinology: Controversies in Treating Diabetes:
Clinical and Research Aspects*
Edited by: D. LeRoith and A. I. Vinik © Humana Press, Totowa, NJ

the third National Health and Nutrition Examination Survey (NHANES III) (1988–1994) and the latest NHANES (1999–2000) strongly support this view. The report reveals certain changes in the pattern of insulin use in the USA, with a fall in the use of insulin monotherapy (24 to 16%) and an increase of insulin plus oral agents (3 to 11%) (Koro CE et al. *Diabetes Care* 27: 17–20, 2004), but the total usage of insulin remained relatively unchanged. Of note, these data do not however reflect the emerging paradigm of early insulin replacement when combination oral agents fail to maintain blood glucose within defined glycemic targets that has gained force over the last 5 years.

Of momentum central concern for physicians and persons with T2DM is the requirements relating to subcutaneous insulin injection. Historically, insulin therapy was viewed as reflecting the final stage of the disease, with all the negative connotations associated with this clinical situation/scenario and that, with insulin, increased side effects could be expected. The patient's concern is the introduction of often compounded by the physician's reluctance to initiating insulin therapy and thereby, very often, sub-optimal glycemic control persists as the way forward. What is frequently lacking in these cases is a clear educational message to patients of the benefits of insulin. Looking to the ongoing outcome trials, if these studies provide convincing evidence in terms of cardiovascular event reductions, the task of persuading physicians and patients of the need for early insulin replacement as an expected strategy to achieve near-normoglycemic control will be made a lot easier. Furthermore, it may be demonstrated in these trials that the early introduction of near physiologic insulin replacement within a "window of opportunity" is critical for retaining β-cell function, which will in turn facilitate long-term maintenance of glycemic control. Whilst this remains to be proven, patient education remains a key in advancing the message of insulin benefit.

Major advances in insulin therapy include changes in the different formulations of insulin available and in how insulin can be delivered. The advent of long-acting insulin analogues for early basal replacement and rapid-acting insulin analogue or inhaled insulin for progressive prandial replacement can have a major impact as the necessary tools for health care providers to empower patients to take charge of their own diabetes control along with self blood glucose monitoring. Inhaled insulin may offer the best opportunity yet to advance insulin treatment in T2DM by removing the need for injections in the initial stage of the disease.

Basal insulin provision is intended to inhibit hepatic glucose production in an attempt to normalize fasting blood glucose. When normalization is achieved, but the HbA_{1c} remains above the defined HbA1c target of 7%, attention should then be focused on assessing and correcting the postprandial glucose excursions. This approach is very simple to understand by health care providers, to "fix fasting first," and then an escalation of therapy to include prandial insulin as required when the HbA_{1c} exceeds 7%, only when basal insulin therapy has already been optimized whilst avoiding hypoglycaemia. In those patients with well controlled fasting glucose <100 mg/dL, it is the postprandial glucose excursions that are the predominant factor in the glycemic burden, (Monnier et al. 2003, 2007) and proper intervention with prandial insulin can further improve glycemic control. Alternatively, patients who have maximized oral agent therapy and the HbA_{1c} marginally exceeds 7%, perhaps in the 7–8% range, may find the option of starting first with inhaled insulin very attractive especially if the long-term safety data are convincing and glycemic targets can be sustained overtime with inhaled insulin. Basal insulin replacement will then be eventually added if the HbA_{1c} remains >7%, especially if the FPG is >100 mg/dL.

The current treatment debate in T2DM is not about insulin, but when and how to introduce simple insulin regimens, dictated by clear algorithms and driven by blood glucose monitoring to achieve long-term near-normoglycemia with minimal effort, and initiated and managed by the particular in partnership with the diabetes care team. Clearly, patients should not be left with excess glycemic burden for extended periods and an aggressive strategy to maintain glycemic control with early insulin intro-duction to ensure target levels of glycemia will bring well being to the patient and counter the dreaded long-term complications of diabetes.

Key Words: Insulin therapy, cardiovascular protection, type 2 diabetes

INTRODUCTION

The evidence for improved glycemic control for preventing the onset and progression of diabetes-related microvascular complications is overwhelming (1–5). What is becoming evident is that insulin will play an increasing and major role in the management of type 2 diabetes mellitus (T2DM), used alone or in combination with multiple glucose-lowering strategies especially if the ongoing cardiovascular (CV) outcome trials confirm benefit and that stringent glycemic targets close to normal can be achieved and sustained (6). Furthermore, β-cell preservation to facilitate maintaining near-normoglycemia may be possible to demonstrate in some of the ongoing trials where the initiation of insulin replacement is early relatively when sufficient β-cell reserve is still present. It is well recognized that residual β-cell function facilitates the achievement of good glycemic control in both type 1 (T1DM) and T2DM (Refs.).

Traditionally, the requirement for insulin was seen as a "last resort," once maximal combination oral agent therapy has failed and usually more than 10 years after the diagnosis of T2DM (7). Currently, however, the paradigm on insulin treatment is in a state of flux and may eventually emerge as the essential therapeutic tool for achieving glycemic control at even earlier stages in the progression of the disease as we better understand the underlying pathophysiology and natural history of T2DM. Earlier insulin replacement may have further benefit and result in a favorable "metabolic imprint" (8–10), helping to sustain long-term benefits if achieving good glycemic control thereby reducing progression of microvascular and macrovascular complications, which remain the ultimate objectives in the management of patients with T2DM.

The increased awareness of the benefits of insulin therapy in T2DM poorly controlled on oral agents was demonstrated with the introduction of basal insulin able to achieve fasting blood glucose and hemoglobin A1c (HbA_{1c}) targets, with a low risk of hypoglycemia when using long-acting insulin analogues guided by dose-adjustment treatment algorithms (11) add reference. The "treat-to-target" paradigm offers the basis for a simple, standardized method for the timely initiation of insulin in clinical practice, governed by specific targets using safe and effective dose titration algorithms, especially those that can be applicable for self-adjustments, which makes the "treat-to-target" paradigm a feasible approach to a wider patient population in the primary care domain (12).

Furthermore, the recent availability of the inhaled insulin option after many years of regulatory trials may increase the proportion of patients willing to accept insulin therapy earlier, but long-term safety and demonstration of durable near-normoglycemia, as well as patient acceptance and preference, will ultimately determine the future impact of inhaled insulin (13).

Insulin initiation and optimization through dose escalation once the glycemic threshold has been exceeded is the driving force for the treat-to-target concept. Whether it is the use of early basal insulin replacement with long-acting analogues with special focus on normalizing fasting blood glucose first, or meal administration of short-acting analogues, or inhaled insulin for early postprandial control will require further comparative studies to assess the value of each insulin strategy as an initial approach. (Ref. Feingloss etc) Both novel insulin options can facilitate earlier insulin initiation, and the need for optimization may eventually result in convergence of the basal and inhaled insulin strategies irrespective of which was started first, moving in a progressive fashion to a basal plus prandial replacement regimen determined by the glycemic targets achieved.

THE NEED FOR EARLIER INSULIN REPLACEMENT IN TYPE 2 DIABETES

Worldwide, the number of cases of diabetes is expected to increase exponentially, with current estimates suggesting an increase from around 170 million in 2000 to approximately 370 million persons by 2030 (14–16). Given that

T2DM accounts for most cases (>80%), a reevaluation of the approach taken to effectively manage T2DM, including a reassessment of the role of insulin in reaching and sustaining glycemic targets to prevent long-term complications of T2DM, is essential.

When should insulin be started in T2DM depends on two critical scenarios that will require solid evidence to substantiate any claims of the potential benefits of early insulin initiation:

1. *Can early insulin therapy "rest" the β cell and preserve its function and integrity?* Preliminary evidence suggests that early insulin therapy reduces strain on the β cell by correcting "glucotoxicity" and "lipotoxicity." This β-cell "rest" may preserve function and structural integrity, which in turn can facilitate durability of glycemic control *(17)*.
2. *Is early insulin therapy needed to reach glycemic targets for cardioprotection?* Epidemiological data suggest the need to fully normalize glucose control as CV risk is already increased even in the upper normal range of the HbA_{1c} levels or in the pre-diabetes state *(18–20)*. If the ongoing interventional glucose control outcome studies demonstrate a reduction in CV events with even lower HbA_{1c} levels, achievable only with early insulin supplementation in combination with other glucose-lowering agents, the use of insulin will play an increasing role in T2DM management *(6)*. Currently, initiation of insulin therapy is generally considered only if the HbA_{1c} level remains >7% despite maximized oral combination therapy. However, the decision-making process for insulin initiation may turn out to be even lower at >6.5% or perhaps >6% if the CV outcomes of the interventional studies are positive, which will necessitate insulin therapy in most patients with T2DM.

Early Insulin Therapy and β-Cell Preservation

β-CELL DYSFUNCTION AND β-CELL LOSS: KEY DEFECTS IN TYPE 2 DIABETES

There is strong evidence that β-cell dysfunction is a fundamental underlying genetic abnormality in the pathogenesis of T2DM that cannot develop solely because of insulin resistance. Early β-Cell dysfunction the progression from normal glucose tolerance (NGT) to impaired glucose tolerance (IGT) and finally to T2DM *(21)*. Thereafter, deteriorating glycemic control results from predominantly a progressive decline in pancreatic β-cell function determines along with insulin insensitivity right resulting in increased hepatic glucose production and impaired peripheral glucose uptake *(7,22)*. As insulin fails to suppress lipolysis, the increased concentrations of free fatty acids (FFAs) combined with progressive hyperglycemia act negatively on pancreatic β cells and insulin-sensitive tissues to further inhibit both insulin secretion and peripheral action *(23)*.

Recent evidence has suggested that the progressive insulin deficiency in T2DM is not only a functional defect of the β cell but a decrease in β-cell mass (Ref) because of increased apoptosis. In a study of pancreatic tissue from 124 autopsies, relative β-cell volume, frequency of β-cell apoptosis, β-cell replication, and the formation of new islets from exocrine ducts were measured *(24)*. Relative β-cell volume was decreased by 63 and 44% in both obese and lean persons with T2DM respectively, in comparison with healthy age- and weight-matched non-diabetic controls. In addition, subjects with pre-diabetes also exhibited a 40% decreased relative β-cell volume, suggesting this is etiologically important in the development of T2DM due to a predominance of β-cell apoptosis, which was increased 10-fold in lean subjects and threefold in obese subjects with T2DM. It appears that β-cell loss is an early feature of the pathogenesis of T2DM, and this finding is probably independent from the rate of new islet formation. The implications for treating T2DM from this perspective of β-cell dysfunction and progressive β-cell loss are that strategies that limit glucotoxicity and lipotoxicity can potentially reduce the increased rate of β-cell apoptosis, and therefore, at least partial restoration of β-cell mass may be possible as islet neogenesis remains intact resulting in increased functional β-cell mass.

Indeed, insulin therapy in T2DM can improve peripheral insulin action by correcting glucotoxicity and lipotoxicity and, by also inducing "β-cell rest," can potentially enhance insulin secretion and thereby potentially reduce β-cell loss and/or preserve β-cell integrity (Fig. 1). There is some preliminary evidence, reviewed below, suggesting β-cell preservation with early insulin therapy, but long-term controlled studies, such as Outcome Reduction with Initial Glargine Intervention (ORIGIN), will be needed to demonstrate that the proposed strategy of very early insulin replacement for β-cell preservation can facilitate the maintenance of glycemic control *(17)*.

THE TIMING OF INSULIN INITIATION: A "WINDOW OF OPPORTUNITY"

The concept of the possible existence of a "window of opportunity," such that failure to improve glucose control early can result in long-term detrimental effects on diabetes-related complications. Despite later restoration of glycemic control because of "metabolic or vascular imprinting." This is important to consider in the context of early insulin intervention in T2DM. As reported in the long-term follow-up of Diabetes Control and Complications Trial (DCCT) in the Epidemiology of Diabetes Intervention and Complications (EDIC) study, early improvement of glycemic control through intensive insulin treatment intervention in patients with T1DM is associated with long-term reductions in major diabetes-related complications, despite equivalent glycemic control during the extended observation time *(8–10)*. Whether the same phenomenon

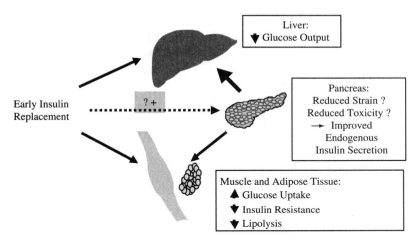

Fig. 1. Early insulin therapy in type 2 diabetes mellitus (T2DM)—"resting" the β cell by replacing insulin. Early insulin therapy may contribute to improved insulin secretion by pancreatic β cells, which contributes to improved insulin-mediated suppression of glucose production and peripheral tissue-mediated glucose uptake and clearance. (Modified from *17*).

applies in T2DM requires long-term follow up on the currently ongoing CV outcome studies assessing the impact of glycemic control.

In addition, the concept of a "window of opportunity" may also apply to the key contribution of the β-cell dysfunction that goes undetected for several years before the diagnosis of T2DM, as classically illustrated by the 6-year follow-up data of the UK Prospective Diabetes Study (UKPDS). This report demonstrated that by the time of diagnosis, patients may have already lost as much as 50% of their β-cell function with a subsequent inexorable decline in β-cell function *(25)*.

Of interest is the UKPDS 57 report on a modified protocol for the last eight UKPDS centers known as the "Glucose Study 2" that tested whether insulin therapy used alone from the time of diagnosis or as an early supplementation to oral agent therapy according to a specific FPG target could avoid progressive deterioration of glycemic control. Insulin therapy was added to sulfonylurea therapy if maximal doses did not maintain FPG levels <108 mg/dL (6.0 mmol/L) *(26)*. Most of the patients were initiated on insulin around 2–3 years after diagnosis, and over half of those newly diagnosed patients treated with a sulfonylurea eventually required early insulin replacement that achieved a median HbA_{1c} level of 6.6% at 6 years. This study provided the first proof of concept in newly diagnosed patients that prompt addition of insulin replacement, when oral therapy is inadequate to reach glycemic targets, can achieve sustain near-normoglycemic control in T2DM.

Conceivably, early insulin replacement can offer sustained improvements in glycemic control. Preliminary support for the hypothesis of insulin-mediated "β-cell rest" is provided by the several studies, as reviewed below, in which newly diagnosed patients with severe hyperglycemia treated only with short-term intensive insulin therapy were subsequently able to maintain near-normoglycemic control without any pharmacologic intervention for prolonged periods of time.

The rationale for such an approach in T2DM came originally from short-term intensive insulin therapy studies performed over the last 20 years that demonstrated improved insulin action and increased endogenous insulin secretion probably induced by reversing glucotoxicity and lipotoxicity (27–31). Further preliminary support for this "β-cell rest" hypothesis is provided by a small uncontrolled Israeli study in newly diagnosed hyperglycemic patients with T2DM subjected to a short, 2-week period of intensive insulin therapy, resulting in near-normoglycemia.Once the intensive insulin therapy was stopped, most of the patients continued with sustained adequate glycemic control for long periods of time (9 to >50 months with a median of 26 months) without pharmacologic intervention to reduce blood glucose (32).

A similar principle was applied in a larger, but still uncontrolled 16-month Korean trial in 92 patients with T2DM of longer duration disease (33). Overall, 34% of the patients went into "remission" that lasted an average of 14 months after 54 ± 39 days on intensive insulin therapy using an insulin pump. The criteria for remission was sustained FPG of <108 mg/dL (6.0 mmol/L) and postprandial glucose (PPG) of <180 mg/dL (10.0 mmol/L). It is important to note that remission rates were higher when patients started intensive insulin therapy with a shorter diabetes duration (3.3 ± 3 years vs. 9.1 ± 4 years for the remission and non-remission groups, respectively; $p < 0.001$) and with lower postprandial blood glucose levels and higher C-peptide responses, strongly suggesting better β-cell reserve.

Of interest, a small Scandinavian trial in newly diagnosed islet cell antibody-negative T2DM patients, randomized to either glyburide or two daily injections of pre-mixed insulin, demonstrated similar significant reductions of HbA_{1c} levels during the first year in both groups, but, by the end of the second year, HbA_{1c} had deteriorated in the glyburide group but not in the insulin-treated group (34). Of note, at 1 and 2 years, the glucagon-stimulated C-peptide response was increased in the insulin-treated group, whereas it was decreased in the sulfonylurea group. Fasting insulin levels after 2 years were higher subsequent to treatment withdrawal in the insulin-treated group compared with the sulfonylurea-treated group. It is conceivable that sulfonylurea treatment might have had a deleterious effect on the β cell or alternatively the early insulin replacement protected and prolonged endogenous insulin secretion resulting in better metabolic control.

Similarly, a recent Canadian study demonstrated that treating newly diagnosed hyperglycemic patients with T2DM to a short (2- to 3-week) course of intensive insulin therapy can successfully lay the foundation for prolonged good glycemic control *(35)*. The authors indicated that the ease with which normoglycemia was achieved may predict those patients who can later succeed in controlling glucose levels with attention to diet alone.

These intriguing findings, albeit with relatively few patients, suggest that the earlier introduction of insulin treatment in T2DM might halt disease progression and the increased endogenous insulin secretion may permit the use of simpler insulin-replacement regimens alone or in combination with oral agents for long-term maintenance of near-normoglycemic control and impact on the prevention of costly complications.

Early Insulin Therapy and Cardioprotection

Sustained near-normoglycemia is the primary treatment goal in the prevention of diabetes-related complications. Epidemiological analysis of the UKPDS data showed a continuous association between the risk of CV complications and glycemia and showed that for each 1% decrease in HbA_{1c} there were significant reductions in major DM-related endpoints, that is, a 37% reduction in microvascular endpoints, a significant 43% reduction in amputation or death from peripheral vascular disease, and a significant 14% reduction in combined fatal and non-fatal myocardial infarction *(5)*. Of note, no glycemic threshold for these complications above normal glucose levels was evident, suggesting that any improvement is beneficial, but these epidemiological data require full validation with interventional studies to define how close to normal the HbA_{1c} should be lowered.

COMPLETED CV OUTCOME TRIALS IN TYPE 2 DIABETES

Despite the importance of the health problems posed by T2DM and the findings of the UKPDS, there is little definitive data on the effects of intensive control of glycemia on CV event rates in patients with DM.

The Kumamoto study was a relatively small, long-term trial, not powered for CV outcomes, but demonstrated a non-significant 44% reduction in CV events, in addition to reduced microvascular complications in the intensive insulin therapy group who achieved HbA_{1c} levels of 7.1% compared with the conventional insulin therapy who had an HbA_{1c} 9.4% *(3)*. In contrast, the VA feasibility trial reported a non-significant 40% higher rate of CV events in the intensive insulin plus combination oral agents group, who achieved an HbA_{1c} of 7.1% compared with the control group with an HbA_{1c} of 9.3% *(36)*.

The Steno-2 Study compared the effect of intensive, multifactorial intervention with that of conventional treatment on modifiable risk factors for cardiovascular disease (CVD) in patients with T2DM and microalbuminuria *(37)*. Eighty patients were randomly assigned to receive conventional treatment in accordance with national guidelines and 80 patients to receive intensive treatment, which was characterized by a stepwise implementation of behaviour modification, followed by multiple drug therapy targeting hyperglycemia, hypertension, dyslipidemia, and microalbuminuria, along with secondary prevention of CVD with aspirin. The principal findings are shown in Fig. 2.

These findings from the Steno-2 study offer important insights into the value of a multi-targeted approach to DM management although the glycemic targets were only reached by few patients, which emphasizes the need for the important ongoing long-term outcome studies designed to provide more answers to these important health care questions.

ONGOING CV OUTCOME TRIALS IN TYPE 2 DIABETES

There are multiple ongoing trials testing different hypothesis with different study designs and pharmacologic interventions attempting to demonstrate benefits on hard CV event reductions *(17,38)*. Among these three important studies can potentially have a major impact to define the role of early insulin

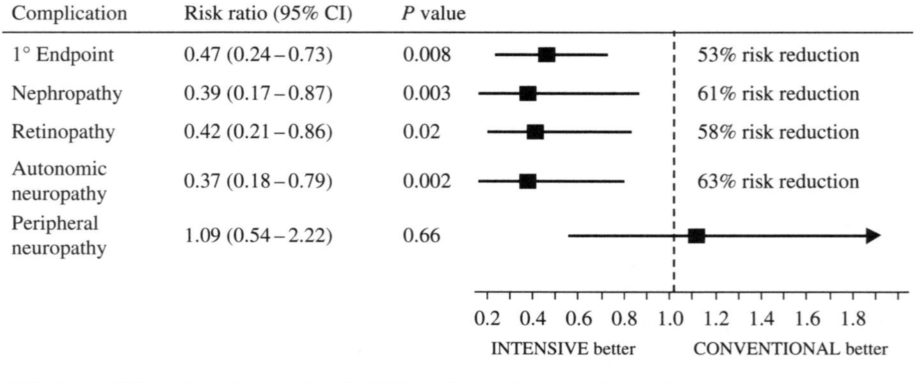

Complication	Risk ratio (95% CI)	P value		
1° Endpoint	0.47 (0.24–0.73)	0.008	■	53% risk reduction
Nephropathy	0.39 (0.17–0.87)	0.003	■	61% risk reduction
Retinopathy	0.42 (0.21–0.86)	0.02	■	58% risk reduction
Autonomic neuropathy	0.37 (0.18–0.79)	0.002	■	63% risk reduction
Peripheral neuropathy	1.09 (0.54–2.22)	0.66	■	

```
         0.2  0.4  0.6  0.8  1.0  1.2  1.4  1.6  1.8
         INTENSIVE better          CONVENTIONAL better
```

1° Endpoint: CVD death, nonfatal MI, CABG, PTCA, nonfatal stroke, amputation, any bypass

Fig. 2. Steno-2 Multifactorial Intervention Study. The relative risk of the development or progression of nephropathy, retinopathy, and autonomic and peripheral neuropathy during the average follow-up of 7.8 years in the intensive-therapy group compared with that in the conventional-therapy group. (Reproduced from *37*; ©2003 Massachusetts Medical Society).

initiation in T2DM: the Veterans Affairs Diabetes Trial (VADT), the Action to Control Cardiovascular Risk in Diabetes (ACCORD) study and the ORIGIN trial (Table 1).

VADT is a 5 to 7 year, randomized, multicenter trial following 1792 older patients with T2DM in the VA System in the USA *(38)*. The study has been designed to answer these specific questions: (i) in older VA patients with established T2DM, what are the relative effects of conventional versus intensive glycemic control on CV morbidity and mortality? (ii) in this population, what is the risk-to-benefit ratio associated with intensive glycemic control? and (iii) should treatment efforts be directed toward intensive glycemic control or other areas (e.g., BP management, lipid therapy, supportive care)? The primary outcome measures are major CV events (CV death, stroke, congestive heart failure), amputation, CAD, and peripheral vascular disease. Secondary outcome measures are angina, transient ischemic attack, critical limb ischemia, total mortality, retinopathy, nephropathy, neuropathy, quality of life, cognitive function, and cost-effectiveness.

ACCORD is a 5-year, randomized, multicenter, double 2×2 factorial design trial following 10,000 patients with T2DM and high CVD risk. The study has been designed to answer these specific questions: (i) does a strategy that targets HbA_{1c} to <6.0% reduce CVD events compared with HbA_{1c} 7.0–7.9%? (ii) in

Table 1
Interventional Studies on Cardiovascular (CV) Outcomes

>Study	Participants (n)	Follow-Up (years)	A1c Target		Expected Results
			Intensive	Standard	
VADT	~1700	5–7	<6%	8–9%	2007
ACCORD	~10,000	4–8 (average 5.6)	<6%	7.0–7.9% (expected mean 7.5%)	2010
ORIGIN	~12,500	4–8	FPG[<95 mg/dL (glargine)]	<7%A1C (standard care with no insulin)	2008

[a] Three ongoing, long-term clinical trials will help to define the role of early insulin initiation in type 2 diabetes mellitus (T2DM): the Veterans Affairs Diabetes Trial (VADT), the Action to Control Cardiovascular Risk in Diabetes (ACCORD) Study, and the Outcome Reduction with Initial Glargine Intervention (ORIGIN) Trial.

the context of good glycemic control, does using a fibrate and a statin reduce CVD events compared with statin treatment alone? (iii) in the context of good glycemic control, does targeting systolic BP to <120 mm Hg reduce CVD events compared with a systolic BP <140 mm Hg? The primary outcome measure is CVD morbidity and mortality. Secondary outcome measures are other CV outcomes, total mortality, microvascular outcomes, quality of life, and cost-effectiveness.

ORIGIN is a 5-year, randomized, open-label, multicenter, 2 × 2 factorial design trial following approximately 12,500 patients ≥ 50 years of age with at least one CVD risk factor (to state the risk factors) and pre-diabetes (IFG, IGT) or early T2DM. The study has been designed to answer these specific questions: (i) does early supplementation with insulin glargine targeting fasting plasma glucose <95 mg/dL (5.3 mmol/L) reduce CV morbidity and/or mortality in high-risk patients with pre-diabetes (IFG, IGT) or early T2DM? (ii) do omega-3 fatty acid supplements reduce CV mortality in patients with pre-diabetes (IFG, IGT) or early T2DM? The primary outcome measures are CV morbidity and/or mortality. Secondary outcome measures are myocardial infarction (MI), stroke, death, coronary artery bypass and/or coronary angioplasty, hospitalization for congestive heart failure, microvascular complications, and new T2DM.

These trials are designed to achieve glycemic targets very close to normal, which are well below those levels reported in previous interventional clinical trials. Clearly, the patients randomized to the intensive regimens in VADT and ACCORD will be on multiple oral agents, but insulin will be required by most to attain and sustain long-term near-normoglycemia. Positive outcomes demonstrating a reduction in the risk of CV events with these trials will determine the new targets for glycemic control. Insulin will then possibly need to be considered much earlier in the course of the disease if alternative glucose-lowering strategies fail to achieve the new glycemic targets that could be set as low as an HbA_{1c} <6%. Furthermore, if the ORIGIN trial is also positive in demonstrating a reduction in CV events, then considerations should be given to basal insulin as a first line therapy to correct dysglycemia (FPG >95 mg/dL) in early diabetes and/or pre-diabetes in patients with evidence of CV disease. Clearly, any potential positive results will result in an overwhelming burden to the health care system and potentially an increased risk of hypoglycemia, which hopefully will be outweighed by a meaningful risk reduction of CV events.

WOULD THE NEW INSULINS OVERCOME COMPLEXITY BARRIERS FOR EARLY INSULIN INITIATION?

Even if the rationale for earlier insulin initiation is correct and well validated, the critical issues will firstly be acceptance by patients and secondly by physicians in general practice. The preceding evidence offers support to the concept of insulin-mediated cessation of disease progression with early insulin intervention to preserve β cells, especially if insulin is to be initiated much earlier to achieve more stringent glycemic targets. The current treatment debate is not about the introduction of intensive short-term insulin regimens as in the pilot studies described above, but how to introduce simple insulin regimens, dictated by clear algorithms and driven by blood glucose monitoring to achieve long-term near-normoglycemia with minimal effort, but initiated and managed in partnership with the patient early in the course of the disease. The concept of early introduction of insulin in combination with oral agents should occur as soon as the threshold target of HbA_{1c} is exceeded; today, that target is 7%, but in future that may well be 6% *(39)*.

However, treatment inertia prevails in clinical practice, and the overall glycemic burden to which patients are exposed reflects the delay in adjusting therapy to meet the increasing requirements for intervention over time. On average, patients accumulate 10 HbA_{1c}-years of glycemic burden of more than 7% before insulin is initiated *(40)*. This clinical inertia, with a failure to promptly advance treatment and dosages of the various oral agents and insulin therapy, results in chronic hyperglycemia. The option of insulin therapy has often emergest at an advanced stage of the disease *(41,42)*. In addition, the multiple barriers to insulin therapy will need to be addressed so that the introduction of early insulin supplementation can become a feasible option for the patient, in line with a physiological approach to supporting the endogenous insulin deficit.

The postponement of insulin therapy in persons with T2DM is because of many well-recognized barriers *(12,43)*. The requirement for subcutaneous insulin injections and the stigma of having to inject insulin cannot be underestimated, as the need for insulin is perceived by the patients and physician as a personal failure and or seen as a terminal phase of the condition. The Diabetes Attitude, Wishes and Needs (DAWN) study emphasized the need to consider patients' and health care providers' attitudes and environment in addition to therapy when attempting to improve the patients' overall health status and well being *(44)*. The DAWN study clearly concluded that "patient and provider resistance to insulin is substantial and for providers it is part of a larger pattern of reluctance to prescribe blood glucose-lowering medications. Interventions to facilitate timely initiation of insulin therapy will need to address factors associated with this resistance." The patient's concerns are often compounded by the physician's resistance to initiating insulin therapy and thereby very often accept sub-optimal glycemic control for prolonged persists of time. Physicians' usual concerns include the complexity and limitations of current insulin preparations, the fear of hypoglycemia, weight gain, and the misconception that the introduction of insulin can potentially increase insulin resistance and CV risk as well as the time needed to educate the prevent above insulin administration and self-maintaing of blood glucose. As discussed above, the evidence does not support insulin therapy increasing insulin resistance (27–31) or having an unfavorable influence on other known CV risk factors; in fact, the opposite may be turn out to be true.

Among all insulin barriers, the fear of hypoglycemia remains the main barrier that explains why patients and physicians are both reluctant to its initiation and also sub-optimally utilizing insulin in T2DM. Indeed, achieving and maintaining euglycemia has been an elusive goal because of the pharmacokinetic imperfections of old human insulins and the resulting barrier of hypoglycemia (45,46). The unpredictable kinetics of the previously available long-acting insulin preparations, in particular NPH insulin, has been a key component in the decision to delay insulin intervention (39). NPH is not an ideal once-daily insulin, with a peak of activity 4–6 h after subcutaneous injection an inadequate duration of action (12–16 h) and variability in absorption due to the need for resuspension prior to injection. The need for more complex insulin treatment algorithms to account for the poor kinetic characteristics is a major barrier to insulin initiation.

Progress has been made, however, with the introduction of more predictable short- and long-acting insulin analogues, which have partially overcome some of the insulin barriers by reducing the risk of hypoglycemia (47,48).

An additional, important barrier for physicians has been the hitherto complex nature of insulin regimens and algorithms, which are difficult to implement under the current limited time and logistical constraints of clinical practice. Even if the reasons to start insulin earlier, as discussed above, are to be proven correct, still any attempt to change the paradigm for earlier insulin replacement will need to overcome the complexity barrier with simpler, safer, and more effective strategies that are easy to implement in general practice. Initiation with basal insulin by using long-acting insulin analogues or initiation with prandial insulin by using short-acting insulin analogues or inhaled insulin will be the focus of future discussions, and different comparative strategies will require further study (39).

"Overcoming Complexity Barriers"—Starting with Basal Insulin

The use of a basal insulin injection to supplement ongoing treatment with oral agents has been demonstrated to offer a simple and practical approach to overcome the complexities of introducing insulin therapy in persons with type 2 diabetes. This strategy has the advantage that only once-daily insulin injection is required and titration can be accomplished effectively in a relatively safe and simple manner by the patient based on daily FPG monitoring (12).

Basal insulin replacement has gained considerable clinical research experience and is increasingly being positioned as a first line insulin initiation approach in T2DM. New consensus guidelines (ADA/EASD) Nathan et al. Proof of concept was initially demonstrated by the 24-week treat-to-target study that enrolled 756 insulin naïve patients on oral agents with mean HbA_{1c} of 8.6% (entry values of 7.5–10%) and 8–9 years diabetes duration (49). Patients continued to receive oral agents and were also treated with either once-daily bedtime NPH insulin or insulin glargine, a long-acting insulin analogue with a relatively flat action profile and up to 24-h duration of action. The insulin dose was force-titrated weekly to an FPG target of ≤100 mg/dL following a structured insulin titration algorithm according to FPG and evidence of hypoglycemia. Similar reductions in HbA_{1c} levels (6.96 versus 6.97%, respectively) were achieved by study end, and approximately 60% of the patients achieved HbA_{1c} values of ≤ 7% with both insulin regimens. However, treatment with insulin glargine was associated with a significantly lower incidence of nocturnal hypoglycemia. Similar results, in the same type of patient population, have been achieved with insulin detemir, another long-acting insulin analogue with a smooth, protracted time-action profile with a duration of action of approximately 14–16 h when compared with NPH (50) when both insulins were given twice daily. Similar improvements of HbA_{1c} <7%, were seen but there was also a reduced risk of nocturnal hypoglycemia and less weight gain with detemir compared with NPH.

A common consideration as therapy is escalated is the option of adding a third oral agent, as opposed to initiating insulin (51). Important concerns with three oral agents include the potential for an additive risk of adverse events, dose adjustments that may become complex, and cost considerations. Recently, the efficacy, safety, and cost of adding a third agent, a thiazolidinedione or insulin glargine, were tested in T2DM patients who previously failed a regimen of two oral agents, sulfonylurea and metformin (52). The average diabetes duration was 8–9 years, and the baseline HbA_{1c} of approximately 8.8% was very similar to the treat-to-target study, but the insulin titration algorithm was less stringent. Both strategies, add-on low-dose insulin glargine or add-on maximum-dose rosiglitazone (RSG), resulted in similar HbA_{1c} reductions of 1.7 and 1.5%, respectively, with a final HbA_{1c} of approximately 7.1% (Fig. 3A). Greater improvements in HbA_{1c} were seen with insulin glargine when baseline HbA_{1c} was ≥ 9.5% (Fig. 3B). Insulin glargine resulted in more hypoglycemia but with less weight gain and no edema at a lower cost than RSG. Perhaps, any of these triple agent strategies if used much earlier in the course of the disease, at a lower baseline HbA_{1c} level, just above 7%, and not like in most studies with higher HbA_{1c} 8.5%, then the chances of most patients

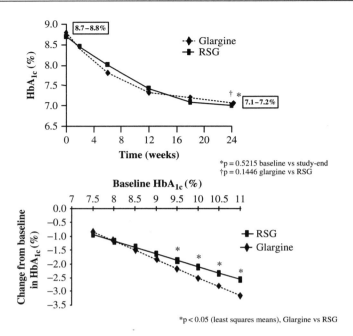

Fig. 3. Triple agent therapy in type 2 diabetes mellitus (T2DM). In a randomized comparison of rosiglitazone (RSG) or insulin glargine as add-on therapy to sulfonylurea and metformin, mean hemoglobin A1c (HbA_{1c}) levels from baseline to end point showed a similar decrease for both insulin glargine (–1.66%) and RSG (–1.51%; $p = 0.1446$). In the comparison of RSG or insulin glargine as add-on therapy, improvement in HbA_{1c} was significantly greater for insulin glargine-treated patients versus RSG-treated patients if baseline HbA_{1c} was >9.5%.

sustaining the HbA_{1c} target of <7.0% would be considerably greater, but this approach requires further long-term, controlled studies.

The original "treat-to-target" structured insulin algorithm is not only effective but also simple to understand and implement and has been satisfactorily applied in multiple other studies (*39*). However, how widely effective has it been when adopted in clinical practice remains controversial as patients do not have the same level of support and interaction with the health care providers as in the setting of clinical research studies. Often, patients are sub-optimally titrated on these "clinic-driven" algorithms taking lower insulin sub-optimal doses without achieving glycemic targets if they are not closely supervised.

The LANMET study in patients with T2DM who were inadequately controlled on oral agents (mean HbA_{1c} 9.5%) took the treat-to-target concept one step further in terms of simplicity to facilitate patient involvement with self-titration of insulin *(53)*. This study demonstrated the feasibility of achieving tight glycemic control using a very simple forced-titration regimen consisting of increments of 2 IU insulin dose every 3 days if FPG was >100 mg/dL coupled with infrequent (3-monthly) physician contact. The study design required patients to remain on metformin (2 g) and were randomized to insulin glargine or NPH. Patients consistently self-monitored FPG levels and also were empowered to self-adjust their insulin dose, which resulted in significant in HbA$_{1c}$ of 2.4% reductions with a final HbA$_{1c}$ of 7.1% across both groups but those patients receiving insulin glargine had a lower incidence of hypoglycemia (Fig. 4).

Furthermore, the safety and efficacy of the two insulin glargine-forced titration algorithms have been tested comparing the original algorithm from the treat-to-target study, which was "clinic-driven" to direct weekly dose escalations of 2–8 units according to different FPG values versus the self-titration algorithm from the LANMET study, which was "patient-driven" for adjustments of 2 units every 3 days if the mean FPG was greater than 100 mg/dL *(54)*. Interestingly, the "patient-driven" self-titration algorithm achieved slightly better reductions in FPG and HbA$_{1c}$ levels and allowed titration to higher insulin doses and with no difference in the frequency of hypoglycemia between the two insulin regimens.

Results of these studies therefore clearly demonstrate that basal insulin replacement can be easily implemented with long-acting insulin analogues to

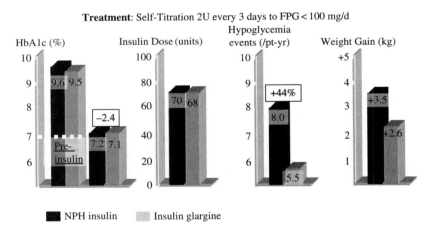

Fig. 4. The LANMET Study. In this randomized, open-label trial, good glycemic control was achieved with both insulin glargine and NPH insulin when using home glucose monitoring. Insulin glargine was associated with reduced symptomatic hypoglycemia during the first 12 weeks and dinner-time hyperglycemia compared with NPH insulin.

achieve FPG and HbA$_{1c}$ targets using forced titration algorithms that can be driven by patients themselves, with no increase in the risk of hypoglycemia and with the potential of reducing the burden on health care system utilization. The novel strategy of empowering the patients to self-adjust their basal insulin dose adds a further dimension to achieving normal fasting blood glucose targets as an early strategy in this treatment paradigm (*fix fasting first*) facilitated by the use of long-acting insulin analogues with reduced risk of hypoglycemia.

However, if the target HbA$_{1c}$ level is not achieved after basal insulin is effectively titrated to correct FPG levels to <100 mg/dL, then further benefit can be attained by advancing the insulin regimen with progressive additions of pre-meal short-acting insulin analogues or with inhaled insulin to control postprandial glycemic peaks. Other options, not subject to this review, include parenteral GLP-1 derivatives, pramlintide, or the oral agents such as the DPP-4 inhibitors.

Recent evidence provides some insight into the relative contributions of fasting and postprandial hyperglycemia to the glycemic burden in patients treated on oral agents without insulin (*55*). When the HbA$_{1c}$ is close to 7%, the postprandial glucose excursions are the predominant factor in the glycemic burden, and proper intervention with prandial insulin to escalate therapy can further improve glycemic control when basal insulin therapy has already been maximized. Coverage with basal insulin plus the stepwise introduction of prandial inhaled insulin or short-acting insulin analogues at the main meal or at the meal with the maximum glucose excursion first and then followed over time with covering additional meals will be determined according to blood glucose monitoring and the target HbA$_{1c}$ achieved.

"Overcoming Complexity Barriers"—Starting with Prandial Insulin

Mealtime insulin supplementation to limit postprandial hyperglycemic excursions in combination with oral agents is an attractive and physiologic approach for the early initiation of insulin therapy. The administration of pre-meal doses of a short-acting insulin analogue (bolus) to control postprandial hyperglycemic peaks has been successfully demonstrated in patients whose HbA$_{1c}$ levels remain elevated despite the use of oral agents and the achievement of normal fasting blood glucose (*56,57*). At the end of a 12-week study (*57*), treatment with three injections of mealtime lispro insulin added to a sulfonylurea achieved lower HbA$_{1c}$ than sulfonylurea in combination with bedtime NPH or with metformin. HbA$_{1c}$ improved with all therapies but was significantly lower for the lispro plus sulfonylurea compared with sulfonylurea combination with metformin or added bedtime NPH to the sulfonylurea (7.7, 8.3, and 8.5%, respectively). Clearly, still away from target values probably because of inadequate titration, the increased complexity of this insulin regimen and the need for multiple daily prandial insulin injections are major barriers for non-adherence, and the potential acceptance by the patients is understandably low.

However, now that inhaled insulin, Exubera™, recently obtained FDA approval, a prandial regimen using non-injectable pre-meal insulin replacement may facilitate initiation of insulin therapy and has the potential to become a valid option for first-line insulin intervention if on-going and future studies demonstrate longer-term safety with sustained glycemic effects over time. Currently, sustained efficacy and safety up to 4 years has been reported in a small group of patients remaining from the original phase II studies who were offered long-term inhaled insulin therapy after they completed the initial 12-week randomized, controlled trials (58).

The main efficacy and safety data on inhaled insulin in patients with T2DM on oral agents come from a carefully controlled study that demonstrated sustained glycemic effects, and the early small changes in pulmonary function detected in FEV_1 and DLco, did not lead to increased rates of lung function loss over a 2-year period, and resolved upon discontinuation of therapy (59). Similar findings were recently reported in T2DM patients on previous insulin therapy, comparing prandial coverage with inhaled insulin versus a subcutaneous insulin. Treatment group differences in changes from baseline in FEV_1 and DLco were small (<1.5% of mean baseline) and remained stable with no progression for 2 years. Furthermore, HbA_{1c} improved from 7.7 and 7.8% to 7.3 and 7.3% with inhaled and subcutaneous insulin, respectively, but inhaled insulin resulted in greater FPG reductions from 151 to 136 mg/dL versus 148 to 147 mg/dL, respectively (60).

Regarding the potential for early initiation with inhaled insulin, the efficacy of adding pre-prandial inhaled insulin to oral therapy was recently demonstrated in a 3-month clinical trial (61). Patients with T2DM ($n = 309$) with mean baseline HbA_{1c} of 9.5% (entry criteria 8–11%) on combination oral therapy with two agents (insulin secretagogue plus metformin or a thiazolidinedione) were randomized to three different arms: (i) addition of prandial inhaled insulin to the current doses of oral agents; (ii) discontinuation of oral agents and initiation of prandial inhaled insulin as monotherapy; (iii) continuation of oral agents with no changes (control group). The results were particularly notable in that inhaled insulin added to oral agents showed a significant effect on both the postprandial glucose increments and the FPG levels, with mean decreases of 76 mg/dL in PPG and 53 mg/dL in FPG at 12 weeks (Fig. 5A). The glycemic effects observed with inhaled human insulin extended beyond the predicted pharmacokinetic activity by substantially improving FPG levels, which probably contributes to the impressive reductions of HbA_{1c} levels. The largest decrease in HbA_{1c} (1.9%) was demonstrated in the group receiving combination oral agents plus supplementation with inhaled insulin whereas

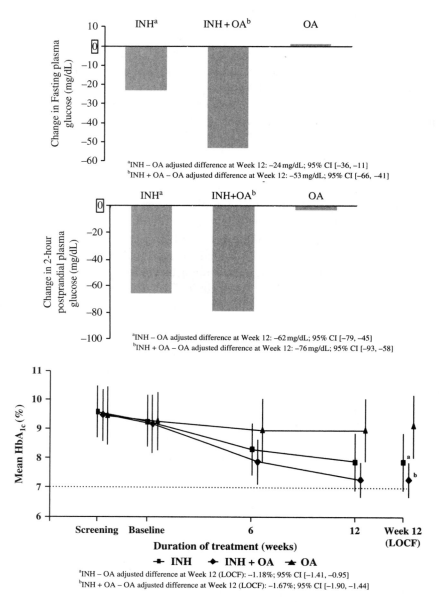

Fig. 5. Inhaled insulin supplementation to oral agents. Adjusted mean change in fasting plasma glucose concentration from baseline to study end after 12 weeks of inhaled insulin treatment. Adjusted mean change in fasting plasma glucose concentration from baseline to study end after 12 weeks of inhaled insulin treatment. Reductions in hemoglobin A1c level were greatest with inhaled insulin. Adjusted treatment group differences for inhaled insulin plus oral agents and inhaled insulin alone compared with continued oral agent therapy were 1.67 and 1.18%, respectively.

the group on inhaled insulin alone and the control group achieved a lesser reduction in HbA$_{1c}$ of 1.4 and 0.2%, respectively (Fig. 5B).

Patient acceptance and preference will ultimately determine the future use of inhaled insulin. Several studies have shown that patients receiving inhaled insulin prefer this therapy and experience greater short- and longer-term satisfaction than patients taking subcutaneous insulin (62,63). The availability of inhaled insulin could therefore have a major impact if physicians can convince patients with T2DM to begin using insulin much earlier. It would be reasonable to consider the option of starting insulin therapy at each meal, targeting premeal blood glucose levels, which can be basically considered late PPG levels, as the first step in insulin therapy, challenging our current standard practice of starting with a basal insulin replacement.

As we move to more stringent HbA$_{1c}$ targets (64,65), it is highly conceivable that in the future we may consider, for those patients who are "well controlled" with two or three oral agents but whose HbA$_{1c}$ are just above target 7%, perhaps in the 7.1–7.5% range, the option of supplementing with inhaled insulin. This strategy will be most appropriate and could facilitate initiation of insulin at those mildly elevated HbA$_{1c}$ values that otherwise physicians and patients have been very reluctant to start insulin. Perhaps, one dose of inhaled

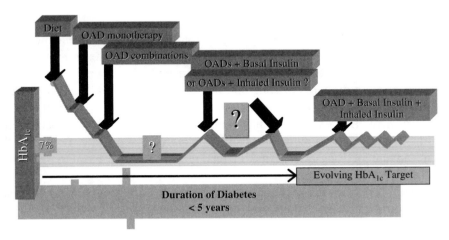

Fig. 6. The evolving management of type 2 diabetes mellitus (T2DM). The early, aggressive approach to type 2 diabetes management avoids the risk of early treatment failure by adopting an intensive therapeutic strategy immediately upon diagnosis. Early combinations of agents with complementary modes of action targeting the dual defects underlying type 2 diabetes (insulin resistance and (-cell dysfunction) are most likely to support tight, long-term glycemic control. Stringent hemoglobin A1c (HbA$_{1c}$) targets will determine the prompt initiation and optimization of insulin replacement with either basal or inhaled insulin, and eventually both, to supplement oral agents.

insulin before the main meal of the day, in combination with oral agents, may suffice to achieve an HbA_{1c} reduction of 0.4–0.5% that may be enough to attain the HbA_{1c} goal of <7%. It would be essential to start inhaled insulin where an excessive glucose excursion is present [delta blood glucose >40 mg/dL (>2.2 mmol/L)]. Otherwise, if the initial HbA_{1c} is considerably higher or remains above 7% then further prandial coverage at each meal would be advisable with insulin adjustments based on the PPG levels measured at the following pre-meal time and/or based on the 2 h post pradical glucose level.

Eventually, patients may require supplementation of basal insulin if target FPG and HbA_{1c} are not achieved. Regardless of what insulin is initiated first, it is likely that, eventually, a combination of basal and pradical insulin increased on subentaneous will be required for long-term maintenance of near-normoglycemic control (Fig. 6).

CONCLUSIONS

The evidence for improved glycemic control for preventing the onset and progression of diabetes-related microvascular complications is overwhelming.

The concept of the possible existence of a "window of opportunity" for improved glycemic control, because of a "metabolic" or "vascular" imprinting, is gaining credence.

It may be that the early timing of physiologic insulin replacement within a "window of opportunity" is critical for potential β-cell preservation, which may in turn can facilitate long-term maintenance of glycemic control.

Although the rationale is strong and the data clearly justify the early use of insulin, the issues of implementation and overcoming perceive insulin barriers remain critical. However, there has been a major change with respect to the insulins available and how insulin can be delivered.

The advent of long-acting insulin analogues for early basal replacement with inhaled insulin on rapid-acting insulin analogue, for progressive prandial replacement provides the necessary tools for health care providers to empower patients to take charge of their own diabetes control.

Ongoing trials, designed to achieve glycemic targets very close to normal, may provide convincing evidence in terms of CV risk reductions, the task of persuading physicians and patients of the need for early insulin replacement as an expected strategy to achieve near-normoglycemic control will be lessened.

The advances outlined contribute greatly to addressing the multiple barriers to insulin therapy so that the option of early insulin replacement can become a feasible option for the patient, in line with a physiologic approach to supplement and possibly sustain the remaining endogenous insulin secretion.

REFERENCES

1. DCCT Research Group. The effect of intensive treatment of diabetes on the development and progression of long-term complications in insulin-dependent diabetes mellitus. The Diabetes Control and Complications Trial Research Group. *N Engl J Med* 329: 977–986, 1993.

2. DCCT Research Group. The relationship of glycemic exposure (HbA$_{1c}$) to the risk of development and progression of retinopathy in the diabetes control and complications trial. *Diabetes* 44: 968–983, 1995.

3. Ohkubo Y, Kishikawa H, Araki E, Miyata T, Isami S, Motoyoshi S, Kojima Y, Furuyoshi N, Shichiri M. Intensive insulin therapy prevents the progression of diabetic microvascular complications in Japanese patients with non-insulin-dependent diabetes mellitus: a randomized prospective 6-year study. *Diabetes Res Clin Pract* 28: 103–117, 1995.

4. U.K. Prospective Diabetes Study (UKPDS) Group. Intensive blood-glucose control with sulphonylureas or insulin compared with conventional treatment and risk of complications in patients with type 2 diabetes (UKPDS 33). *Lancet* 352: 837–853, 1998.

5. Stratton IM, Adler AI, Neil HA, Matthews DR, Manley SE, Cull CA, Hadden D, Turner RC, Holman RR. Association of glycaemia with macrovascular and microvascular complications of type 2 diabetes (UKPDS 35): prospective observational study. *BMJ* 321: 405–412, 2000.

6. Buse JB, Rosenstock J. Prevention of Cardiovascular Outcomes in Type 2 Diabetes Mellitus: Trials on the Horizon. *Endocrinol Metab Clin North Am* 34: 221–235, 2005.

7. Rosenstock J, Wyne K. Insulin Treatment in Type 2 Diabetes. In: Goldstein BJ, Muller-Wieland D (Eds). *Textbook of Type 2 Diabetes* 2003, pp 131–154.

8. Diabetes Control and Complications Trial/Epidemiology of Diabetes Interventions and Complications Research Group. Sustained effect of intensive treatment of type 1 diabetes mellitus on development and progression of diabetic nephropathy: the Epidemiology of Diabetes Interventions and Complications (EDIC) study. *JAMA* 290: 2159–2267, 2003.

9. Diabetes Control and Complications Trial/Epidemiology of Diabetes Interventions and Complications Research Group (DCCT/EDIC). Intensive diabetes therapy and carotid intima-media thickness in type 1 diabetes mellitus. *N Engl J Med* 348: 2294–2303, 2003.

10. Diabetes Control and Complications Trial/Epidemiology of Diabetes Interventions and Complications (DCCT/EDIC) Study Research Group. Intensive diabetes therapy and cardiovascular disease in patients with type 1 diabetes. *N Engl J Med* 353: 2643–2653, 2005.

11. Rosenstock J. Basal insulin supplementation in type 2 diabetes: Refining the tactics. *Am J Med* 116: 10S–16S, 2004.

12. Rosenstock J, Riddle M. Insulin Therapy in Type 2 Diabetes. In: Cefalu WT, Gerich JE, LeRoith D (Eds). *The Cadre Handbook of Diabetes Management*. New York: Medical Information Press; 2004.

13. Bindra S, Rosenstock J, Cefalu W. Inhaled insulin: a novel route for insulin delivery. *Expert Opin Investig Drugs* 11: 687–691, 2002.

14. King H, Aubert RE, Herman WH. Global burden of diabetes, 1995–2025: prevalence, numerical estimates, and projections. *Diabetes Care* 21: 1414–1431, 1998.

15. Green A, Hirsch NC, Pramming SK. The changing world demography of type 2 diabetes. *Diabetes Metab Res Rev* 19: 3–7, 2003.

16. Wild S, Roglic G, Green A, Sicree R, King H. Global prevalence of diabetes: estimates for the year 2000 and projections for 2030. *Diabetes Care* 27: 1047–1053, 2004.

17. Gerstein HC, Rosenstock J. Insulin therapy in people who have dysglycemia and type 2 diabetes mellitus: can if offer both cardiovascular protection and beta cell preservation. *Endocrinol Metab Clin North Am* 34: 137–154, 2005.

18. Khaw KT, Wareham N, Luben R, Bingham S, Oakes S, Welch A, Day N. Glycated haemoglobin, diabetes, and mortality in men in Norfolk cohort of European prospective investigation of cancer and nutrition (EPIC-Norfolk). *BMJ* 322: 15–18, 2001.

19. Meigs JB, Nathan DM, D'Agostino RB, Wilson PW, Framingham Offspring Study. Fasting and postchallenge glycemia and cardiovascular disease risk: the Framingham Offspring Study. *Diabetes Care* 25: 1845–1850, 2002.

20. Coutinho M, Gerstein HC, Wang Y, Yusuf S. The relationship between glucose and incident cardiovascular events. A metaregression analysis of published data from 20 studies of 95,783 individuals followed for 12.4 years. *Diabetes Care* 22: 233–40, 1999.

21. Weyer C, Bogardus C, Mott DM, Pratley RE. The natural history of insulin secretory dysfunction and insulin resistance in the pathogenesis of type 2 diabetes mellitus. *J Clin Invest* 104: 787–794, 1999.

22. Kahn SE. The importance of β-cell failure in the development and progression of type 2 diabetes mellitus. *J Clin Endocrinol Metab* 86: 4047–58, 2001.

23. McGarry JD. Banting Lecture 2001: dysregulation of fatty acid metabolism in the etiology of type 2 diabetes. *Diabetes* 51: 7–18, 2002.

24. Butler AE, Janson J, Bonner-Weir S, Ritzel R, Rizza RA, Butler PC. Beta-cell deficit and increased betacell apoptosis in humans with type 2 diabetes. *Diabetes* 52: 102–110, 2003.

25. UK Prospective Diabetes Study 16. Overview of 6 years' therapy of type II diabetes: a progressive disease. *Diabetes* 44: 1249–1258, 1995.

26. Wright A, Burden AC, Paisey RB, Cull CA, Holman RR, U.K. Prospective Diabetes Study Group. Sulfonylurea inadequacy: efficacy of addition of insulin over 6 years in patients with type 2 diabetes in the U.K. Prospective Diabetes Study (UKPDS 57). *Diabetes Care* 25: 330–336, 2002.

27. Scarlett JA, Gray RS, Griffin J, Olefsky JM, Kolterman OG. Insulin treatment reverses the insulin resistance of type II diabetes mellitus. *Diabetes Care* 5: 353–363, 1982.

28. Andrews WJ, Vasquez B, Nagulesparan M, Klimes I, Foley J, Unger R, Reaven GM. Insulin therapy in obese, non-insulin-dependent diabetes induces improvements in insulin action and secretion that are maintained for two weeks after insulin withdrawal. *Diabetes* 33: 634–642, 1984.

29. Garvey WT, Olefsky JM, Griffin J, Hamman RF, Kolterman OG. The effect of insulin treatment on insulin secretion and insulin action in type II diabetes mellitus. *Diabetes* 34: 222–234, 1985.

30. Henry RR, Gumbiner B, Ditzler T, Wallace P, Lyon R, Glauber HS. Intensive conventional insulin therapy for type II diabetes. *Diabetes Care* 16: 21–31, 1993.

31. Pratipanawatr T, Cusi K, Ngo P, Pratipanawatr W, Mandarino LJ, DeFronzo RA. Normalization of plasma glucose concentration by insulin therapy improves insulin-stimulated glycogen synthesis in type 2 diabetes. *Diabetes* 51: 462–468, 2002.

32. Ilkova H, Glaser B, Tunckale A, Bagriacik N, Cerasi E. Induction of long-term glycemic control in newly diagnosed type 2 diabetic patients by transient intensive insulin treatment. *Diabetes Care* 20: 1353–6, 1997.

33. Park S, Choi SB. Induction of long-term normoglycemia without medication in Korean type 2 diabetes patients after continuous subcutaneous insulin infusion therapy. *Diabetes Metab Res Rev* 19: 124–130, 2003.

34. Alvarsson M, Sundkvist G, Lager I, Henricsson M, Berntorp K, Fernqvist-Forbes E, Steen L, Westermark G, Westermark P, Orn T, Grill V. Beneficial effects of insulin versus

sulphonylurea on insulin secretion and metabolic control in recently diagnosed type 2 diabetic patients. *Diabetes Care* 26: 2231–2237, 2003.

35. Ryan EA, Imes S, Wallace C. Short-term intensive insulin therapy in newly diagnosed type 2 diabetes. *Diabetes Care* 27: 1028–1032, 2004.

36. Abraira C, Colwell JA, Nuttall F, Sawin CT, Henderson W, Comstock JP, Emanuele NV, Levin SR, Pacold I, Lee HS. Cardiovascular events and correlates in the veterans affairs diabetes feasibility trial. *Arch Intern Med* 157: 181–188, 1997.

37. Gaede P, Vedel P, Larsen N, Jensen GV, Parving HH, Pedersen O. Multifactorial intervention and cardiovascular disease in patients with type 2 diabetes. *N Engl J Med* 348: 383–93, 2003.

38. Abraira C, Duckworth W, McCarren M, Emanuele N, Arca D, Reda D, Henderson W. Design of the cooperative study on glycemic control and complications in diabetes mellitus type 2: Veterans Affairs Diabetes Trial. *J Diabetes Complications* 17: 314–322, 2003.

39. Rosenstock J, Banarer S, Owens D. Insulin Strategies in Type 1 and Type 2 Diabetes Mellitus. In: Fonseca V (Ed). *Clinical Diabetes: Translating Research into Practice.* Saunders Elsevier, 2006, pp 371–394.

40. Brown JB, Nichols GA, Perry A. The burden of treatment failure in type 2 diabetes. *Diabetes Care* 27: 1535–1540, 2004.

41. Grant RW, Cagliero E, Dubey AK. Clinical inertia in the management of type 2 diabetes metabolic risk factors. *Diabet Med* 21: 150–155, 2004.

42. Shah BR, Hux JE, Laupacis A, Zinman B, van Walraven C. Clinical inertia in response to inadequate glycemic control. *Diabetes Care* 28: 600–606, 2005.

43. Korytkowski M. When oral agents fail: practical barriers to starting insulin. *Int J Obes* 26: S18–S24, 2002.

44. Peyrot M, Rubin RR, Lauritzen T, Skovlund SE, Snoek FJ, Matthews DR, Landgraf R, Kleinebreil L. Resistance to insulin therapy among patients and providers. Results of the cross-national Diabetes Attitudes, Wishes and Needs (DAWN) study. *Diabetes Care* 28: 2673–2679, 2005.

45. Cryer PE. Hypoglycaemia: the limiting factor in the glycaemic management of type I and type II diabetes. *Diabetologia* 45: 937–48, 2002.

46. Cryer PE. Diverse causes of hypoglycemia-associated autonomic failure in diabetes. *N Engl J Med* 350: 2272–2279, 2004.

47. Owens DR, Zinman B, Bolli GB. Insulins today and beyond. *Lancet* 358: 739–746, 2001.

48. DeWitt DE, Hirsch IB. Outpatient insulin therapy in type 1 and type 2 diabetes mellitus: scientific review. *JAMA* 289: 2254–2264, 2003.

49. Riddle MC, Rosenstock J, Gerich J, Insulin Glargine 4002 Study Investigators. The treat-to-target trial: randomized addition of glargine or human NPH insulin to oral therapy of type 2 diabetic patients. *Diabetes Care* 26: 3080–3086, 2003.

50. Hermansen K, Derezinski T, Kim H, Gall M-A. Treatment with insulin detemir in combination with oral agents is associated with less risk of hypoglycemia and less weight gain than NPH insulin at comparable levels of glycaemic improvement in people with type 2 diabetes. *Diabetologia* 47(Suppl 1): A273, 2004. (Abstract)

51. Riddle M, Rosenstock J. Type 2 Diabetes: Oral Monotherapy and Combination Therapy. In: Cefalu WT, Gerich JE, LeRoith D (Eds). *The Cadre Handbook of Diabetes Management.* New York: Medical Information Press; 2004.

52. Rosenstock J, Sugimoto D, Strange P, Stewart JA, Soltes-Rak E, Dailey G. Triple therapy in type 2 diabetes: Insulin glargine or rosiglitazone added to combination therapy of sulfonylurea plus metformin in insulin-naive patients. *Diabetes Care* 29: 554–559, 2006.

53. Yki-Järvinen H, Kauppinen- Mäkelin R, Tiikkainen M, Vahatalo M, Virtamo H, Nikkilä K, Tulokas T, Hulme S, Hardy K, McNulty S, Hänninen J, Levanen H, Lahdenperä S, Lehtonen R, Ryysy L. Insulin glargine or NPH combined with metformin in type 2 diabetes: the LANMET study. *Diabetologia* 49: 442–451, 2006.

54. Davies M, Storms F, Shutler S, Bianchi-Biscay M, Gomis R. Improvement of glycemic control in subjects with poorly controlled type 2 diabetes. *Diabetes Care* 28: 1282–1288, 2005.

55. Monnier L, Lapinski H, Colette C. Contributions of fasting and postprandial plasma glucose increments to the overall diurnal hyperglycemia of type 2 diabetic patients: variations with increasing levels of HbA1c. *Diabetes Care* 26: 881–885, 2003.

56. Woerle HJ, Pimenta WP, Meyer C, Gosmanov NR, Szoke E, Szombathy T, Mitrakou A, Gerich JE. Diagnostic and therapeutic implications of relationships between fasting, 2-hour postchallenge plasma glucose and hemoglobin a1c values. *Arch Intern Med* 164: 1627–32, 2004.

57. Bastyr E, Stuart C, Brodows R, Schwartz S, Graf CJ, Zagar A, Robertson KE. Therapy focused on lowering postprandial glucose, not fasting glucose, may be superior for lowering HbA$_{1c}$. IOEZ Study Group. *Diabetes Care* 23: 1236–1241, 2000.

58. Skyler J, for the Exubera® Phase II Study Group. Sustained long-term efficacy and safety of inhaled insulin (Exubera®) during 4 years of continuous therapy. *Diabetes* 53(Suppl 2): A115, 2004. (Abstract)

59. Dreyer M, for the Exubera Phase 3 Study Group. Efficacy and 2-year pulmonary safety data of inhaled insulin as adjunctive therapy with metformin or glibenclamide in type 2 diabetes patients poorly controlled with oral monotherapy. *Diabetologia* 47(1 Suppl): A44, 2004. (Abstract)

60. Rosenstock J, Klioze S, Ogawa M, Aubin LS, Duggan W, the Exubera 1029 Study Group. Inhaled human insulin (Exubera®) therapy shows sustained efficacy and is well tolerated over a 2-year period in patients with type 2 diabetes (T2DM). *Diabetes* 55(Suppl 2): 2006. (Abstract)

61. Rosenstock J, Zinman B, Murphy Clement LJSC, Moore P, Bowering CK, Hendler R, Lan SP, Cefalu WT. Inhaled insulin improves glycemic control when substituted for or added to oral combination therapy in type 2 diabetes. *Ann Intern Med* 143: 459–558, 2005.

62. Cappelleri JC, Cefalu WT, Rosenstock J, Kourides IA, Gerber RA. Treatment satisfaction in type 2 diabetes: a comparison between an inhaled insulin regimen and a subcutaneous regimen. *Clin Ther* 24: 552–564, 2002.

63. Rosenstock J, Cappelleri JC, Bolinder B, Gerber RA. Patient satisfaction and glycemic control after 1 year with inhaled insulin (Exubera) in patients with type 1 or type 2 diabetes. *Diabetes Care* 27: 1318–1323, 2004.

64. European Diabetes Policy Group. A desktop guide to type 2 diabetes mellitus. *Diabet Med* 16: 716–730, 1999.

65. American Diabetes Association. Standards of medical care in diabetes—2006. *Diabetes Care* 29: S4–S42, 2006.

6 Diabetic Retinopathy

Can it be Prevented?

Emily Y. Chew, MD

CONTENTS

SUMMARY

The intensive medical management of persons with diabetes, especially both glycemic control as well as blood pressure control, has been proven by randomized controlled clinical trials to be highly beneficial in reducing both the development and progression of diabetic retinopathy in both types 1 and 2 diabetes. It is possible that aggressive therapy of dyslipidemia in this population may also play an important role in the treatment of diabetic retinopathy. This is to be proven in the randomized controlled trial called Actions to Control Cardiovascular Risks in Diabetes (ACCORD) which is designed to evaluate the role of treatment of intensive control of glycemia and blood pressure and treatment of dyslipidemia. Other medical conditions such as pregnancy may also have an effect on the progression of diabetic retinopathy.

From: *Contemporary Endocrinology: Controversies in Treating Diabetes:*
Clinical and Research Aspects
Edited by: D. LeRoith and A. I. Vinik © Humana Press, Totowa, NJ

Key Words: Diabetic retinopathy, glycemia, blood pressure, dyslipidemia aspirin use, pregnancy, diabetic macular edema

INTRODUCTION

Diabetic retinopathy is one of the leading causes of blindness in the USA and in the developed world *(1)*. In 2004, over 411 million persons were estimated to have diabetic retinopathy with 899,000 affected with vision-threatening diabetic retinopathy *(2)*. With the increase in the survival of the aging population and the increase in the prevalence in diabetes, the number of individual affected with diabetic retinopathy will increase as a major public health disease. Any preventive measure may lessen the impact on the potential toll this disease may take in terms of health care cost, personal loss in productivity, and societal cost and burden.

The two main causes of vision loss associated with diabetic retinopathy are diabetic macular edema and proliferative diabetic retinopathy. The risk factors known to be associated with the development and progression of sight-threatening diabetic retinopathy are varied and numerous *(3–6)*. However, some of these factors are not yet proven conclusively to be associated with the development and progression of retinopathy because there are either inconsistent findings across various studies or the nature of the supportive data is only observational. This chapter will explore some of these controversial factors and will emphasize the potential approach to validating some of the results. We will also emphasize the risk factors that are well known to be associated with the development and progression of diabetic retinopathy.

GLYCEMIC CONTROL

Tight glycemic control has been proven to be an important factor the progression of diabetic retinopathy. This risk factor, however, was considered controversial when it was introduced by Dr. Elliot Joslin *(7,8)*. He emphasized the importance of intensive treatment to attain near-normal glucose control in the treatment of diabetes for the prevention of diabetic complications in his clinical practice in the 1950s and 1960s with great resistance from the medical community of his times. In the late 1970s and throughout the 1980s, the baseline hemoglobin A1C (HbA1C) level of the participants of Early Treatment Diabetic Retinopathy was 9.8%, the Diabetes Control and Complications Trial (DCCT) was 9.1%, and the United Kingdom Prospective Diabetes Trial (UKPDS) whose participants were recently diagnosed with diabetes, was 7.1%. The relatively higher HbA1C in the earlier studies reflect the tendency of medical practice to have less intensive glycemic control in these earlier years.

Dr. Joslin was eventually proven to be correct a number of decades later in the 1990's when the results of randomized controlled clinical trials showed that tight or intensive glucose control compared with standard care prevented progression or development of diabetic retinopathy and other microvascular abnormalities. This was found for persons with type 1 or type 2 diabetes. The results of these studies will be presented.

TYPE 1 DIABETES

In the DCCT, 1441 patients with type 1 diabetes were randomly assigned to either conventional or intensive insulin treatment, and followed for a period of 4–9 years (9–13). The DCCT demonstrated that intensive insulin treatment is associated with a decreased risk of either the development of or progression of diabetic retinopathy in patients with type 1 diabetes. In patients without any visible retinopathy when enrolled in the DCCT, the 3-year risk of developing retinopathy was reduced by 75% in the intensive insulin treatment group compared with the standard treatment group. However, even in the intensively treated group, retinopathy could not be completely prevented over the 9-year course of the study. The benefit of the strict control was also evident in patients with existing retinopathy (50% reduction in the rate of progression of retinopathy compared with controls). At 6- and 12-month visits, a small adverse affect of intensive treatment on retinopathy progression was seen, similar to that described in other trials of glucose control. However, in eyes with little or no retinopathy at that time of initiating intensive glucose control, this early worsening of retinopathy is unlikely to threaten vision. When the DCCT results were stratified by HbA1C levels, there was a 35–40% reduction in the risk of retinopathy progression for every 10% decrease in HbA1C (e.g., from 8 to 7%). This represented a fivefold increase in the risk for patients with HbA1C.

The beneficial effects of intensive therapy were evident after 3 years of therapy on all different severities of retinopathy evaluated in the DCCT (9). Intensive therapy reduced the risk of any retinopathy by 27% ($p = 0.002$). The risk of developing retinopathy or progression to clinically significant degrees was reduced by 34–76% by intensive treatment of the glycemia. It was most effective when initiated early in the course of the disease, and it had beneficial effect over the entire range of retinopathy and in all patient subgroups. This reduction in risk resulted in reduced need for laser treatment and saved sight.

After 6.5 years of follow-up, the DCCT ended, and all patients were encouraged to maintain strict control of blood sugar. These patients are followed in the Epidemiology of Diabetes Interventions and Complications trial (EDIC), which includes 95% of DCCT subjects, half from each treatment group. A total of 1294–1335 patients have been examined annually in the EDIC.

Further progression of diabetic retinopathy during the first 4 years of the EDIC was 66–77% less in the former intensive treatment group than in the former conventional treatment group *(10)*. The benefit persists even at 7 years *(11)*. This benefit included an effect on severe diabetic retinopathy, including severe nonproliferative diabetic retinopathy, proliferative diabetic retinopathy, clinically significant macular edema, and the need for focal or scatter laser therapy. The decrease in the mean HbA1C from 9 to $\sim 8\%$ did not drastically reduce the progression of diabetic retinopathy in the former conventional treatment group nor did the increase in HbA1c from ~ 7 to $\sim 8\%$ drastically accelerate diabetic retinopathy in the former intensive treatment group. Thus, it takes time for improvements in control to negate the long-lasting effects of prior prolonged hyperglycemia, and once the biological effects of prolonged improved control are manifest, the benefits are long lasting. Furthermore, the total glycemic exposure of the patient (i.e., degree and duration) determines the degree of retinopathy observed at any one time.

TYPE 2 DIABETES

Would similar results be seen in people with type 2 diabetes? The role of intensive glucose control in type 2 diabetes was evaluated in a controlled, randomized, controlled clinical trial, the United Kingdom Prospective Diabetes Study (UKPDS). The effect of glycemic control on the incidence and progression of diabetic retinopathy is similar in patients with type 2 diabetes, as assessed in observational studies and randomized studies conducted in Japan and the UK *(12–15)*. Findings in- a study of Japanese patients with type 2 diabetes have shown that multiple insulin-injection treatment reduced the onset of retinopathy from 32 to 8% and reduced a two-step progression retinopathy from 44 to 19% compared with people receiving conventional insulin treatments over 6 years *(13)*. In the UKPDS, the largest and longest study of 4209 patients with type 2 diabetes followed for 15 years and there was a 25% reduction in the risk of the "any diabetes-related microvascular endpoint," including the need for retinal photocoagulation in the intensive treatment group compared with the conventional treatment group. After 6 years of follow-up, a smaller proportion of patients in the intensive treatment group than in the conventional group had a two-step progression (worsening) in diabetic retinopathy ($p < 0.01$). Epidemiologic analysis of the UKPDS data showed a continuous relationship between the risk of microvascular complications and glycemia, such that for every percentage point decrease in HbA1C (e.g., 9–8%), there was a 35% reduction in the risk of microvascular complications.

There is no longer a controversy regarding the importance of glycemic control in the progression of diabetic retinopathy. The results of both the DCCT and the UKPDS show that while intensive therapy of glucose reduces the risk of the development and progression of diabetic retinopathy, it does not prevent retinopathy completely. This still can be translated clinically to both preservation of vision and reduction in therapy such as laser photocoagulation.

HYPERTENSION

The findings of observational studies assessing the importance of blood pressure in the progression of nonproliferative diabetic retinopathy are inconsistent. However, in the UKPDS, a randomized comparison of more intensive blood pressure control versus less intensive blood pressure control in persons with type 2 diabetes demonstrated that intensive blood pressure control was associated with a decreased risk of retinopathy progression (16). Of the 1148 hypertensive patients in the UKPDS, 758 were allocated to tight control of blood pressure and 390 to less tight control with a median follow-up of 8.4 years. The target for the intensive treatment was a blood pressure <150/85 mm Hg versus a less tight blood pressure control goal of <180/105 mm Hg. The outcome measures included the deterioration of diabetic retinopathy of two or more steps along the modified Early Treatment Diabetic Retinopathy Study (ETDRS) final scale, photocoagulation, vitreous hemorrhage, and cataract extraction, and analysis of specific retinal lesions (microaneurysms, hard exudates, and cotton-wool spots). Visual acuity was assessed at 3-year intervals.

Tight blood pressure control resulted in a 37% reduction in microvascular diseases, predominantly reduced risk of retinal photocoagulation, when compared with less tight control. Retinal hard exudates increased from a prevalence of 11.2–18.3% at 7.5 years after randomization with fewer lesions found in the tight blood pressure (BP) control group [relative risk (RR), 0.53; $p < 0.001$]. Cotton-wool spots increased in both groups but less so in the tight BP control group which had fewer cotton-wool spots at 7.5 years (RR, 0.53; $p < 0.001$). A two-step or more deterioration on the ETDRS scale was significantly different at 4.5 years with fewer people in the tight BP control group progressing two steps or more (RR, 0.75; $p = 0.02$). Patients assigned to tight BP control were less likely to undergo photocoagulation (RR, 0.65; $p = 0.03$). This difference was mainly in photocoagulation for diabetic macular edema (RR, 0.58; $p = 0.02$). There was a 50% reduction in the risk of moderate vision loss as well with decrease in blindness or vision of 20/200 or worse. The decreased vision of 20/200 or worse in one eye was found in 18 of 758 for the tight BP control group compared with 12 of 390 for less-tight BP control group. The absolute risks of such poor vision was of 3.1–4.1 per 1000 patient-years, respectively ($p = 0.046$; RR, 0.76; 99% CI, 0.29–1.99).

A previously published study of blood pressure medication in diabetic retinopathy suggested that there might be a specific benefit of angiotensin-converting enzyme (ACE) inhibition and blood pressure reduction, even in "normo-tensive" persons, on the progression of diabetic retinopathy *(17)*. The UKPDS included a randomized comparison of beta-blockers and ACE inhibitors in the tight blood pressure control arm of that study. Benefits from tight blood pressure control were present in both the beta-blocker and ACE inhibitor treatment groups, with no statistically significant difference between them. The results of the UKPDS suggest that the treatment effect is more likely to be secondary to blood pressure reduction than to a specific effect of ACE inhibitors *(18)*.

SERUM LIPIDS

Although observational data suggest that serum lipids may be important in the progression of diabetic retinopathy and development of diabetic macular edema and retinal hard exudate, no clinical trial has proven the role of lowering elevated serum cholesterol in the management of diabetic retinopathy. The Wisconsin Epidemiologic Study of Diabetic Retinopathy, a population-based study, and the ETDRS found that elevated levels of serum cholesterol were associated with increased severity of retinal hard exudates (Fig. 1) *(19,20)*. A study of diabetic retinopathy in African Americans with type 1 diabetes also showed the association of macular edema and retinal hard exudates

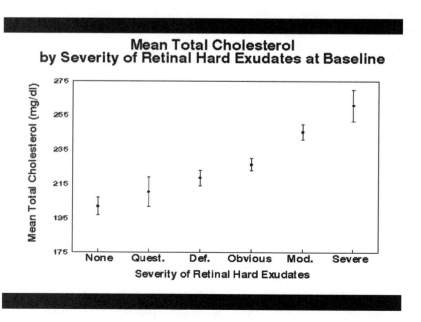

Fig. 1. The baseline data from the Early Treatment Diabetic Retinopathy Study (ETDRS) demonstrate that serum total cholesterol is directly associated with the severity of retinal hard exudate patients with diabetic retinopathy.

with elevated serum lipids *(21)*. Patients with a total cholesterol–high density lipoprotein cholesterol (HDL-C) ratio of 4.5 or greater were almost twice as likely to have retinal hard exudates compared with those with a ratio of < 4.5. Higher quartile of total cholesterol or low-density lipoprotein cholesterol (LDL-C) levels were 5–6 times more likely to have retinal hard exudates than those in the lowest quartiles. In the ETDRS, elevated total cholesterol (240 mg/dL or 6.21 mmol/L) was twice as likely to have retinal hard exudates at baseline [odds ratio (OR): 2.00, 99% CI of 1.35–2.95). Similar results were found when comparing elevated LDL levels (160 mg/dL or 1.14 mmol/L) with the lowest level of LDL (130 mg/dL or 3.37 mmol/L) and the OR was 1.97, 99% CI of 1.3–2.96. Patients with elevated cholesterol and triglyceride levels were 50% more likely to develop retinal hard exudates. Independent of the accompanying macular edema, the severity of retinal hard exudates at baseline was associated with decreased visual acuity in the ETDRS (Fig. 2). The severity of retinal hard exudates was also a significant risk factor for moderate visual loss (15 or more letter loss) during the course of the study. Patients with the most severe level of retinal hard exudates had double the risk of experiencing moderate visual loss.

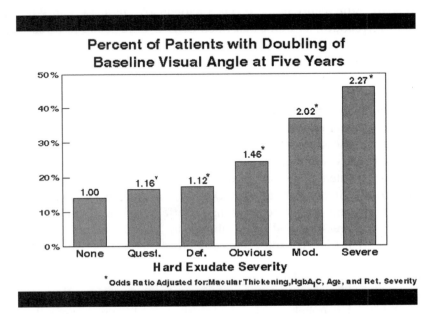

Fig. 2. Multivariable logistic regression demonstrated that the risk of losing visual acuity over five years of follow-up in the Early Treatment Diabetic Retinopathy Study (ETDRS) was associated with both the presence and increasing severity of hard exudate at baseline, adjusted for the presence and increasing severity of macular edema.

Although the intensive treatment of hyperglycemia substantially reduced the development and progression of diabetic retinopathy in the DCCT/EDIC study, there was no statistically significant effect on macular edema. The investigators evaluated the correlation of serum lipids and the incidence of macular edema and retinal hard exudates in this cohort *(22)*. Elevated LDL was associated with an increased risk of macular edema. The comparison of the highest quintile versus the lowest quintile of LDL resulted in an RR of 1.95 (*p* for trend = 0.03). The total-to-HDL cholesterol ratio was also a significant predictor for incident or new cases of clinically significant macular edema with a RR of 3.84 (*p* for trend = 0.03). Similar findings were found for association of serum lipids with the development of retinal hard exudates. After adjusting for all known potential risk factors, the following were statistically significant predictors of retinal hard exudates: total cholesterol: RR = 2.37, *p* for trend = 0.001; LDL-C: 2.77, *p* for trend = 0.002; total-to-HDL cholesterol ratio: 2.44, *p* for trend = 0.0004; and triglycerides: 3.20, *p* for trend = 0.006. These findings were similar to those found in the ETDRS.

In a study of the risk factors associated with the development of subretinal fibrosis in ETDRS patients with diabetic macular edema, the presence of severe hard exudates was the strongest risk factor *(23)*. Elevated serum triglyceride levels were also associated with a greater risk of developing high-risk proliferative diabetic retinopathy in the ETDRS patients *(6)*. In a study in Pittsburgh, elevated triglycerides, as well as elevated LDL-C were found to be associated with proliferative diabetic retinopathy *(3)*.

These are all observational findings with compelling data. It is certainly important to recommend lowering elevated serum lipids in patients with diabetes to reduce the risk of cardiovascular disease (CVD). The risk of vision loss, as seen in the observational studies, should be another motivating factor for patients to lower elevated serum lipids. The effects of treating dyslipidemia require further assessment. Currently, the hypothesis that treatment of dyslipidemia may be very important in the role of progression of diabetic retinopathy is currently evaluated in the Actions to Control Cardiovascular Risk in Diabetes (ACCORD) Eye Study. In brief, ACCORD is a randomized, controlled clinical trial with three components, determining the effects of lowering blood glucose, lowering blood pressure, and using fibrates to lower serum triglycerides and raise serum HDL-C levels (on a background of statin treatment) on CVD in patients with type 2 diabetes. A subset of participants with this study will be evaluated with a standardized protocol for comprehensive eye exams and fundus photography consisting of the seven stereoscopic fields. We hope this study will yield data to help resolve the controversy of the role and will confirm the results of the observational studies of dyslipidemia and diabetic retinopathy. The ACCORD will also help to confirm the effects of tight glycemic and blood pressure control on the development and progression of diabetic retinopathy.

ASPIRIN AND ANTIPLATELET TREATMENTS

There was interest in the past to retard the development and progression of diabetic retinopathy with antiplatelet treatment because of studies of patients with rheumatoid arthritis. Three randomized controlled clinical trials of antiplatelet treatments have been performed in patients with diabetic retinopathy. None has demonstrated a clinical beneficial effect of treatment. The Dipyridamole Aspirin Microangiopathy of Diabetes (DAMAD) study (24) and Ticlopidine Microangiopathy of Diabetes Study (25) enrolled 475 and 435 patients, respectively. These two studies found similar results with little difference in change in retinopathy severity as judged by visual acuity measurements or ophthalmoscopy. There was a difference observed in counts of microaneurysms on fluorescein angiograms, with the increase greater in the placebo group, and less in the aspirin group, the aspirin plus dipyridamole group, and the ticlopidine group. These small differences were of borderline statistical significance and uncertain clinical importance.

In the ETDRS, all patients were randomly assigned to 650 mg of aspirin per day or placebo, and one eye of each patient was randomly assigned to immediate photocoagulation, while the other eye was assigned to deferral of photocoagulation, i.e., careful follow-up and prompt scatter photocoagulation if high risk retinopathy developed. The eyes assigned to deferral of laser photocoagulation were assessed for the effects of aspirin on the progression of diabetic retinopathy (26). Aspirin use did not affect the progression of retinopathy, nor did it affect the risk of visual loss (27). Perhaps surprisingly, aspirin use did not increase the risk of vitreous hemorrhage in patients with AQ8 proliferative retinopathy (28). Aspirin use was associated with a 17% reduction in the morbidity and mortality from CVD (29). Therefore, aspirin should be considered for persons with diabetes, not because of any effect on their diabetic retinopathy, but because of the benefits of aspirin that have been demonstrated for persons at increased risk of CVD. The presence of proliferative diabetic retinopathy should not be considered a contraindication to aspirin use.

DIABETES AND PREGNANCY

The effects of pregnancy on the development and the rate of progression of underlying diabetic retinopathy have been controversial. Although many studies have suggested a worsening of retinopathy during pregnancy (30–33), others have not (34,35). Diabetic retinopathy can worsen during pregnancy because of the pregnancy itself or the changes in metabolic control, usually a marked improvement in glucose control.

The DCCT is the largest prospective study to assess the effect of pregnancy on the development and progression of diabetic retinopathy and other microvascular abnormalities *(36)*. The women in the DCCT were generally younger and had shorter duration of diabetes with fewer or less-severe diabetic complications than those previously reported in other studies. Women in the intensive treatment group had HbA1C levels that were near normal for a mean of 3 years before conception. When the analyses were stratified by the treatment group, both the intensive and the conventional groups showed a short-term deterioration of retinopathy during pregnancy that persisted through the first year post-partum. In the conventional treatment group, there was a 2.5-fold increase in the risk of retinopathy progression when compared with nonpregnant women. This was statistically significant and not affected by other risk factors. In the intensive treatment group, the adjusted risks were not as great whereas the risk of retinopathy progression was nominally statistically significant. However, there were fewer events in the early treatment group.

There was a significant trend toward greater worsening of retinopathy with greater reductions in HbA1C. This progression may be similar to that of the early worsening that has been shown to be related to the magnitude of the decrease of HbA1C with the intensive therapy of glycemia. However, when the recent changes in retinopathy were compared between the pregnant and the nonpregnant women, adjusted for the recent changes in HbA1C, the increased worsening of retinopathy during pregnancy persisted. It would appear that both the effects of pregnancy as well as the effects of intensive therapy are important in the progression (worsening) of retinopathy. The follow-up examinations showed that the effects of pregnancy on retinopathy continued to increase over the first year following delivery of the baby. In addition, there were no long-term consequences of this worsening of retinopathy as both pregnant and nonpregnant women had similar severity of retinopathy at the end of the study. Patients with diabetes who are planning to become pregnant are encouraged to achieve as tight glucose control as possible to reduce the risk of malformations and other genetic abnormalities. Patients with diabetes who are planning to become pregnant are encouraged to have their eyes examined before conception, to be counseled on the risk of development and/or progression of diabetic retinopathy. During the first trimester, another eye examination should be performed; subsequent follow-up will depend on the level of retinopathy found; and post-partum examination may be also important.

CONCLUSIONS

Although diabetic retinopathy cannot be completely prevented, tight glycemic and blood pressure control reduce both the rates of development and the progression of diabetic retinopathy. Although observational data are compelling for recommending aggressive treatment for dyslipidemia, especially for prevention of CVD, there is no randomized controlled trial to suggest that such treatment would be beneficial for preventing or retarding the progression of diabetic retinopathy. The ACCORD study data will address this issue in the future. Antiplatelet treatment has not been effective in the treatment of diabetic retinopathy, but they can also be safely administered to persons with diabetic retinopathy. No harmful effects were seen.

Pregnancy may increase the risk of progression of diabetic retinopathy secondary to improvement in glycemic control and to the pregnancy itself. Again, tight glycemic control, especially before conception, may decrease many adverse side effects such as increased genetic abnormalities and malformations. Tight glucose control plays an important role in the prevention of diabetic retinopathy progression in all clinical situations. Future research may assess genetic associations in patients with diabetic retinopathy.

REFERENCES

1. The Eye Diseases Prevalence Research Group. Causes and prevalence of visual impairment among adults in the United States. *Arch Ophthalmol* 2004;122:477–485.
2. The Eye Diseases Prevalence Research Group. The prevalence of diabetic retinopathy among adults in the U.S. *Arch Ophthalmol* 2004;122:522–536.
3. Janka HU, Warram JH, Rand LI, Krolewski AS. Risk factors for progression of background retinopathy in long-standing IDDM. *Diabetes* 1989;38:460–464.
4. Klein R, Klein BE, Moss SE, et al. The Wisconsin epidemiologic study of diabetic retinopathy. II. Prevalence and risk of diabetic retinopathy when age at diagnosis is less than 30 years. *Arch Ophthalmol* 1984;102:520–526.
5. Klein R, Klein BE, Moss SE, et al. The Wisconsin epidemiologic study of diabetic retinopathy. III. Prevalence and risk of diabetic retinopathy when age of diagnosis of 30 or more years. *Arch Ophthalmol* 1984;102:527–532.
6. Davis MD, Fisher MR, Gangnon RE, et al. Risk factors for high-risk proliferative diabetic retinopathy and severe visual loss: Early Treatment Diabetic Retinopathy Study Report 18. *Invest Opthalmol Vis Sci* 1998;39:233–252.
7. Joslin EP. The younger diabetic and the control of his disease with the help of the hospital teaching clinic. *J Okla State Med Assoc* 1951;44(8):304–308.
8. Joslin EP. How to treat the diabetic patient. *GP.* 1962;52:82–88.
9. The Diabetes Control and Complications Trial Research Group. Progression of retinopathy with intensive versus conventional treatment in the Diabetes Control and Complications Trial. *Ophthalmology* 1994;103:647–661.
10. The Diabetes Control and Complications Trial/Epidemiology of Diabetes Intervention and Complications Research Group. Retinopathy and nephropathy in patients with type 1 diabetes four years after a trial of intensive therapy. *N Engl J Med* 2000;342:381–389.
11. The Diabetes Control and Complications Trial/Epidemiology of Diabetes Intervention and Complications Research Group. Effect of intensive therapy on the microvascular complications of type 1 diabetes mellitus. *JAMA* 2002;287:2563–2569.
12. Klein R, Klein B, Moss S. Relation of glycemic control to diabetic microvascular complications in diabetes mellitus. *Ann Intern Med* 1996;124:90–96.

13. Ohkubo Y, Hideke K, Eiichi A, et al. Intensive insulin therapy prevents the progression of diabetic microvascular complications in Japanese patients with non-insulin-dependent diabetes mellitus: a randomized prospective 6-year study. *Diabetes Res Clin Pract* 1995;28:103–117.

14. UK Prospective Diabetes Study Group. Intensive blood-glucose control with sulphonylureas or insulin compared with conventional treatment and risk of complications in patients with type 2 diabetes (UKPDS 33). *Lancet* 1998;352:837–853.

15. UK Prospective Diabetes Study Group. Effect of intensive blood-glucose control with metformin on complications in overweight patients with type 2 diabetes (UKPDS 34). *Lancet* 1998;352:854–865.

16. UK Prospective Diabetes Study Group. Tight blood pressure control and risk of macrovascular and microvascular complications in Type 2 diabetes (UKPDS 38). *BMJ* 1998;317:703–713.

17. Chaturvedi N, Sjolie AK, Stephen JM, et al. and the EUCLID Study Group. Effect of lisinopril on progression of retinopathy in normotensive people with type 1 diabetes. *Lancet* 1998;351:28–31.

18. Matthews DR, Stratton IM, Aldington SJ, Holman RR, Kohner EM; UK Prospective Diabetes Study Group. Risks of progression of retinopathy and vision loss related to tight blood pressure control in type 2 diabetes mellitus: UKPDS 69. *Arch Ophthalmol* 2004;122:1707–1709.

19. Klein BEK, Moss SE, Klein R, Surawicz TS. The Wisconsin Epidemiologic Study of Diabetic Retinopathy, X: relationship of serum cholesterol to retinopathy and hard exudates. *Ophthalmology* 1991;98:1261–1265.

20. Chew EY, Klein ML, Ferris III FL, et al.; for the ETDRS Research Group. Association of elevated serum lipid levels with retinal hard exudates in diabetic retinopathy. *Arch Ophthalmol* 1996;114:1079–1084.

21. Roy MS, Klein R. Macular edema and retinal hard exudates in African Americans with type 1 diabetes. The New Jersey 725. *Arch Ophthalmol* 2001;119:251–259.

22. Miljanovic B, Glynn RJ, Nathan DM, et al. A prospective study of serum lipids and risk of diabetic macular edema in type 1 diabetes. *Diabetes* 2004;53:2883–2892.

23. Fong DS, Segal PP, Myers F, et al. Subretinal fibrosis in diabetic macular edema, ETDRS Report No. 23. *Arch Ophthalmol* 1997;115:873–877.

24. The DAMAD Study Group. Effects of aspiring alone and aspirin plus dipyridamole in early diabetic retinopathy. A multicenter randomized controlled clinical trial. Diabetes 1989;38:491–8.

25. TIMAD Study Group. Ticlopidine treatment reduces the progression of nonproliferative diabetic retinopathy. Arch Ophthalmol 1990;108:1577–83.

26. Early Treatment Diabetic Retinopathy Study Research Group. Early photocoagulation for diabetic retinopathy. ETDRS Report number 9. Ophthalmol 1991;998:766–785.

27. Early Treatment Diabetic Retinopathy Study Research Group. Effects of aspiring treatment on diabetic retinopathy. ETDRS Report number 8. Ophthalmol 1991;998:757–765.

28. Chew EY, Klein ML, Murphy RP, Remale NA, Ferris FL for the Early Treatment Diabetic Retinopathy Study Research Group. Effects of aspirin on vitreous/preretinal hemorrhage in patients with diabetes mellitus. Arch Ophthalmol 1995;113:52–55.

29. Early Treatment Diabetic Retinopathy Study Research Group. Aspirin effects on mortality and morbidity in patients with diabetes mellitus. ETDRS report no. 14. JAMA 1992;268:1292–1300.

30. Phelps Rl, Sakol P, Metzger BE, et al. Changes in diabetic retinopathy during pregnancy: correlation with regulation of hyperglycemia. *Arch Ophthalmol* 1986;104:1806–1810.

31. Klein BE, Moss SE, Klein R. Effect of pregnancy on progression of diabetic retinopathy. *Diabetes Care* 1990;13:34–40.
32. Chew EY, Mills JL, Metzger BE, et al. Metabolic control and progression of retinopathy. The Diabetes in Early Pregnancy Study. National Institute of Child Health and Human Development Diabetes in Early Pregnancy Study. *Diabetes Care* 1995;18:631–637.
33. Axer-Stegel R, Hod M, Fink-Cohen A, et al. Diabetic retinopathy during pregnancy. *Ophthalmology* 1996;103:1815–1819.
34. Lovestam-Adrian M, Agardh C-D, Aberg A, Agardh E. Pre-eclampsia is a potent risk factor for deterioration of retinopathy during pregnancy in type 1 diabetic patients. *Diabet Med* 1997;14:1059–1065.
35. Lapolla A, Cardone C, Negrin P, et al. Pregnancy does not induce or worsen retinal or peripheral nerve dysfunction in insulin-dependent diabetic women. *J Diabetes Complications* 1998;12:74–80.
36. The Diabetes Control and Complications Trial Research Group. Effect of pregnancy on microvascular complications in the Diabetes Control and Complications Trial. *Diabetes Care* 2000;23:1084–1091.

7 Diabetic Neuropathies
Evaluation, Management and Controversies in Treatment Options

Aaron I. Vinik, MD, PhD, FCP, FACP

CONTENTS

INTRODUCTION
DEFINITION
CLASSIFICATION
CLINICAL MANIFESTATIONS
TREATMENT
CONCLUSIONS
REFERENCES

SUMMARY

Diabetic neuropathies (DN) are a heterogeneous group of disorders that include a wide range of abnormalities. They can be focal or diffuse, proximal or distal, affecting both peripheral and autonomic nervous systems, causing morbidity with significant impact on the quality of life of the person with diabetes, resulting in early mortality. Distal symmetric polyneuropathy, the most common form of DN, usually involves small and large nerve fibers. Small nerve fiber neuropathy often presents with pain *without* objective signs or electrophysiologic evidence of nerve damage. However, there are now measures enabling early recognition of this type of neuropathy as a component of the impaired glucose tolerance and metabolic syndromes. The greatest risk of small fiber neuropathy is foot ulceration and subsequent gangrene and amputation. Large nerve fiber neuropathies produce numbness, ataxia and incoordination, impairing activities of daily living and causing falls and fractures. A careful history and detailed physical examination is

From: *Contemporary Endocrinology: Controversies in Treating Diabetes: Clinical and Research Aspects*
Edited by: D. LeRoith and A. I. Vinik © Humana Press, Totowa, NJ

essential for the diagnosis. Symptomatic therapy has become available, and newer and better treatment modalities based on etiologic factors are being explored with potential for significant impact on morbidity and mortality. Preventive strategies and patient education still remain key factors in reducing complication rates and mortality. A number of mechanical measures for the treatment of neuropathy have been examined, and it is currently unclear whether or not these have salutary effects over and above those of placebo, and longer, well-controlled clinical trials are anticipated. In addition, there is the suggestion that surgical unentrapment of nerves in DN may confer symptomatic relief, but outside of clear applications in proven entrapments, this form of intervention has not been endorsed universally. We now have two drugs approved for the treatment of neuropathic pain in diabetes that is a first, and it remains to be seen whether the evidence-based approach will supersede the need for cost containment and the tried and tested approaches to pain management in the clinic. Finally, the American Diabetes Association have included somatic and autonomic guidelines in their 2006 issue of clinical recommendations, which has come as a welcome relief to the Cinderella of diabetic complications, DN.

Key Words: Diabetes mellitus; diabetic neuropathy; diabetic autonomic neuropathy; treatment; pain.

INTRODUCTION

Diabetic neuropathies (DN) are amongst the most frequent complications of diabetes mellitus (DM), affecting up to 50% of patients, leading to increased morbidity and mortality, and economic burden. DN is the most common form of neuropathy in developed countries and is responsible for 50–75% of non-traumatic amputations. The major morbidity is foot ulceration, which can lead to gangrene and ultimately to limb loss. Every year, 86,000 amputations are performed on diabetic patients in the USA; yet, up to 75% of them are preventable *(1)*. DN also has a tremendous impact on patient's quality of life (QOL) *(2)*.

DN are a heterogeneous group of conditions that involve different components of the somatic and autonomic nervous systems. They can be focal or diffuse, proximal or distal. Causative factors include persistent hyperglycemia, microvascular insufficiency, oxidative stress, nitrosative stress, defective neurotrophism, and autoimmune-mediated nerve destruction *(3)*.

The epidemiology and natural history of DN remains poorly defined, in part because of variable criteria for the diagnosis, failure of many physicians to recognize and diagnose the disease and lack of standardized methodologies used for the evaluation of these patients*(4)*. Nonetheless, it has been estimated that 50% of patients with diabetes have DN, and 2.7 million have painful neuropathy. DN is grossly underdiagnosed and untreated by endocrinologists and non-endocrinologists alike *(5)*.

Here we will focus on the clinical manifestations of DN and its symptomatic treatment, with special emphasis on new therapies aimed at the underlying pathogenesis and controversies in management.

DEFINITION

DN is the presence of symptoms and/or signs of peripheral nerve dysfunction in people with diabetes after the exclusion of other causes. A careful clinical examination is also needed for the diagnosis, because asymptomatic neuropathy is common *(4)*. A minimum of two abnormalities (symptoms, signs, nerve conduction abnormalities, quantitative sensory tests, or quantitative autonomic tests) are required for diagnosis and, for clinical studies, one of theses two abnormalities should include quantitative tests or electrophysiology *(4,6)*.

CLASSIFICATION

Table 1 describes the classification proposed by Thomas and modified by us *(7,8,9)*. It is important to note that different forms of DN often coexist in the same patient (e.g., DPN and proximal neuropathy, or entrapments such as carpal tunnel syndrome).

Table 1
Classification of Diabetic Neuropathies *(8,9)*

Somatic	
Rapidly reversible	• Hyperglycemic neuropathy
Focal and multifocal neuropathies	• Cranial
	• Thoracolumbar radiculoneuropathy
	• Focal limb
	• Proximal motor (amyotrophy)
	• Coexisting CIDP[a]
Generalized symmetrical PN	• Acute sensory
	• Chronic sensorimotor (DPN)
	− Small fiber neuropathy
	− Large fiber neuropathy
Autonomic	• Cardiovascular, GI, Genitourinary, papillary, metabolic

[a]CIDP, chronic inflammatory demyelinating neuropathy.

CLINICAL MANIFESTATIONS
Somatic
FOCAL AND MULTIFOCAL NEUROPATHIES

Focal limb neuropathies are usually due to entrapment, and mononeuropathies must be distinguished from entrapment syndromes *(9,10)*. Mononeuropathies often occur in the older population with an acute onset, associated with pain, and a self-limiting course, resolving in 6–8 weeks. These can involve the median (5.8% of all DN), ulnar (2.1%), radial (0.6%), and common peroneal nerves *(11)*. Cranial neuropathies in diabetic patients are extremely rare (0.05%) and occur in older individuals with a long duration of diabetes *(12)*. Entrapment syndromes start slowly, progress and persist without intervention. Carpal tunnel syndrome occurs three times as frequently in diabetics compared with healthy populations *(13)* and is found in up to one-third of patients with diabetes *(10)*. The diagnosis is confirmed by electrophysiological studies. Treatment consists of resting aided by placement of wrist splint in a neutral position to avoid repetitive trauma. Anti-inflammatory medications and steroid injections are sometimes useful. The role of surgery is not clearly established for the different entrapments, for example, good outcome with carpal tunnel syndrome and poor outcome with ulnar entrapment but should be considered if weakness appears and medical treatment fails *(4,9)*.

PROXIMAL NEUROPATHIES

Typically occurs in older patients (50–60 years) with type 2 diabetes and presents with severe pain and uni- or bilateral muscle weakness and atrophy in proximal thighs. Pathogenesis is still unclear, although immune-mediated epineurial microvasculitis is the culprit in some cases. Controversy exists as to whether or not immunosuppressive therapy should be recommended because there are no double-blind placebo-controlled studies but using high-dose steroids or intravenous immunoglobulin has proved successful in several small studies*(14)*.

DIABETIC TRUNCAL RADICULONEUROPATHY

Diabetic truncal radiculoneuropathy affects middle-aged to elderly patients, especially males. Pain is the most important symptom, occurring in a girdle-like distribution over the lower thoracic or abdominal wall, uni- or bilaterally distributed. Motor weakness is rare. Resolution generally occurs within 4–6 months. It is not clear that any form of intervention changes the natural history of this condition.

CHRONIC INFLAMMATORY DEMYELINATING POLYNEUROPATHY

When an unusually severe, predominantly motor and progressive polyneuropathy develops in diabetic patients, chronic inflammatory demyelinating polyneuropathy (CIDP) should be considered. Progressive motor deficit, progressive sensory neuropathy despite optimal glycemic control together with typical NCV findings and an unusually high CSF protein level suggest the possibility of an underlying demyelinating neuropathy. The diagnosis is often overlooked, although recognition is very important, because, unlike DN, it is treatable. It occurs 11 times more frequently in the diabetic than non-diabetic patient (15,16). Immunomodulatory therapy can produce a relatively rapid and substantial improvement (17), but there are those who believe that there is little to be gained over time and spontaneous resolution.

DISTAL POLYNEUROPATHIES

Rapidly Reversible Hyperglycemic Neuropathy Reversible abnormalities of nerve function with distal sensory symptoms may occur in patients with recently diagnosed or poorly controlled diabetes. Recovery soon follows restoration of euglycemia (4). However, it is also apparent that acute normalization of blood glucose with insulin or oral agents may actually accentuate pain in this syndrome (see below).

Acute Sensory Neuropathy Acute painful sensory neuropathy (ASN) is a distinctive variant of DPN and is characterized by severe pain, cachexia, weight loss, depression, and, in males, erectile dysfunction (7). Patients report unremitting burning, deep pain, and hyperesthesia especially in the feet. Other symptoms include sharp stabbing or "electric shock-like" sensations in the lower limbs that appear more frequently during the night. Signs are usually absent with a relatively normal clinical examination, except for allodynia and, occasionally, absent or reduced ankle reflexes.

ASN is usually associated with poor glycemic control but may also appear after rapid improvement of hyperglycemia (18). It has been hypothesized that changes in blood glucose flux produces alterations in epineurial blood flow, leading to ischemia (19). Other authors propose an immune-mediated mechanism (20).

The key to the management of this syndrome is achieving blood glucose stability. Most patients also require medication for neuropathic pain. The natural history of this disease is resolution of symptoms within 6 months to 1 year (18). There are insufficient information on trials of immunotherapy to define its role here.

Distal Symmetric Polyneuropathy

Clinical Presentation Distal symmetric polyneuropathy (DPN) is probably the most common form of DN *(4,20)*. It is seen in both type 1 and type 2 DM with similar frequency, and it may be already present at the time of diagnosis of type 2 DM *(18)*. A population survey reported that 30% of type 1 and 36–40% of type 2 diabetic patients experienced neuropathic symptoms *(21)* but an American Diabetes Association Omnibus survey of 8119 patients reported symptoms compatible with neuropathy in 75% of patients illustrating the need for specificity with regard to symptom attribution to neuropathy. Several studies have suggested that impaired glucose tolerance (IGT), and the metabolic syndrome may account for 30–50% of "idiopathic neuropathies" *(22,25)*.

Sensory symptoms are more prominent than motor and usually involve the lower limbs. These include pain, paresthesiae, and hyperaesthesia, deep aching, burning, and sharp stabbing sensations. In addition, patients may experience negative symptoms such as numbness in feet and legs leading in time to painless foot ulcers and subsequent amputations, if the neuropathy is not promptly recognized and treated. Unsteadiness frequently occurs because of abnormal proprioception and muscle sensory function *(26,27)*. Some patients may be completely asymptomatic and signs may be only discovered by a detailed neurological examination.

On physical examination, there is usually a symmetrical stocking-like distribution of sensory abnormalities in both lower limbs. In severe cases, the hands may be involved. All sensory modalities can be affected, particularly loss of vibration, touch, and position perception (large A α/β fiber damage); and abnormal heat and cold temperature perception (small A δ and unmyelinated C fiber damage). Ankle and knee reflexes may be absent or reduced. Mild muscle wasting may be observed, but severe weakness is rare and, if present, should raise the question of a possible non- DN *(4,20,28)*. DPN is frequently accompanied by autonomic neuropathy (AN). All patients with DPN are at increased risk of foot ulceration and Charcot´s neuroarthropathy.

Diagnosis of DPNs

History and Physical Examination. Symptoms of neuropathy are personal experiences and vary markedly from one patient to another. Symptom questionnaires with similar scoring systems have been developed. These are useful to assess responses to treatment. The Neurologic Symptom Score (NSS) *(29)* has 38 items that capture symptoms of muscle weakness, sensory disturbances, and autonomic dysfunction.

A comprehensive clinical examination is key to the diagnosis of DPN. Feet must be examined in detail to detect ulcers, calluses, and deformities, and footwear inspected at every visit. The American Diabetes Association (ADA) recommends that all type 2 diabetic patients should be screened for DN at diagnosis, and all type 1 diabetic patients 5 years after diagnosis. Thereafter, screening should be repeated annually and must include sensory examination of the feet and ankle reflexes *(8)*. One or more of the following can be used to assess sensory function: pinprick, temperature, vibration perception (using 128-Hz tuning fork), and 10-G monofilament pressure perception at the distal halluces. Combinations of more than one test have more than 87% sensitivity in detecting DPN *(8,30)*. Longitudinal studies have shown that these simple tests are good predictors of foot ulcer risk *(31)*. Numerous composite scores to evaluate clinical signs of DN such as the nerve impairment score (NIS) are useful in documenting and monitoring neuropathic deficits *(32)*.

Quantitative Sensory Testing. Quantitative Sensory Testing (QST) may be of value in the detection of subclinical neuropathy, assessment of progression, and the prediction of risk for foot ulceration *(30,33)*. These standardized measures of vibration and thermal thresholds also play an important role in multicenter clinical trials as primary efficacy endpoints as discussed below *(2)*.

Nerve Conduction Studies. The use of electrophysiologic measures (NCV) in both clinical practice and multicenter clinical trials is recommended *(34,35)*, but their global use in the clinical arena is not universally agreed on. There are however specific situations where NCS may be of particular help. In type 2 diabetes patients *(36)*, NCV abnormalities in the lower limbs increased from 8% at baseline to 42% after 10 years of disease. A slow progression of NCV abnormalities in type 1 diabetes was observed in the Diabetes Control and Complication Trial (DCCT) *(37)*. The sural and peroneal nerve conduction velocities diminished by 2.8 and 2.7 m/s, respectively, over a 5-year period. Patients who were free of neuropathy at baseline had a 40% incidence of abnormal NCV in the conventionally treated group versus 16% in the intensive therapy treated group after 5 years. Small, unmyelinated nerve fibers are affected early in DM and are not reflected in NCV studies. Other methods that do not depend on conduction such as QST or skin biopsy with quantification of IENF are necessary to identify these patients *(20)*. Nevertheless, NCV plays a key role in ruling out other causes of neuropathy and is essential for the identification of focal and multifocal neuropathies *(4,10)*.

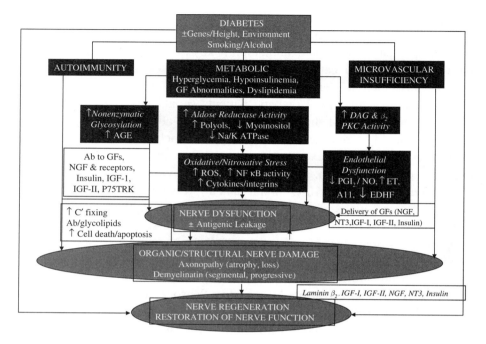

Fig. 1. Modified pathogenesis of diabetic neuropathies from Vinik et al. *(95,96)*

Skin Biopsy and Quantification of Intraepidermal Nerve Fibers. The importance of the skin biopsy as a diagnostic tool for DPN is increasingly being recognized *(38,39,40)*. This technique quantitates small epidermal nerve fibers through antibody staining of the pan axonal marker protein gene product 9.5 (PGP 9.5). Although minimally invasive (3-mm diameter punch biopsies), it enables a direct study of small fibers, which cannot be evaluated by NCV studies (Fig. 1).

Quality of Life in DN. It is widely recognized that neuropathy per se can affect the QOL of the diabetic patient. The Norfolk QOL questionnaire for DN is a validated tool addressing specific symptoms and impact of large, small, and autonomic nerve fiber functions. The tool has been used in clinical trials and is available in several validated language versions *(2)*. The NeuroQoL *(41)* measures patients' perceptions of the impact of neuropathy and foot ulcers.

The diagnosis of DPN is mainly clinical, aided by specific diagnostic tests according to the type and severity of the neuropathy. However, non-diabetic causes of neuropathy must always be excluded, depending on the clinical findings (Fig. 2).

Conceptualization of the Generation of
Neuropathic Pain

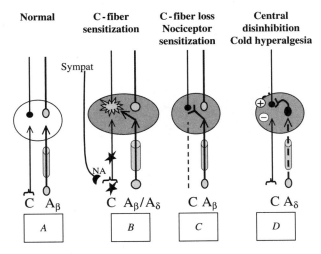

Fig. 2. Schematic representation of the generation of pain. (A) Central terminals of c-afferents project into the dorsal horn and make contact with secondary pain-signaling neurons. Mechanoreceptive Aβ afferents project without synaptic transmission into the dorsal columns (not shown) and also contact secondary afferent dorsal horn neurons. (B) Spontaneous activity in peripheral nociceptors (*peripheral sensitization, black stars*) induces changes in the central sensory processing, leading to spinal cord hyperexcitability (*central sensitization, white star*) that causes input from mechanoreceptive Aβ (light touch) and Aδ fibers (punctuate stimuli) to be perceived as pain (allodynia). (C) C-nociceptor degeneration and novel synaptic contacts of Aβ fibers with "free" central nociceptive neurons, causing dynamic mechanical allodynia. (D) Selective damage of cold-sensitive Aδ fibers that leads to central disinhibition, resulting in cold hyperalgesia *(9)*.

Autonomic Neuropathy

Diabetic autonomic neuropathy (DAN) is a serious and common complication of diabetes but remains among the least recognized and understood. It has a significant negative impact on survival and QOL. Furthermore, cardiovascular autonomic neuropathy (CAN) increases risk of mortality. A meta-analysis, evaluating 15 clinical studies, found a relative risk for mortality of 3.45 (95% CI 2.66–4.47; $p < 0.001$) in studies that used two or more measures to define CAN *(42)*. The reported prevalence of DAN varies widely depending on the cohort studied and the methods used for the diagnosis (7.7–90%) *(43,44)*. The most common clinical features, diagnostic methods, and treatment options are presented in Table 2 Management of hyperglycemia, lipids, blood pressure,

Table 2
Clinical Features, Diagnosis and Treatment of DAN (44)

Symptoms	Tests	Treatments
Cardiac		
Resting tachycardia, exercise intolerance	HRV, MUGA thallium scan, MIBG scan	Graded supervised exercise, ACE inhibitors, β-Blockers
Postural hypotension, dizziness, weakness, fatigue, syncope	HRV, supine and standing BP, catecholamines	Mechanical measures, clonidine, midodrine, octreotide, erythropoietin
Gastrointestinal		
Gastroparesis, erratic glucose control	Gastric emptying study, barium study	Frequent small meals, prokinetic agents (metoclopramide, domperidone, erythromycin)
Abdominal pain, early satiety, nausea, vomiting, bloating, belching	Endoscopy, manometry, electrogastrogram	Antibiotics, antiemetics, bulking agents, tricyclic antidepressants, pyloric botox, gastric pacing
Constipation	Endoscopy	High-fiber diet, and bulking agents, osmotic laxatives, lubricating agents
Diarrhea (often nocturnal alternating with constipation)		Soluble fiber, gluten, and lactose restriction, anticholinergic agents, cholestyramine, antibiotics, somatostatin, pancreatic enzyme supplements

Symptom/Dysfunction	Diagnostic test	Treatment
Sexual dysfunction		
Erectile dysfunction	H&P, HRV, penile-brachial pressure index, nocturnal penile tumes	Sex therapy, psychological counseling, 5'-phosphodiesterase inhibitors, PG E1 injections, devices or prostheses
Vaginal dryness		Vaginal lubricants
Bladder dysfunction		
Frequency, urgency, nocturia, urinary retention, incontinence	Cystometrogram, postvoiding sonography	Bethanechol, intermittent catheterization
Sudomotor dysfunction		
Anhidrosis, heat intolerance, dry skin, hyperhidrosis	Quantitative sudomotor axon reflex, sweat test, skin blood flow	Emollients and skin lubricants, scopolamine, glycopyrrolate, botulinum toxin, vasodilators
Pupillomotor and visceral dysfunction		
Visual blurring, impaired adaptation to ambient light, Argyll- Robertson pupil	Pupillometry, HRV	Care with driving at night
Impaired visceral sensation: silent MI, hypoglycemia unawareness		Recognition of unusual presentation of MI, control of risk factors, control of plasma glucose levels

HRV, heart rate variability; MUGA, multigated angiography; MIBG, metaiodobenzlyguanidine; H & P, history and physical examination; MI, myocardial infarction.

and use of antioxidants *(45)* and ACE inhibitors *(46)* reduce the odds ratio for AN to 0.32 *(47)*.

TREATMENT

Treatment of DN should be targeted toward a number of different aspects:

1. Treatment of specific underlying pathogenic mechanisms.
2. Treatment of symptoms and improvement in QOL.
3. Prevention of progression and treatment of complications of neuropathy.

Treatment of Specific Underlying Pathogenic Mechanisms

GLYCEMIC AND METABOLIC CONTROL

Numerous studies have shown a relationship between hyperglycemia and the development and severity of DN. The DCCT research group reported that clinical and electrophysiological evidence of neuropathy was reduced by 50% in those treated intensively with insulin *(48)*. In the UK Prospective Diabetes Study (UKPDS), control of blood glucose was associated with improvement in vibration perception *(49,50)*. The Steno trial using multifactorial intervention *(51)* reported a reduction in the odds ratio to 0.32 for the development of AN. Furthermore, the EURODIAB, a prospective study that included 3250 patients across Europe *(52)* has shown that the incidence of neuropathy is also associated with potentially modifiable cardiovascular risk factors, including a raised triglyceride level, body mass index, smoking, and hypertension. Therefore, treatment of neuropathy should include measures to reduce macrovascular risk factors, including hyperglycemia, blood pressure, and lipid control and lifestyle modifications including exercise and weight reduction, smoking cessation, a diet rich in omega-3 fatty acids and avoidance of excess alcohol consumption *(51)*.

OXIDATIVE STRESS

A number of studies have shown that hyperglycemia causes oxidative stress in tissues that are susceptible to complications of diabetes, including peripheral nerves. Figure 1 presents our current understanding of the mechanisms and potential therapeutic pathways for oxidative stress-induced nerve damage. Studies show that hyperglycemia induces an increased presence of markers of oxidative stress, such as superoxide and peroxynitrite ions, and that antioxidant defense moieties are reduced in patients with diabetic peripheral neuropathy *(53)*. Therefore, therapies known to reduce oxidative stress are recommended but do not have evidence-based support of large-scale clinical trials but rather meta-analysis of several smaller trials.*(54)*.

Investigational therapies include Aldose Reductase inhibitors (ARIs), alpha lipoic acid, gamma linolenic acid, benfotiamine, and protein kinase C inhibitors. ARIs reduce the flux of glucose through the polyol pathway, inhibiting tissue accumulation of sorbitol and fructose. Newer ARIs are currently being explored (55), but it is becoming clear that these agents may be insufficient per se and combinations of treatments may be needed (9).

Gamma-Linolenic acid has been reported to cause significant improvement in clinical and electrophysiological tests for neuropathy (56), but there are no large-scale clinical trials to support its use alone or in combination in patients with neuropathy.

Alpha-Lipoic acid or Thioctic acid has been used for its antioxidant properties and for its thiol replenishing redox-modulating properties. A number of studies show its favorable influence on microcirculation and reversal of some symptoms of neuropathy (57). While there appears to be some skepticism with regard to the strengths of the meta-analysis ongoing studies will examine its long-term effects on electrophysiology and clinical assessments.

PROTEIN KINASE C BETA (PKC-B) INHIBITION

PKC activation is a critical step in the pathway to diabetic microvascular complications (58). It is activated by both hyperglycemia and disordered fatty acid metabolism resulting in increased production of vasoconstrictive, angiogenic, and chemotactic cytokines including transforming growth factor-β, vascular endothelial growth factor (VEGF), endothelin (ET-1), and intercellular adhesion molecules (ICAMs). Preliminary results of a multinational, randomized, phase-2, double-blind, placebo-controlled trial with ruboxistaurin (a PKC-β inhibitor) failed to achieve the endpoints. Nevertheless, it showed a statistically significant improvement in symptoms in the ruboxistaurin (RBX)-treated neuropathy groups with a sural nerve action potential (SNAP) greater than 0.5 µV at baseline, (59) as compared with placebo (60). The change from baseline for vibratory detection threshold (VDT) was statistically significantly improved in the treated groups. While one phase-3 study failed to meet the endpoint of reduction in symptoms, phase-3 studies are currently taking place, which include objective measures of neuropathy that may confirm or refute the above findings.

NEUROTROPHIC FACTORS

There is increasing evidence that there is a deficiency of nerve growth factor (NGF) in diabetes, as well as the dependent neuropeptides substance P (SP) and calcitonin gene-related peptide (CGRP) and that this contributes to the clinical perturbations in small fiber function (61). Clinical trials with NGF have not been successful but are subject to certain caveats with regard to design (see below), and NGF may still hold promise for sensory and autonomic neuropathies *(62)*. The pathogenesis of DN includes loss of vasa nervorum, so it is likely that appropriate application of VEGF would reverse the dysfunction. Introduction of VEGF gene into muscle of DM animal models improved nerve function *(63)*. There are ongoing VEGF gene studies in humans.

IMMUNE THERAPY

Several different autoantibodies in human sera have been reported that can react with epitopes in neuronal cells and have been associated with DN. We have reported a 12% incidence of apredominantly motor form of neuropathy in patients with diabetes associated with monosialoganglioside antibodies *(64)*. Perhaps the clearest link between autoimmunity and neuropathy has been the demonstration of an 11-fold increase likelihood of CIDP, multiple motor polyneuropathy (MMP), vasculitis, and monoclonal gammopathies in diabetes *(15)*. However, new data support a predictive role of the presence of antineuronal antibodies on the later development of neuropathy *(65)*, which may not be innocent bystanders but neurotoxins *(66)*. There may be selected cases, particularly those with AN and antineuronal autoimmunity, and CIDP, that benefit from IVIg *(67)*.

Treatment of Symptoms and Improvement in Quality of Life

Control of pain is one of the most difficult management issues in DN. It often involves different classes of drugs and requires combination therapies. In any painful syndrome, special attention to the underlying condition is essential for the overall management and for differentiation from other conditions that may coexist in patients with diabetes (i.e., claudication, Charcot's neuroarthropathy, fasciitis, osteoarthritis, radiculopathy, Morton's neuroma, tarsal tunnel syndrome). A careful history of the nature of pain, its exact location, and detailed examination of the lower limbs is mandatory to ascertain alternate causes of pain. Pain can be caused by dysfunction of different types of nerve fibers (A-δ vs. C fiber) that are modulated by sympathetic input with spontaneous firing of different neurotransmitters to the dorsal root ganglia (DRG), spinal cord and cerebral cortex. Figure 2 describes the pathophysiological basis for the generation of neuropathic pain. Different types of pain respond to different types of therapies *(9)*. Figure 3 describes the different nerve fibers affected and possible targeted treatments.

C-FIBER PAIN

Small unmyelinated C fiber damage gives rise to burning or lancinating pain often accompanied by hyperalgesia and dysesthesia. Peripheral sympathetic

Pain Targets

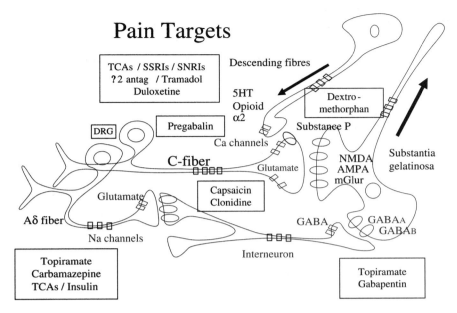

Fig. 3. Different mechanisms of pain and possible treatments: C fibers are modulated by sympathetic input with spontaneous firing of different neurotransmitters to the DRG, spinal cord and cerebral cortex. Sympathetic blockers (clonidine) and depletion of axonal SP used by C-fibers as their neurotransmitter (capsaicin) may improve pain. In contrast, Aδ fibers utilize NA$^+$ channels for their conduction and agents that inhibit Na$^+$ exchange such as antiepileptic drugs, tricyclic antidepressants and insulin may ameliorate this form of pain. Anticonvulsants (Carbamazepine, gabapentin, topiramate) potentiate GABA activity, inhibit Na$^+$ and Ca^{++} channels and inhibit NMDA and AMPA receptors. Pregabalin binds to the $\alpha_2\delta_1$ subunit of the Ca^{++} channel and modifies Ca^{++} uptake. Dextromethorphan blocks NMDA receptors in the spinal cord. TCA, SSRIs, and SNRIs inhibit serotonin and norepinephrine reuptake, enhancing their effect in endogenous pain-inhibitory systems in the brain. Tramadol is a central opioid analgesic Abbreviations: SP: substance P, TCA: tricyclic antidepressants, SSRIs: selective serotonin reuptake inhibitors, SNRIs: serotonin and norepinephrine reuptake inhibitors, NMDA: N-methyl-D-aspartate, AMPA: α-amino-3-hydroxy-5-methyl-4-isoxazole propionic acid, GABA: gamma-aminobutyric acid *(9,96).*

fibers are C-fibers, too, and spontaneous firing or activation exacerbates the pain, which can be blocked with systemic administration of the α_2-adrenergic agonist Clonidine. These nerve fibers are peptidergic carrying substance P as the neurotransmitter. Depletion of substance P with local application of capsaicin abolishes transmission of painful stimuli to higher centers *(68).* Targeting higher levels of pain transmission also helps with C fiber pain *(69,70).*

A-DELTA FIBER PAIN

Pain from A-delta fibers is deep-seated, dull, and aching. It responds to nerve blocks, Tramadol or dextromethorphan, antidepressants and tricyclic agents. Insulin infusion at a rate of 0.8–1 units/h without lowering blood glucose helps in resolution of pain in about 48 h *(71)*. N-methyl-D-aspartate (NMDA) receptor antagonist like dextromethorphan exert an analgesic effect in hyperalgesia and allodynia while centrally acting opioids such as Tramadol achieve symptomatic relief *(72)*.

ANTIDEPRESSANTS IN NEUROPATHY

These drugs inhibit reuptake of norepinephrine and/or serotonin. Anticholinergic effects, orthostatic hypotension, and sexual side effects limit their use. They remain first line agents in many centers, but consideration of their safety and tolerability is important in avoiding adverse effects, a common result of treatment of neuropathic pain. Dosages must be titrated based on positive responses, treatment adherence, and adverse events *(73)*. Among the norepinephrine reuptake inhibitors, desipramine, amitryptylline, and imipramine have been shown to be of benefit. Selective serotonin reuptake inhibitors (SSRIs) that have been used for neuropathic pain are paroxetine, fluoxetine, sertraline, and citalopram. Fluoxetine appears to provide some pain relief *(74)*. Duloxetine has recently been approved for neuropathic pain in the USA. It is a selective, balanced, and potent inhibitor of serotonin (5-HT) and noradrenalin reuptake (SNRIs) in the brain and spinal cord leading to increase neuronal activity in efferent inhibitory pathways. Physicians must be alert to suicidal ideation, exacerbation of autonomic symptoms, as well as aggravation of depression, and should stop the drug immediately *(69)*.

ANTICONVULSANTS IN DN

Anticonvulsants have stood the test of time in treatment of DN. Principal mechanisms of action include sodium channel blockade, potentiation of gamma-amino butyric (GABA) activity, calcium channel blockade, antagonism of glutamate at NMDA receptors or α-amino-3-hydroxy-5-methyl-4-isoxazole propionic acid (AMPA) receptors *(3)*.

Carbamazepine is useful for patients with shooting or electric, shock-like pain. In a placebo-controlled trial, gabapentin-treated patients had significantly lower mean daily pain scores and improvement of all secondary efficacy parameters *(75)*. Gabapentin has the additional benefit of improving sleep *(75)*, which is often compromised in patients with chronic pain *(73)*. In the long term, it is known to produce weight gain, which may complicate diabetes management, and it has not been successful in all trials *(76)*.

Pregabalin produced significant improvements on pain scores within 1 week of treatment ($p < 0.01$), which persisted for the 8 weeks ($p < 0.01$). For the patient global impression of change (PGIC), there was a 67% improvement versus 39% in patients given placebo ($p = 0.001$). Furthermore, 40% of patients receiving Pregabalin reported a $\geq 50\%$ reduction in pain, compared with 14.5% with placebo ($p = 0.001$) (70).

In trials with topiramate, a fructose analog, 50% of patients on topiramate versus 34% on placebo responded to treatment, defined as a >30% reduction in pain score ($p < 0.004$). Topiramate also reduced pain intensity versus placebo ($p < 0.003$) as well as sleep disruption scores ($p < 0.02$) (77). This drug also lowers blood pressure, has a favorable impact on lipids, decreases insulin resistance, and causes growth of intraepidermal nerve fibers (77,78).

As mentioned previously, pain symptoms in neuropathy significantly impact QOL. Neuropathic pain therapy is challenging, and selection of pain medication and dosages must be individualized, with attention to potential side effects and drug interactions.

Adjunctive Management and Treatment of Complications

While small fiber neuropathy presents as different forms of pain, large fiber neuropathy is manifested by reduced vibration perception and position sense, weakness, muscle wasting, and depressed deep tendon reflexes. Diabetic patients with large fiber neuropathies are uncoordinated and ataxic and are 17 times more likely to fall than their non-neuropathic counterparts (79). Therefore, it is important to improve strength and balance in patients with large fiber neuropathy. Patients can benefit from high intensity strength training by increasing muscle strength, improving coordination and balance, and thus reducing fall and fracture risks (80). Low impact activities, which emphasize muscular strength and coordination, and challenge the vestibular system, such as Pilates, yoga, and Tai Chi, may also be particularly helpful. In addition, options to prevent and correct foot deformities are available, for example, orthotics, surgery, and reconstruction.

Basic management of small fiber neuropathies by the patient should be encouraged. These are foot protection and ulcer prevention by wearing padded socks; regular foot inspection using a mirror to examine the soles of the feet daily; selection of proper footwear; scrutiny of shoes for the presence of foreign objects; avoidance of sun-heated surfaces; hot bathwater or sleeping with feet in front of fireplaces or heaters. Patient education should reinforce these strategies and, additionally, discourage soaking feet in water. Education will also promote foot care by encouraging emollient creams to help skin retain moisture and prevent cracking and infection.

Mechanical Measures

TRANSCUTANEOUS NERVE STIMULATION (ELECTROTHERAPY), MAGNETIC FIELD THERAPY, INFRARED LIGHT, AND ELECTRICAL CORD STIMULATION

Transcutaneous nerve stimulation (electrotherapy) occasionally may be helpful and certainly represents one of the more benign therapies for painful neuropathy *(81,82)*. Care should be taken to move the electrodes around to identify sensitive areas and obtain maximal relief.

Static magnetic field therapy *(83)* has been reported to be of benefit, but it was difficult to blind such studies. More recently, Bosi and colleagues used frequency-modulated electromagnetic neural stimulation (FREMS) in 31 patients with painful DN using an ingenious method of 10 applications of placebo versus active treatment using a switch on the device. FREMS induces a significant reduction in daytime and nighttime pain, in addition a significant increase in tactile threshold detected using SMW and lowering of the VDT using a biosthesiometer, improved motor nerve conduction velocity. A significant persistent of the effect was observed after 4 months, and there was an additional benefit in measures of QOL using the SF 36 in terms of general health, physical, and social functioning *(84)*.This finding suggest that FREMS may be an active safe method to improve symptoms of neuropathy with the added possibility of enhancing neurological function.

Similarly the use of infrared light has reportedly had benefit, but this remains to be proven. Leonard and colleagues examined 27 patients; 9 of whom were sensitive to a 6.65 g Semmes Weinstein monofilament (SWM) and 18 who were insensate. Extremities were treated for 2 weeks with sham or active infrared, and there was reportedly a reduction in the number of 5.07 g SWM insensate sites in patients with mild neuropathy but not in those with greater sensory loss and reportedly improved balance, which was not quantified objectively. Clearly these observations need to be extended for longer periods and more objective measure applied to evaluating the responsiveness.

A case series of patients with severe painful neuropathy unresponsive to conventional therapy suggested efficacy of using an implanted spinal cord stimulator *(85)*. However, this cannot be generally recommended except in very resistant cases as it is invasive, expensive, and unproven in controlled studies.

The presence of certain kinds of subclinical noise has been shown to enhance sensitivity in various situations, and sensory neurons exposed to low-level noise have enhanced neurotransmission. Khaodhiar and colleagues *(86)* examined the acute effects of vibration of the sole of the foot below the individual's threshold for 30–60 s in 20 subjects with mild neuropathy and determined the impact on vibration detection and Semmes Weinstein monofilament thresholds. They found that VDT threshold improved, and the ability to detect MF application to the sole of the foot but not the big toe was enhanced. This ability to amplify signals from the neuropathic foot may have relevance to protecting feet from injury and possibly even enhancing postural stability. These studies need to be expanded to longer term to determine the durability of their effects and that hopefully there will be no tachyphyllaxis.

Surgery for the Treatment of Neuropathy

Controversy exists as to the role tarsal tunnel release has in the management of the diabetic patient with a painful foot syndrome. The major problem is the application of tarsal tunnel release to DPN and not specifically for those patients with tarsal tunnel entrapment syndrome (TTS). Because of the intrinsic swelling of peripheral nerves in the diabetic (endoneurial edema secondary to increased sorbitol levels within the peripheral nerve), an increased incidence of compression neuropathy has been well documented. The "double crush syndrome" as described by Upton and McComas *(87)* may be applied to the diabetic patient. This hypothesis states that when multiple "sub-clinical" nerve compressions exist in series; they may be "additive" and give rise to symptoms even though each compression, by itself, would not. The "first crush" would be the peripheral neuropathy of diabetes and the "second crush" compression of the tibial nerve at the tarsal tunnel. TTS *(88)* is a painful lower limb entrapment. Passing through the tarsal tunnel, the tibial nerve innervates only muscles of the sole and clinical signs are mostly sensory. Foot pain may be severe, burning, worse on standing and walking; Tinel sign on underside of medial malleolus, with atrophy of the sole muscles is typical. Weakness is rare, because most of the small foot muscles (flexor hallucis longus) are not damaged in TTS. Pain on the inside of the foot must be distinguished from other causes of pain for example: a Morton's neuroma, plantar fasciitis, heel spurs, arthritis or bone spurs, early Charcot's neuroarthropathy. An MRI of the foot can be very helpful to identify neuromas and shows edema of bones in the midfoot with Charcot's, which presents as a hot foot with increased blood flow *(89)*. It may also be a manifestation of systemic disease *(90)*. Once these are excluded, NCV can be informative in the case of a normal plantar response from one leg and abnormal one from the symptomatic one in unilateral TTS. TTS is not difficult to diagnose clinically when DSPN is not severe and NCV is moderately abnormal. Mild symmetric peroneal and tibial NCV abnormality with intact ankle jerks and sensation of the dorsal aspect of the foot with the abovementioned clinical signs are the most important diagnostic features of TTS. When the neuropathy is severe, then diagnosis may be impossible. A positive Tinel sign, tapping just below the medial malleolus maybe helpful but unfortunately may also simply reflect nerve damage in peripheral neuropathy, a negative sign suggesting that nerve damage predicts a poor outcome of surgery.

If patients are carefully selected, release of the tibial nerve through the tarsal tunnel in the diabetic may improve plantar sensibility and help prevent plantar ulceration and ultimate lower extremity amputation. Several recent studies lend credence to this notion, although study design flaws need to be rectified before universal acceptance of this principle is achieved. Caffee et al. *(91)* presented data on 36 patients collected over a 9-year period from 1989–1997 reviewed retrospectively. The mean follow up was 32 months, and these were patients who had severe disease with foot ulcers in 11 patients and painful paresthesias in 28 cases. Fifty-eight decompressions were done in 36 patients followed for 7–84 months. In these studies, the Semmes Weinstein monofilaments were used to monitor responses. Twenty-four of twenty-eight had complete relief of pain some on the operating table still under anesthetic and 13 of 24 had improved subjective sensation. He concluded that there is some room for optimism but had no objective data of recovery, the only record of change being that reported on by the patients. The failure in 50% of cases is attributed to the advanced status of their disease and that objective testing of sensation is an oxymoron despite the reports by Wiemann and Patel *(92)* and Dellon *(93)* of improved two point discrimination after surgical decompression.

In the Wiemann and Patel *(92)* report on 33 limbs in 26 patients, 32 had a positive Tinel sign yet 19 of 26 responded and 7 with positive Tinel signs did not. Thus, as Dellon *(93)* showed there may be an 80% response in Tinel positive people but failure in 20% would be in agreement with the Wiemann and Patel *(92)* study, suggesting that the sign is not a good predictor of response. Unfortunately, in the Wiemann and Patel *(92)* study, neither foot pressures nor ED showed any changes in the operated patients and only symptoms of pain improved. The objective measures of two point discrimination fell equivalently from15.1 ± 4 to 11.1 ± 3.5 in responders and from 13.7 ± 3 to 11.1 ± 2.5 in non-responders pointing out the lack of validity of this as a test of response to decompression. Thus, these studies have not clearly established the role of decompression in entrapment syndromes, left us floundering with regard to the value of a positive Tinel sign over the ankle and created some consternation amongst those people who are concerned that this is being advocated as a procedure for common or garden DN in the absence of entrapment even when there is no evidence of recoverable nerve function. Indeed, as Carneiro *(94)* pointed out, there is a need to grade the severity of the entrapments using measures of sensory deficits with validated tests, the presence of a Tinel sign, the time taken for Phalen's test to become positive and the presence of motor features and atrophy to identify the best candidates for surgery. We would go further than that and add that a conduction block must be present at the site, that there should not be such severe DN to preclude distinction of this from entrapment, and that controlled sham operations have to be compared with unentrapment for relief of symptoms if this is the only measurement.

CONCLUSIONS

Somatic and autonomic neuropathies (DPN) are amongst the most common long-term complications of diabetes and its precursors, IGT, and the metabolic syndrome. DPN is associated with considerable morbidity and mortality and significant impact on QOL. It is highly prevalent in diabetic populations although often not recognized by physicians. A thorough history and detailed physical examination is essential for the diagnosis. A number of simple tests that can be done in the clinic are useful for detection of DPN and prediction of complications, such as foot ulcers and gangrene. Standardized and validated quantitative measures of disease progression are now available and allow better interpretation of responses to different treatments and study results. Management of the disease is complex and the key to success depends, in part, on discovering the underlying pathological processes in each particular clinical presentation. Studies on new agents that target the pathophysiological mechanisms have lead to a better understanding of the pathogenesis of DPN as well as the pain mechanisms for the different types of pain syndromes. Two drugs have recently been approved in the USA for the treatment of neuropathic pain of diabetes. Two decades ago, physicians could only diagnose DPN and commiserate with the patient. This has changed in the last few years with increasing available therapies as the knowledge of the condition continues to grow.

REFERENCES

1. Caputo, G.M., Cavanagh, P.R., Ulbrecht, J.S., Gibbons, G.W., and Karchmer, A.W. 1994. Assessment and management of foot disease in patients with diabetes. *N Engl J Med* 331:854–860.
2. Vinik, E., Hayes, R., Oglesby, A., Bastyr, E., Barlow, P., Ford-Molvik, S., and Vinik, A. 2005. The development and validation of the Norfolk QOL-DN a new measure of patients' perception of the effects of diabetes and diabetic neuropathy. *Diabetes Technol Ther* 7(3):497–508.
3. Vinik, A.I. 2004. Advances in diabetes for the millennium: new treatments for diabetic neuropathies. *Med Gen Med* 6:13.
4. Boulton, A., Malik, T., Arezzo, J. C., and Sosenko, J. 2004. Diabetic somatic neuropathies: technical review. *Diabetes Care* 27:1458–1486.
5. Herman, W.H. and Kennedy, L. 2005. Underdiagnosis of peripheral neuropathy in type 2 diabetes. *Diabetes Care* 28:1480–1481.
6. Dyck, P.J. 2003. Severity and staging of diabetic polyneuropathy. In *Textbook of Diabetic Neuropathy* (pp. 170–175), Thieme, Stuttgart.

7. Thomas, P.K. 1997. Classification, differential diagnosis and staging of diabetic peripheral neuropathy. *Diabetes* 46(Suppl 2):S54–S57.

8. Boulton, A. J., Vinik, A., Arezzo, J., Bril, V., Feldman, E., Freeman, R., Malik, R., Maser, R., Sosenko, J., Ziegler, D., and American Diabetes Association. 2005. Position statement: diabetic neuropathies. *Diabetes Care* 28(4):956–962.

9. Vinik, A. and Mehrabyan, A. 2004. Diabetic neuropathies. *Med Clin North Am* 88(4): 947–999.

10. Vinik, A., Mehrabyan, A., Colen, L., and Boulton, A. 2004. Focal entrapment neuropathies in diabetes. *Diabetes Care* 27(7):1783–1788.

11. Wilbourn, A.J. 1999. Diabetic entrapment and compression neuropathies. In (Dyck PJ, Thomas PK, eds) *Diabetic Neuropathy* (pp. 481–508), Philadelphia, Saunders.

12. Watanabe, K., Hagura, R., Akanuma, Y., Takasu, T., Kajinuma, H., Kuzuya, N., and Irie, M. 1990. Characteristics of cranial nerve palsies in diabetic patients. *Diabetes Res Clin Pract* 10:19–27.

13. Perkins, B., Olaleye, D., and Bril, V. 2002. Carpal tunnel syndrome in patients with diabetic polyneuropathy. *Diabetes Care* 25:565–569.

14. James, P., Dyck, B., and Windenbank, A. 2002. Diabetic and nondiabetic lumbosacral radiculoplexus neuropathy: new insights into pathophysiology. *Muscle Nerve* 25:477–491.

15. Sharma, K., Cross, J., Farronay, O., Ayyar, D., Sheber, R., and Bradley, W. 2002. Demyelinating neuropathy in diabetes mellitus. *Arch Neurol* 59:758–765.

16. Krendel, D.A., Zacharias, A., and Younger, D.S. 1997. Autoimmune diabetic neuropathy. *Neurol Clin* 15:959–971.

17. Ayyar, D.R. and Sharma, K.R. 2004. Chronic inflammatory demyelinating polyradiculoneuropathy in diabetes mellitus. *Curr Diab Rep* 4:409–412.

18. Oyibo, S.O., Prasad, Y.D., Jackson, N.J., Jude, E.B., and Boulton, A.J. 2002. The relationship between blood glucose excursions and painful diabetic peripheral neuropathy: a pilot study. *Diabet Med* 19:870–873.

19. Tesfaye, S., Malik, R., Harris, N., Jakubowski, J.J., Mody, C., Rennie, I.G., and Ward, J.D. 1996. Arterio-venous shunting and proliferating new vessels in acute painful neuropathy of rapid glycaemic control (insulin neuritis). *Diabetologia* 39:329–335.

20. Sinnreich, M., Taylor, B.V., and Dyck, P.J. 2005. Diabetic neuropathies. Classification, clinical features, and pathophysiological basis. *Neurologist* 11:63–79.

21. Harris, M., Eastman, R., and Cowie, C. 1993. Symptoms of sensory neuropathy in adults with NIDDM in the U.S. population. *Diabetes Care* 16:1446–1452.

22. Singleton, J.R., Smith, A.G., and Bromberg, M.B. 2001. Painful sensory polyneuropathy associated with impaired glucose tolerance. *Muscle Nerve* 24:1225–1228.

23. Singleton, J.R., Smith, A.G., and Bromberg, M.B. 2001. Increased prevalence of impaired glucose tolerance in patients with painful sensory neuropathy. *Diabetes Care* 24: 1448–1453.

24. Sumner, C., Sheth, S., Griffin, J., Cornblath, D., and Polydefkis, M. 2003. The spectrum of neuropathy in diabetes and impaired glucose tolerance. *Neurology* 60:108–111.

25. Pittenger, G., Mehrabyan, A., Simmons, K., Rice, A., Barlow, P., and Vinik, A. 2005. Small fiber neuropathy is associated with the metabolic syndrome. Metab Syndr Relat Disord 3(2), 113–121.

26. Cavanagh, P.R., Simoneau, G.G., and Ulbrecht, J.S. 1993. Ulceration, unsteadiness, and uncertainty: the biomechanical consequences of diabetes mellitus. *J Biomech* 26(Suppl 1):23–40.

27. Katoulis, E.C., Ebdon-Parry, M., Lanshammar, H., Vileikyte, L., Kulkarni, J., and Boulton, A.J. 1997. Gait abnormalities in diabetic neuropathy. *Diabetes Care* 20: 1904–1907.

28. Dyck, P.J., Kratz, K.M., Karnes, J.L., Litchy, W.J., Klein, R., Pach, J.M., Wilson, D.M., O'Brien, P.C., Melton, L.J., III, and Service, F.J. 1993. The prevalence by staged severity of various types of diabetic neuropathy, retinopathy, and nephropathy in a population-based cohort: the Rochester Diabetic Neuropathy Study. *Neurology* 43:817–824.

29. Dyck, P.J. 1988. Detection, characterization and staging of polyneuropathy: assessed in diabetes. *Muscle Nerve* 11:21–32.

30. Vinik, A.I., Suwanwalaikorn, S., Stansberry, K.B., Holland, M.T., McNitt, P.M., and Colen, L.E. 1995. Quantitative measurement of cutaneous perception in diabetic neuropathy. *Muscle Nerve* 18:574–584.

31. Abbott, C.A., Carrington, A.L., Ashe, H., Bath, S., Every, L.C., Griffiths, J., Hann, A.W., Hussein, A., Jackson, N., Johnson, K.E. et al. 2002. The North-West Diabetes Foot Care Study: incidence of, and risk factors for, new diabetic foot ulceration in a community-based patient cohort. *Diabet Med* 19:377–384.

32. Dyck, P.J., Melton, L.J., III, O'Brien, P.C., and Service, F.J. 1997. Approaches to improve epidemiological studies of diabetic neuropathy: insights from the Rochester Diabetic Neuropathy Study. *Diabetes* 46(Suppl 2):S5–S8.

33. Yarnitsky, D. and Sprecher, E. 1994. Thermal testing: normative data and repeatability for various test algorithms. *J Neurol Sci* 125:39–45.

34. Consensus Statement. 1988. Report and recommendations of the San Antonio conference on diabetic neuropathy. American Diabetes Association American Academy of Neurology. *Diabetes Care* 11:592–597.

35. Peripheral Nerve Society. 1995. Diabetic polyneuropathy in controlled clinical trials: Consensus Report of the Peripheral Nerve Society. *Ann Neurol* 38:478–482.

36. Partanen, J., Niskanen, L., Lehtinen, J., Mervaala, E., Siitonen, O., and Uusitupa, M. 1995. Natural history of peripheral neuropathy in patients with non-insulin-dependent diabetes mellitus. *N Engl J Med* 333:89–94.

37. DCCT Research Group. 1995. The effect of intensive diabetes therapy on the development and progression of neuropathy. *Ann Intern Med* 122:561–568.

38. Kennedy, W.R., Wendelschafer-Crabb, G., and Johnson, T. 1996. Quantitation of epidermal nerves in diabetic neuropathy. *Neurology* 47:1042–1048.

39. Polydefkis, M., Hauer, P., Griffin, J.W., and McArthur, J.C. 2001. Skin biopsy as a tool to assess distal small fiber innervation in diabetic neuropathy. *Diabetes Technol Ther* 3:23–28.

40. Pittenger, G.L., Ray, M., Burcus, N.I., McNulty, P., Basta, B., and Vinik, A.I. 2004. Intraepidermal nerve fibers are indicators of small-fiber neuropathy in both diabetic and nondiabetic patients. *Diabetes Care* 27:1974–1979.

41. Vileikyte, L., Peyrot, M., Bundy, C., Rubin, R.R., Leventhal, H., Mora, P., Shaw, J.E., Baker, P., and Boulton, A.J. 2003. The development and validation of a neuropathy- and foot ulcer-specific quality of life instrument. *Diabetes Care* 26:2549–2555.

42. Maser, R. E., Mitchell, B. D., Vinik, A. I., and Freeman, R. 2003. The association between cardiovascular autonomic neuropathy and mortality in individuals with diabetes: a meta-analysis. *Diabetes Care* 26(6):1895–1901.

43. Ziegler, D., Gries, F.A., Spuler, M., and Lessmann, F. 1992. The epidemiology of diabetic neuropathy. Diabetic Cardiovascular Autonomic Neuropathy Multicenter Study Group. *J Diabet Compl* 6:49–57.

44. Vinik, A.I., Maser, R.E., Mitchell, B.D., and Freeman, R. 2003. Diabetic autonomic neuropathy. *Diabetes Care* 26(5):1553–1579.

45. Ziegler, D. and Gries, F.A. 1997. Alpha-lipoic acid in the treatment of diabetic peripheral and cardiac autonomic neuropathy. *Diabetes* 46(Suppl 2):S62–S66.

46. Athyros, V.G., Didangelos, T.P., Karamitsos, D.T., Papageorgiou, A.A., Boudoulas, H., and Kontopoulos, A.G. 1998. Long-term effect of converting enzyme inhibition on circadian sympathetic and parasympathetic modulation in patients with diabetic autonomic neuropathy. *Acta Cardiol* 53:201–209.

47. Gaede, P., Vedel, P., Parving, H.H., and Pedersen, O. 1999. Intensified multifactorial intervention in patients with type 2 diabetes mellitus and microalbuminuria: the Steno type 2 randomized study. *Lancet* 353:617–622.

48. DCCT Research Group. 1993. The effect of intensive treatment of diabetes on the development and progression of long-term complications in insulin dependent diabetes mellitus. *N Engl J Med* 329:977–986.

49. UK Prospective Diabetes Study Group. 1998. Tight blood pressure control and risk of macrovascular and microvascular complications in type 2 diabetes: UKPDS 38. *BMJ* 317:703–713.

50. UK Prospective Diabetes Study (UKPDS) Group. 1998. Effect of intensive blood-glucose control with metformin on complications in overweight patients with type 2 diabetes (UKPDS 34). *Lancet* 352:854–865.

51. Gaede, P., Vedel, P., Larsen, N., Jensen, G., Parving, H., and Pedersen, O. 2003. Multifactorial intervention and cardiovascular disease in patients with type 2 diabetes. *N Engl J Med*383–393.

52. Tesfaye, S., Chaturvedi, N., Eaton, S.E., Ward, J.D., Manes, C., Ionescu-Tirgoviste, C., Witte, D.R., and Fuller, J.H. 2005. Vascular risk factors and diabetic neuropathy. *N Engl J Med* 352:341–350.

53. Ziegler, D., Sohr, C.G., and Nourooz-Zadeh, J. 2004. Oxidative stress and antioxidant defense in relation to the severity of diabetic polyneuropathy and cardiovascular autonomic neuropathy. *Diabetes Care* 27:2178–2183.

54. Vincent, A.M., Russell, J.W., Low, P., and Feldman, E.L. 2004. Oxidative stress in the pathogenesis of diabetic neuropathy. *Endocr Rev* 25:612–628.

55. Bril, V. and Buchanan, R.A. 2004. Aldose reductase inhibition by AS-3201 in sural nerve from patients with diabetic sensorimotor polyneuropathy. *Diabetes Care* 27:2369–2375.

56. Keen, H., Payan, J., Allawi, J., Walker, J., Jamal, G.A., Weir, A.I., Henderson, L.M., Bissessar, E.A., Watkins, P.J., Sampson, M. et al. 1993. Treatment of diabetic neuropathy with g- linolenic acid. *Diabetes Care* 16:8–15.

57. Ziegler, D., Nowak, H., Kempler, P., Vargha, P., and Low, P.A. 2004. Treatment of symptomatic diabetic polyneuropathy with the antioxidant alpha-lipoic acid: a meta-analysis. *Diabet Med* 21:114–121.

58. Vinik, A. and Kles, K. 2005. Microvascular Dysfunction. *Curr Diab Rev.*

59. Vinik, A.I., Bril, V., Litchy, W.J., Price, K.L., and Bastyr, E.J., III. 2005. Sural sensory action potential identifies diabetic peripheral neuropathy responders to therapy. *Muscle Nerve* 32: 619–625.

60. Vinik, A., Bril, V., Kempler, P., Litchy, W., Dyck, P., Tesfaye, S., Price, K., Bastyr, E., and for the MBBQ Study. 2005. Treatment of symptomatic diabetic peripheral neuropathy with protein kinase CB inhibitor ruboxistaurin mesylate during a 1-year randomized, placebo-controlled, double-blind clinical trial. *Clinical Therapeutics* 27:1164–1180s.

61. Vinik, A.I., Pittenger, G., Stansberry K.B., Park, T., and Skeen, M. 2001. Neurotrophic factors in diabetic neuropathy. In *Current Opinion in Endocrinology and Diabetes* (Chapter 8, pp. 205–212), George Thiem Verlag.

62. Vinik, A.I. 1999. Treatment of diabetic polyneuropathy (DPN) with recombinant human nerve growth factor (rhNGF). *Diabetes* 48(Suppl 1):A54–A55 [Abstract].

63. Rivard, A., Silver, M., Chen, D., Kearney, M., Magner, M., Annex, B., Peters, K., and Isner, J.M. 1999. Rescue of diabetes-related impairment of angiogenesis by intramuscular gene therapy with adeno-VEGF. *Am J Pathol* 154:355–363.

64. Milicevic, Z., Newlon, P.G., Pittenger, G.L., Stansberry, K.B., and Vinik, A.I. 1997. Anti-ganglioside GM1 antibody and distal symmetric "diabetic polyneuropathy" with dominant motor features. *Diabetologia* 40:1364–1365.

65. Granberg, V., Ejskjaer, N., Peakman, M., and Sundkvist, G. 2005. Autoantibodies to autonomic nerves associated with cardiac and peripheral autonomic neuropathy. *Diabetes Care* 28:1959–1964.

66. Vinik, A.I., Anandacoomaraswamy, D., and Ullal, J. 2005. Antibodies to neuronal structures: innocent bystanders or neurotoxins? *Diabetes Care* 28:2067–2072.

67. Krendel, D.A., Costigan, D.A., and Hopkins, L.C. 1995. Successful treatment of neuropathies in patients with diabetes mellitus. *Arch Neurol* 52:1053–1061.

68. Rains, C. and Bryson, H.M. 1995. Topical capsaicin. A review of its pharmacological properties and therapeutic potential in post-herpetic neuralgia, diabetic neuropathy and osteoarthritis. *Drugs Aging* 7:317–328.

69. Goldstein, D.J., Lu, Y., Detke, M.J., Lee, T.C., and Iyengar, S. 2005. Duloxetine vs. placebo in patients with painful diabetic neuropathy. *Pain* 116:109–118.

70. Rosenstock, J., Tuchman, M., LaMoreaux, L., and Sharma, U. 2004. Pregabalin for the treatment of painful diabetic peripheral neuropathy: a double-blind, placebo-controlled trial. *Pain* 110:628–638.

71. Said, G., Bigo, A., Ameri, A., Gayno, J.P., Elgrably, F., Chanson, P., and Slama, G. 1998. Uncommon early-onset neuropathy in diabetic patients. *J Neurol* 245:61–68.

72. Harati, Y., Gooch, C., Swenson, M., Edelman, S., Greene, D., Raskin, P., Donofrio, P., Cornblath, D., Sachdeo, R., Siu, C.O. et al. 1998. Double-blind randomized trial of tramadol for the treatment of the pain of diabetic neuropathy. *Neurology* 50:1842–1846.

73. Dworkin, R.H., Backonja, M., Rowbotham, M.C., Allen, R.R., Argoff, C.R., Bennett, G.J., Bushnell, M.C., Farrar, J.T., Galer, B.S., Haythornthwaite, J.A. et al. 2003. Advances in neuropathic pain: diagnosis, mechanisms, and treatment recommendations. *Arch Neurol* 60:1524–1534.

74. Sindrup, S., Gram, L., and Brosen, K. 1990. The selective serotonin reuptake inhibitor paroxetine is effective in treatment of diabetic neuropathy symptoms. *Pain* 42:144.

75. Backonja, M., Beydoun, A., Edwards, K.R., Schwartz, S.L., Fonseca, V., Hes, M., LaMoreaux, L., and Garofalo, E. 1998. Gabapentin for the symptomatic treatment of painful neuropathy in patients with diabetes mellitus: a randomized controlled trial. *JAMA* 280:1831–1836.

76. DeToledo, J.C., Toledo, C., DeCerce, J., and Ramsay, R.E. 1997. Changes in body weight with chronic, high-dose gabapentin therapy. *Ther Drug Monit* 19, 394–396.

77. Raskin, P., Donofrio, P., Rosenthal, N., Hewitt, D., Jordan, D., Xiang, J., and Vinik, A. 2004. Topiramate vs placebo in painful diabetic neuropathy: Analgesic and metabolic effects. *Neurology* 63, 865–873.

78. Vinik, A. 2005. Use of antiepileptic drugs in the treatment of chronic painful diabetic neuropathy. *J Clin Endocrinol Metab* 90(8):4936–4945.

79. Cavanagh, P.R., Derr, J.A., Ulbrecht, J.S., Maser, R.E., and Orchard, T.J. 1992. Problems with gait and posture in neuropathic patients with insulin-dependent diabetes mellitus. *Diabet Med* 9:469–474.

80. Liu-Ambrose, T., Khan, K.M., Eng, J.J., Janssen, P.A., Lord, S.R., and McKay, H.A. 2004. Resistance and agility training reduce fall risk in women aged 75 to 85 with low bone mass: a 6-month randomized, controlled trial. *J Am Geriatr Soc* 52:657–665.

81. Somers, D.L. and Somers, M.F. 1999. Treatment of neuropathic pain in a patient with diabetic neuropathy using transcutaneous electrical nerve stimulation applied to the skin of the lumbar region. *Phys Ther* 79:767–775.
82. Hamza, M.A., White, P.F., Craig, W.F., Ghoname, E.S., Ahmed, H.E., Proctor, T.J., Noe, C.E., Vakharia, A.S., and Gajraj, N. 2000. Percutaneous electrical nerve stimulation: a novel analgesic therapy for diabetic neuropathic pain. *Diabetes Care* 23:365–370.
83. Weintraub, M.I., Wolfe, G.I., Barohn, R.A., Cole, S.P., Parry, G.J., Hayat, G., Cohen, J.A., Page, J.C., Bromberg, M.B., Schwartz, S.L. et al. 2003. Static magnetic field therapy for symptomatic diabetic neuropathy: a randomized, double-blind, placebo-controlled trial. *Arch Phys Med Rehabil* 84:736–746.
84. Bosi, E., Conti, M., Vermigli, C., Cazzetta, G., Peretti, E., Cordoni, M.C., Galimberti, G., and Scionti, L. 2005. Effectiveness of frequency-modulated electromagnetic neural stimulation in the treatment of painful diabetic neuropathy. *Diabetologia* 48:817–823.
85. Tesfaye, S., Watt, J., Benbow, S.J., Pang, K.A., Miles, J., and MacFarlane, I.A. 1996. Electrical spinal-cord stimulation for painful diabetic peripheral neuropathy. *Lancet* 348:1698–1701.
86. Khaodhiar, L., Niemi, J.B., Earnest, R., Lima, C., Harry, J.D., and Veves, A. 2003. Enhancing sensation in diabetic neuropathic foot with mechanical noise. *Diabetes Care* 26:3280–3283.
87. Upton, A.R. and McComas, A.J. 1973. The double crush in nerve entrapment syndromes. *Lancet* 7825:359–362.
88. Sammarco, G., Chalk, D., and Feibel, J. 1993. Tarsal tunnel syndrome and additional nerve lesions in the same limb. *Foot Ankle* 14(2):71–77.
89. Shapiro, S.A., Stansberry, K.B., Hill, M.A., Meyer, M.D., McNitt, P.M., Bhatt, B.A., and Vinik, A.I. 1998. Normal blood flow and vasomotion in the diabetic Charcot foot. *J Diabetes Compl* 12:147–153.
90. Oloff, L., Jacobs, A., and Jaffe, S. 1983. Tarsal tunnel syndrome: a manifestation of systemic disease. *J Foot Surg* 22(4):302–307.
91. Caffee, H. 2000. Treatment of diabetic neuropathy by decompression of the posterior tibial nerve. *Plast Reconstr Surg* 106:813–815.
92. Wieman, T. and Patel, V. 1995. Treatment of hyperesthetic neuropathic pain in diabetics. Decompression of the tarsal tunnel. *Ann Surg* 221(6):660–664.
93. Dellon, A. 1992. Treatment of sympotomatic diabetic neuropathy by surgical decompression of multiple peripheral nerves. *Plast Reconstr Surg* 89(4):689–697.
94. Carneiro, R. 1999. Carpal tunnel syndrome: the cause dictates the treatment. 66(3):159–164.
95. Vinik, A.I. and Milicevic, Z. 1996. Recent advances in the diagnosis and treatment of diabetic neuropathy. *Endocrinologist* 6:443–461.
96. Vinik, A., Ullal, J., Parson, H., and Casellini, C. (in press) Diabetic Neuropathy. Nat Clin Pract Endocrinol Metab.

Diabetic Neuropathies
Endpoints in Clinical Research Studies

Aaron I. Vinik, MD, PhD, FCP, FACP

CONTENTS

INTRODUCTION
SYMPTOMS OF NEUROPATHY AS AN ENDPOINT
    IN CLINICAL STUDIES
QUALITY OF LIFE IN DIABETIC NEUROPATHY
NEUROVASCULAR FUNCTION
IDENTIFICATION OF CANDIDATES FOR
    PARTICIPATION IN RESEARCH STUDIES
CONCLUSIONS
REFERENCES

SUMMARY

Clinical trials of agents for the treatment of diabetic neuropathy have been confronted with a lack of agreement on appropriate endpoints and have generated controversy on why ample demonstration of efficacy of an agent in animal studies has not been readily translated into success in human clinical trials. There has been a failure to recognize that the relief of symptoms does not equate to change in the underlying biological disorder and great disagreement on indices, which can reliably measure changes in nerve function which translate into changes in the quality of life, activities of daily living, and health of the individual. Here, one will focus on the various measures that have been used for the evaluation of symptoms and those that quantify nerve function and compare and contrast the reasons for failure of different measures neurological deficits, prevention of degeneration of specific small fiber, large fiber and autonomic nerve deficits and those that have potential for reversal of these deficits.

From: *Contemporary Endocrinology: Controversies in Treating Diabetes:*
Clinical and Research Aspects
Edited by: D. LeRoith and A. I. Vinik © Humana Press, Totowa, NJ

Key Words: Intensive care unit; intensive insulin therapy; hyper-glycemia; hypoglycemia

INTRODUCTION

Among the challenges for studies of diabetic neuropathy is the selection of the measures that can be used to determine the efficacy of the agents. Common endpoints include (i) questionnaires that allow for quantification of any changes in the signs or symptoms of diabetic neuropathy, or the quality of life (QOL) of the patient, (ii) Objective evaluation of the physical impact of neuropathy, (iii) quantitative tests of sensory, motor, and autonomic modalities that allow more precise measures of nerve function, (iv) electrophysiologic evaluation of nerve conduction, (v) skin biopsy that allows direct observation of the morphology of sensory nerve fibers, and (vi) combinations of these tests that add to the power of being able to detect the impact of any prospective agent for the treatment of neuropathy.

SYMPTOMS OF NEUROPATHY AS AN ENDPOINT IN CLINICAL STUDIES

Systematic questioning regarding family history of nondiabetic neuropathies should be addressed first. If any other causes for peripheral neuropathy are discovered in the family history then other therapeutic approaches should be used. The diagnosis of diabetic neuropathy requires a careful history for which many questionnaires have been developed (1–5). Symptoms are scored according to the Neurologic Symptom Score (NSS). This inventory, modified over time in the Norfolk clinical research center from the original by Dyck (2), captures symptoms of muscle weakness, sensory disturbances, and autonomic function as simply present or absent according to the patient's prompted report. On the basis of patient responses, neuropathy symptoms are scored as follows: 0 = no symptoms; 1 = symptoms present. The NSS is a 38-item inventory of symptoms scored as "yes" or "no" and modified by severity with three levels. These individual points are summed for a final symptom score. We have provided the modified inventory in the appendix.

An ad hoc panel on endpoints for diabetic neuropathy trials suggested that symptoms could be a satisfactory endpoint for epidemiologic studies and controlled trials in diabetic peripheral neuropathy (DPN) (6). Sensory symptoms of neuropathy can be classified into negative (i.e., with a decrease or absent sensory fibers, receptors or central mechanism) or positive (from hyperfunction of the systems). Negative symptoms relate to the patients' reports of decreased ability to feel tactile stimuli, mechanical displacement or movement of hair, skin or other anatomical parts and decreased cognitive function (e.g., recognition of temperature changes or differences in cooling and warming and cold and heat pain or other noxious stimuli). Sensory loss includes imbalance ataxia inability to perform skilled movements. Notably, these are reported quite differently in different ethnic groups and in different countries. For example, in Japan patients will report on unusual sensations in their legs, and in the USA, patients talk of inability to discern different textures, for example, when crossing the floor from a tiled surface to a carpet in going from the bathroom to the bedroom. Loss of position awareness is often very distressing and has a marked impact on QOL and activities of daily living (ADLs), compromising the ability to play sports. In contrast, positive symptoms are sensory experiences that arise spontaneously. Patients describe small fiber symptoms as superficial, prickling, tingling, and burning sensations, such as a fire or bee stinging. This may be accompanied by misinterpretation for nonpainful stimuli as painful, referred to as allodynia, and clinically, this may correspond with hyperesthesia or hyperalgesia. On the contrary, patients with predominantly large fiber disease will report such feelings as: a dog gnawing at the bones of the feet; a toothache in the foot; the feet feel like they are encased in concrete; they feel like cardboard or cotton bunched up in the shoe; they always have a sock on or feel squeezed; and constriction with aching, boring, or throbbing deep-seated pain. A third of pain symptoms are a spontaneous burst of pain such as lightning, which comes and goes and may last but a few minutes. These are regarded as neuropathic pain, and may have an electrical lancinating quality, are short lived, and tend to occur in clusters and in the same anatomical region. Restless leg pain usually is a deep, aching pain, and occurs with inactivity and often responds to mobilization. Pain is often cyclical and usually worse at night. One surprising observation is that when the patient talks of numbness it may not mean a deficit in pain perception, but rather that the patient feels that the limb has gone to sleep or as if they have been given an anesthetic. It is a positive symptom. Perhaps the most distressing symptom relates to the apparent or real perception of weakness. Pain produces anxiety, and weakness causes depression! In diabetes, the small fiber, large fiber, motor and sensory symptoms tend to occur together simultaneously, although there are many instances in which they may be distinct. The hot foot syndrome is one in which pure small fiber symptoms are present with normal strength, reflexes and electrophysiology, and there may be no objective features to confirm neuropathic origin. The advent of skin biopsies has established loss of intraepidermal nerve fibers (IENF) as being the root cause (see below), and these small fiber functions are not measured by electrophysiological tests. For this reason, tools that quantify these symptoms have become critical as endpoints in studies of DPN. Several tools have now been developed which are reproducible, standardized, and valid measurements that address the positive and negative symptoms and provide measurements of the constancy, severity, distributions, and frequency of the symptoms. In the Total Symptom Score, the severity (mild, moderate, or severe) and frequency (infrequent, frequent, and constant) are scored *(4)*. The nerve symptom change (NSC), the positive and negative symptoms are characterized as absent, mild, moderate and severe by anatomical location are quantitated by number, severity and change by comparison with a previous examination *(7)*. For pain, discussed elsewhere in this book, different pain questionnaires or visual analog scales are used, and the questions address the most severe pain in the last 24 h as a single day's recall or a week's recall *(8,9)*. The newest tool that had been used successfully in clinical trial is the Neuropathy Total symptom Score-6 (NTSS-6) *(10,11)*. The NTSS-6 questionnaire was developed conceptually to evaluate the frequency and intensity of individual neuropathy sensory symptoms identified frequently in patients with DPN (numbness and/or insensitivity, prickling and/or tingling sensation, aching pain, burning pain, lancinating pain, and allodynia and/or hyperalgesia). The NTSS-6 was administered eight times over a 1-year period to 205 DPN patients. The NTSS-6 reliability (determined by internal consistency and test–retest reproducibility), construct (convergent) validity, clinical responsiveness, clinical relevance (interpretability) and minimally clinically important differences (MCID) were determined. Internal consistency was demonstrated at all eight visits (Cronbach's $p > 0.7$). Test–retest reproducibility (intraclass correlation coefficient >0.9) was observed during the baseline period and at endpoint. Construct validity was demonstrated by a statistically significant correlation between the NTSS-6 score and the Neuropathy Symptoms and Change (NSC) score ($p < 0.01$). Clinical responsiveness was demonstrated by significant correlations between change in the NTSS-6 and (i) change in the NSC score ($p < 0.01$); (ii) change in the Neuropathy Impairment Score of the Lower Limbs; and (iii) composite nerve function scores ($p < 0.007$). Clinical relevance was demonstrated by a statistically significant association between the change in the NTSS-6 score and the Clinical Global Impression (r = 0.402, $p < 0.01$). The within- and between-groups MCID for the total NTSS-6 scores were -1.26 and 0.97, respectively. The authors conclude that the NTSS-6 is a valid and reliable instrument for assessing clinically meaningful changes in neuropathic sensory symptoms in DPN patients.

Distinction of neuropathic pain from various other causes is important in study design. Failure to do so was the cause of failure of three studies of topiramate in DPN, whereas the successful trial *(12)* specified the origin of the pain, so that it was not confused with entrapment, fasciitis, or gout arthritis to name a few. Four criteria help to define this: (i) Several symptoms occur together, for example, numbness and pain with weakness; (ii) They occur in the known distribution of DPN; (iii) They conform to the anatomy of the peripheral nervous system; and (iv) They conform to the areas found on clinical examination to have nerve damage, although this may be very misleading. Whatever the case, a physical examination remains mandatory to define the nature of the underlying pathology.

For therapeutic trials, the distinction between symptomatic therapy and therapy addressing the basic biology of the disease must be made. For example, a simple analgesic does not alter nerve function. It must also be shown that the agent used does not relieve the symptoms by damaging the nerves. For this reason, the agency insists that electrophysiological studies are done and the days of the 28-day pain trial are over and 3–6 months trial are now required. To demonstrate that the agent does not hurt the nervous system requires demonstration of no deleterious effects on nerve physiology, and to show that there is indeed a biologic effect, the changes must outlast the period of treatment or go beyond the pharmacological action of the drug. With this in mind, the studies need to be powered adequately on these endpoints, and the design power and execution of the study must be adequate. Thus, the following requirements should be met:

1. The symptom must improve to a significant degree.
2. The improvement must not be due to worsening of neuropathy.
3. The change, if possible, should correlate with evidence of improved nerve function (electrophysiology, IENF, Quantitative sensory testing [QST] and QAFT).
4. The change should be biologically relevant (e.g., if the scale is three intervals, mild, moderate or severe, or infrequent, frequent or constant, then a 1.667 on one of the three scales would be biologically relevant. If more than one descriptor is used for the symptom, then this can be reduced to 0.834 points.), based on the view that this is what patients interpret as clinically meaningful (6).
5. The drug being evaluated should have a low number needed to treat (NNT) to achieve response in a single patient, i.e., a high responder rate and a very low number needed to harm (NNH) (13).
6. The effects are greater than those of placebo. Assuming placebo effects can yield a 30% improvement in 30% of patients, a 50% improvement in 50% of patients seems ideal.
7. Adequate masking should have been achieved. For example, NGF caused local site pain when administered, which is difficult to conceal and clouds judgment. Certain ARI pills had a bitter taste not matched by placebo.

Neurological Examination

The neurological examination is carried out in a standardized manner by a trained neurologist or diabetologist who has undergone specialized instruction on the degree of precision required to obtain reproducible results and to use judgment for the size and strength of the individual. Results are scored on a 5-point Likert scale using the Neurologic Impairment Score (NIS) tool, a 37-item inventory that measures motor and sensory function bilaterally on a 0–4 or 0–2 scale as judged by the clinician in the neurological exam. The motor neurological examination measures cranial nerve weakness, pupillary reflexes, muscle weakness, muscle wasting, and reflexes. The sensory neurological evaluation measures sensation in the right and left index and little fingers and great and little toes to touch, prickling pain, vibration, joint position, and pressure (using 1- and 10-g monofilaments). The NIS tool for lower limbs (NIS-LL) reflects only abnormalities in the lower limbs. The total neuropathy score (TNS) reflects a summation of the symptoms, sensory, and motor scores. A score of =1 is no neuropathy, 2–9 mild, 10–19 moderate, and >20 severe neuropathy.

All the signs and symptoms of neuropathy can be scored and recorded allowing changes in response to treatment to be monitored longitudinally. In addition, there have been similar forms developed for quantitation of the disabilities related to nerve dysfunction and even forms for quantitation of the impact on the patient's QOL. Unfortunately, such questionnaires are quite subjective and may not be sensitive enough to discern small changes in nerve fiber functions in a small test group over a short period of time. Unless a study includes a large number of subjects and a sufficient period of time, significant changes may not be detectable, particularly in the short time periods that most efficacy trials are designed for.

Quantitative Sensory Tests

QST is performed to assess somatosensory function using established, validated methods and algorithms for measuring both large and small fiber somatosensory function. These include vibration thresholds, light touch (Semmes-Weinstein monofilaments), cold and warm thermal sensation, and cold- and heat-induced pain thresholds at the dominant great toe *(14)*. Generally, for each of these non-noxious sensations, we use the method of limits, six ascending trials with an inter-stimulus interval randomly varying from 4 to 20 s using the Medoc TSA 2001/VSA 3000 (Medoc Advanced Medical, Minneapolis, MN, USA) or the Case IV device *(15)*, although there are others in use. The thresholds are calculated as the mean stimulus intensity level over all six responses.

QUALITY OF LIFE IN DIABETIC NEUROPATHY

In previous studies, patients' perceptions of the effects of DPN have been assessed using generic instruments *(16–18)* or a symptom checklist *(19)*. These instruments do not capture the entire spectrum of unique aspects of DPN, particularly those related to specific somatic and autonomic nerve fibers. We previously reported data on health-related QOL and ADL in relation to specific nerve fiber function *(20)*. Subsequently, the NeuroQol *(21)*, which measures patients' perceptions of the impact of neuropathy and foot ulcers, has been published. While focusing on peripheral neuropathy outcomes, specifically foot ulcers, it does not cover the full scope of neuropathy related to large fiber, small fiber, and autonomic neuropathy function. In contrast, we have developed a comprehensive questionnaire that captures the entire spectrum of DPN, including the concentration of symptoms in the extremities, subtle loss of function such as fine motor impairments and slight sensory changes, unique problems with proprioception and balance, and autonomic symptoms that are not captured in existing instruments. This instrument has the ability to discriminate the presence of neuropathy as well as the different levels of neuropathy and the specific nerve fibers involved *(20)*. It can be used to monitor disease progression as well as evaluate treatment modalities *(22,23)*. Since its development and preliminary validation, the tool has been used in clinical trials providing further validation opportunities as well as psychometric evaluation *(22)*.

A caveat is our findings that the Norfolk QOL-DN identifies symptoms in patients with diabetes who do not have established neuropathy. The symptom complex of diabetes in patients with diabetes without neuropathy characterized by highly variable blood sugar levels together with the effects of other factors of the metabolic syndrome such as high blood pressure, insulin resistance, and dyslipidemia appears to manifest health-related problems not entirely dissimilar to their neuropathic counterparts. Further research is necessary to fully understand these contributions to patients' perception of QOL. As such, future modifications to these items in the Norfolk QOL-DN may be necessary.

We believe that QOL is an important tool for measuring patients' perception of the impact of diabetes and neuropathy on their physical and psychosocial functioning and may act as a guide in decision-making toward altering apparent health and functional status.

Quantitative Electrophysiology

Nerve conduction studies (NCS) are the most reproducible, reliable, and objective measure of peripheral neuropathy available currently to document peripheral neuropathy. NCS in DPN has demonstrated small changes in nerve function (conduction velocity) with treatment in well-controlled studies *(24, 25)*. The translation of small changes in NCS into clinical relevance has raised doubts *(26)*. The natural progression of DPN is a decline of peroneal motor conduction velocity of only 0.2–0.4 m/s per year *(27)*. A clinically meaningful improvement of 1.5 m/s therefore generally requires about 3 years. Most recently, this has been achieved in the study of an ARI in which the participants were carefully selected to have positive sural sensory nerve action potentials (SNAPs) *(28)*. There is a strong correlation between myelinated fiber density and SNAP and a loss of 1 μv in SNAP correlates with a loss of about 150 nerve fibers/mm². There is about a 5% loss per year in SNAP, supporting the notion that selection of patients for entry into studies who have mild neuropathy or those of relatively short duration with the greatest likelihood of responding. Alternatively, a 50% prevention of the expected deterioration in a given time interval has been considered evidence of positive efficacy *(27)*.

F waves detect any abnormality in the antidromic conduction of the compound neural wave generated by electrical stimulation distally reaching the spinal cord, activating a subpopulation of spinal cord motor neurons, followed by the orthodromic conduction of the newly established wave and postsynaptic activation of muscle fibers in the appropriate distribution. The long loop of this measure increases the likelihood of identifying an abnormality at any of several sites, and it has been shown to be the most reproducible measure in NCS of diabetic neuropathy *(29)*. NCS of course does not measure small fibers and for this reason alone cannot be the sole endpoint in clinical studies.

A key role for electrophysiological assessment is to rule out other causes of neuropathy or to identify neuropathies superimposed on DPN. Unilateral conditions, such as entrapments, are far more common in the patients with diabetes *(30)*. The principal factors that influence the speed of NCV are (i) the integrity and degree of myelination of the largest diameter fibers, (ii) the mean cross-sectional diameter of the responding axons, (iii) the representative internodal distance in the segment under study, and (iv) the micro-environment at the nodes, including the distribution of ion channels. Thus, small unmyelinated fibers and the changes cannot be evaluated using NCS and must rely on measures such as skin biopsies and QST! Furthermore, demyelinating conditions affect conduction velocities, whereas diabetes primarily reduces amplitudes, thus the finding of a profound reduction in conduction velocity strongly supports the occurrence in a diabetic patient of an alternative condition. Indeed, the odds of occurrence of CIDP were 11 times higher among diabetic than nondiabetic patients *(31)*. With the recognition of the limitations of NCS for the evaluation of neuropathy in diabetes, it remains a robust measure in clinical trials and serves to exclude entrapments, demyelinating conditions, and responsiveness to interventions can be based on the identification of potential responders with mild neuropathy based on the presence of sural nerve responses.

Quantitative Sensory Tests

Because diabetic neuropathy virtually always exhibits compromise of sensory nerve function and often includes autonomic dysfunction, quantitative sensory and autonomic measures are an attractive alternative to the question-naire scoring approach. Over the past 15–20 years, there has been progressive development of protocols and devices for quantitatively measuring thermal sensation, vibration, and pressure detection. In 2002, an international group of experts in diabetic neuropathy held a consensus meeting to develop guide-lines for the management of DPN by the practicing clinician using quantitative function tests *(32)*. Combined, these tests cover a range of sensory modal-ities, including vibratory, proprioceptive, tactile, pain, thermal, and autonomic function. These measurements are geared for evaluation of sensory functions at specific points on the body with relative accuracy and precision. The strengths of QST are well documented *(33)*, but the investigator must also be aware of the limitations of QST. No matter what the instrument or procedure used, QST can be considered only a semi-objective measure, because the results are affected by the subject's attention, motivation, and cooperation, as well as by anthropometric variables such as age, gender, body mass, and history of smoking and alcohol consumption. Expectancy and subject bias are additional factors that can exert a powerful influence on QST findings. In addition, QST is sensitive to changes in structure or function along the entire neuro-axis from nerve to cortex; it is not a specific measure of peripheral nerve function *(33)*. The American Academy of Neurology reported that QST could be used as an ancillary measure for clinical and research purposes *(34)* but were not suffi-ciently robust for routine clinical use. Nevertheless, quantitative sensory and autonomic testing, under the right conditions, provides a means for evaluation of the efficacy of treatments for diabetic neuropathy. QST is a psychophysical measure of polyneuropathy but is much more variable and unpredictable than NCS in the diabetic neuropathy population.

The most reliable QST is quantitative vibration perception threshold by various techniques *(35)*. QST of vibration (vibration detection threshold [VDT]) is particularly useful as a sensitive and specific measure of large fiber function because it can be done quickly, is noninvasive, simple, painless, and reproducible *(14)*. VDT reflects the activation of mechanoreceptors and conduction in large fiber nerves that are important for proprioception, position, ataxia, balance, and gait as well as muscle strength. VDT correlated with the neuropathy disability score *(36)*, lack of reflex in the lower extremities, and symptoms of DPN *(37,38)* and nerve conduction changes *(39)*. A strong correlation was noted between VDT and a number of microvessel abnormal-ities *(40)*. Loss of vibration perception predisposes individuals with diabetes to instability, falling, and decreased QOL *(41,42)*. Prospective studies have established impaired vibration sensation as a positive predictor of long-term complications such as ulcers and amputations *(43–45)*.

The improvement found in VDT in the recently reported ruboxystaurin study *(11)* is unique in that it demonstrates that directly the drug impacts the pathophysiology of the peripheral nerve rather than acting centrally to reduce pain through analgesic pathways. Thus, there are many reasons to believe that QST particularly of VDT can be used in the evaluation of responses to intervention in clinical trials.

However, patients followed in research trials frequently have more abnormality of small fiber function, (46), and the variability of small fiber QST testing is even greater than that of large fiber QST testing in the clinic setting and has not proven useful save for possibly the cooling detection threshold in the NGF study (47).

Quantitative Autonomic Function Tests

Diabetic autonomic neuropathy (DAN) is a serious and common complication of diabetes (48). Major clinical manifestations of DAN include resting tachycardia, exercise intolerance, orthostatic hypotension, constipation, gastroparesis, erectile dysfunction, sudomotor dysfunction, impaired neurovascular function, "brittle diabetes," and hypoglycemic autonomic failure. DAN may affect many organ systems throughout the body (e.g., gastrointestinal, genitourinary, and cardiovascular). Gastrointestinal disturbances (e.g., esophageal enteropathy, gastroparesis, constipation, diarrhea, and fecal incontinence) are common, and any section of the gastrointestinal tract may be affected. Gastroparesis should be suspected in individuals with erratic glucose control. Upper gastrointestinal symptoms should lead to consideration of all possible causes including autonomic dysfunction. Although a radiographic gastric emptying study can definitively establish the diagnosis of gastroparesis, a reasonable approach is to exclude autonomic dysfunction and other known causes of these upper GI symptoms. Constipation is the most common lower gastrointestinal symptom but can alternate with episodes of diarrhea. Diagnostic approaches should rule out autonomic dysfunction and the well-known causes such as neoplasia. Occasionally, anorectal manometry and other specialized tests typically performed by the gastroenterologist may be helpful.

DAN is also associated with genitourinary tract disturbances including bladder and/or sexual dysfunction. Evaluation of bladder dysfunction should be performed for individuals with diabetes who have recurrent urinary tract infections, pyelonephritis, incontinence, or a palpable bladder. Specialized assessment of bladder dysfunction typically is performed by an urologist. In men, DAN may cause loss of penile erection and/or retrograde ejaculation. A complete work-up for impotence in men should include history (medical and sexual), psychological evaluation, hormone levels, measurement of nocturnal penile tumescence, tests to assess penile, pelvic, and spinal nerve function, cardiovascular autonomic function tests, and measurement of penile and brachial blood pressure. Neurovascular dysfunction resulting from DAN contributes to a wide spectrum of clinical disorders, including erectile dysfunction, loss of skin integrity, and abnormal vascular reflexes. Disruption of microvascular skin flow and sudomotor function may occur as among the earliest results of DAN and lead to dry skin, loss of sweating and the development of fissures and cracks that allow microorganisms to enter. These changes ultimately contribute to the development of ulcers, gangrene, and limb loss. Various aspects of neurovascular function can be evaluated with specialized tests, but generally these have not been well standardized and have limited clinical utility.

Cardiovascular autonomic neuropathy (CAN) is the most studied and clinically important form of DAN. Meta-analyses of published data demonstrate that reduced cardiovascular autonomic function as measured by heart rate variability (HRV) is strongly (i.e., relative risk is doubled) associated with increased risk of silent myocardial ischemia and mortality. The determination of the presence of CAN is usually based on a battery of autonomic function tests rather than just on one test. Proceedings from a consensus conference in 1992 and re-affirmed in ref. *13* recommended that three tests (R-R variation, Valsalva maneuver, and postural blood pressure testing) be used for longitudinal testing of the cardiovascular autonomic system. Other forms of autonomic neuropathy can be evaluated with specialized tests, but these are less standardized and less available than commonly used tests of cardiovascular autonomic function, which quantify loss of HRV. Interpretability of serial HRV testing requires accurate, precise, and reproducible procedures that employ established physiologic maneuvers. The battery of three recommended tests for assessing CAN is readily performed in the average clinic, hospital, or diagnostic center with the use of available technology. Measurement of HRV at time of diagnosis of type 2 diabetes and within 5 years after diagnosis of type 1 diabetes (unless an individual has symptoms suggestive of autonomic dysfunction earlier) serves to establish a baseline, with which 1-year interval tests can be compared. Regular HRV testing provides early detection and thereby promotes timely diagnostic and therapeutic interventions. HRV testing may also facilitate differential diagnosis and the attribution of symptoms (e.g., erectile dysfunction, dyspepsia, and dizziness) to autonomic dysfunction. Finally, knowledge of early autonomic dysfunction can encourage patient and physician to improve metabolic control and to use therapies such as angiotensin-converting enzyme inhibitors and beta-blockers proven to be effective for patients with CAN.

Low and colleagues examined 231 patients with diabetes (type 1, n = 83; type 2, n = 148) and 245 healthy subjects using a self-report instrument (Autonomic Symptom Profile *[49]*) and evaluated the severity and distribution of autonomic deficits (cardiovagal, sudomotor, and adrenergic) with the objective laboratory-based composite autonomic severity score (CASS). CASS is a screening carried out in the Mayo Autonomic Laboratory that evaluates the severity and distribution of post-ganglionic autonomic nerve fiber function. Using the CASS, Philip Low (50) made the statement that autonomic symptoms and deficits are common in diabetes; yet, mild in severity, the correlation between symptoms and deficits is overall weak, emphasizing the need to separately identify autonomic symptoms. In our factor analysis, three autonomic features were identified as constituting the autonomic factor. These features included orthostasis, diarrhea, sudomotor, adrenergic, and cardiovagal functions. Sympathetic postganglionic cholinergic function is assessed using the quantitative sudomotor axon-reflex test at the forearm and three lower extremity sites. Sympathetic adrenergic function is carried out by the measurement of the beat-to-beat blood pressure and heart rate responses to head up tilt and the Valsalva maneuver. Cardiovagal function is evaluated by heart rate response to deep breathing and the Valsalva maneuver. Results are compared to a normative database of 557 normal subjects. On the basis of the results of the screen, a 10-point composite score can be derived (CASS) that corrects for the compounding effects of age and sex. The 10-point scale is divided into three subscales: adrenergic (range 0–4), sudomotor (range 0–3), and cardiovagal (range 0–3). The ASP includes orthostasis, secretomotor, urinary, diarrhea, constipation, sleep, pupillomotor, male sexual function, vasomotor, upper gastrointestinal, and syncope as symptoms. Although symptoms were frequent and there appeared to be a difference in patients with type 1 and type 2 diabetes, Spearman rank correlations showed no relationships between the CASS and the ASP in patients with type 2 diabetes. The authors concluded that autonomic symptoms and deficits are common in diabetes, but mild in severity, and the correlation between symptom scores and overall deficits is weak in mild diabetic neuropathy, emphasizing the need to separately evaluate autonomic symptoms.

Vinik et al. have reported on the use of their NSS, which contains 11 questions pertinent to the same areas of dysfunction that the ASP covers (51). In 350 patients with mild (Dyck Stage 1) neuropathy, symptoms were present, but there were significant floor effects, so that the autonomic domain of the Norfolk QOL-DN tool did not identify this as a major factor. However, in a German population with advance neuropathy and a history of present of foot ulcers or an amputation, autonomic symptoms were clearly present and related to autonomic function. These were orthostasis, constipation, and vomiting. In the mild population, these are not features. However, they appear in patients with more advanced neuropathy. Clearly, further studies are needed to determine what the optimum tool is for the evaluation of responses of autonomic symptoms and objective measures to intervention will be.

NEUROVASCULAR FUNCTION

There is now widespread recognition that type 2 diabetes is one manifestation of a constellation comprising insulin resistance, dyslipidemia, obesity, hypertension, and hypercoagulability referred to as the "dysmetabolic syndrome" (52–54). Recently, yet another component has been added: altered blood flow in various organs including skin, muscle, gut, pancreas, corpora cavernosa, and so on. There is even the suggestion that disturbed blood flow may be a major contributor to apparent resistance to the action of insulin (52–58). Recently, there has been more direct evidence that disturbed blood flow in skin precedes the development of diabetes and is part of an "inflammatory syndrome," but the precise mechanisms of disturbance in blood flow has escaped resolution (59).

We have previously demonstrated several neurovascular abnormalities that occur in diabetes (60,61). There is both impaired peripheral vasoconstriction and vasodilatation in cutaneous vessels that strongly resembles an enhancement of normal aging effects seen in peripheral vasculature (60). There is a correlation between the reduction in blood flow and reduced C-fiber function in the toes. The abnormalities in blood flow in the fingers was found in the absence of disordered sensory perception, suggesting that it may be a more sensitive measure of neurovascular function and does not reflect permanent structural damage to neurons. We devised a simple stimulus for vessel distension that relies on the effects of local heating and purely on the hydrostatic gradient imposed by elevation and lowering of the upper limb, that is, reflecting the degree of microvascular distensibility (61,62). In hairy skin (the hand dorsum), there is an active vasodilative mechanism that is dependent on C-fiber nociceptors that accounts for 75% of vascular dilative capacity when heated. There were, in addition, significant inverse correlations between systolic blood pressure and hyperemic response to ischemia ($r = -0.76$, $p < 0.01$) and the heated arm lowering ($r = -0.52$, $p < 0.05$). There were also significant correlations between blood flow at 35°C and the LDL cholesterol ($r = -0.62$, $p < 0.001$), C-peptide ($r = -0.65$, $p < 0.05$), and triglycerides ($r = -0.47$, $p < 0.05$). Thus, there is a disorder of the whole neurovascular unit in type 2 diabetes that co-segregates with elements of the metabolic syndrome particularly insulin resistance.

We have shown that the neurovascular response can be used as an endpoint in studies of topiramate (63,64), and the tests are now being used in studies of other agents that are prospective candidates for the treatment and prevention of neuropathy.

Skin Biopsy for the Evaluation of Nerve Fiber Morphology

Another potential endpoint for diabetic neuropathy treatment studies is skin biopsy for the evaluation of peripheral nerve fibers in the affected areas.

In common practice, a small punch biopsy is collected from affected sites and subsequent immunochemical staining with antibody to PGP 9.5; a panneuronal marker reveals the epidermal nerve fibers. Good results have been obtained with both light microscopy and confocal microscopy for evaluation of the density, length, and integrity of IENF. These techniques have been used to describe a loss of nerve fiber density and fiber length in diabetic neuropathy (65–67). Our own data shows that there is a decrease in IENF length in patients with metabolic syndrome, considered a pre-diabetic state (68). However, evaluation may be complicated by an apparent increase in fiber density in the years immediately surrounding the diagnosis of diabetes (67). Although further work needs to be done to verify this observation in a larger population, it is possible that this represents an initial attempt to maintain sensory system function in the face of nerves that are failing physiologically.

Demonstrating how quickly changes in epidermal nerve fibers can be detected by the skin biopsy technique, it has been used to observe the loss of fiber density just 2 weeks after topical exposure to capsaicin, a noxious agent that depletes substance P from C fibers (69,70). Subsequent recovery of fiber density over a similarly short period of time after removal of capsaicin has also been demonstrated by skin biopsy (71). Their studies of IENF embrace the use of capsaicin-induced fiber loss and measurement of the rate of regeneration in a study of 31 healthy controls and 20 subjects with diabetes. Although the rate of regeneration in diabetes was highly variable, it was correlated with the baseline IENF density but not age, gender, or epidermal thickness. They report that the normal rate of regeneration is 0.177 ± 0.075 fibers/mm/day after adjusting for initial fiber density, in diabetes was reduced to 0.1 ± 0.07 fibers/mm/day, and that concomitant neuropathy reduced this further to 0.04 ± 0.03 fibers/mm/day and was independent of diabetes type, control, or duration. They suggest that their results have significant implications for study design with the ability to measure regenerative capacity over a few months and that this would reduce the length of trials as well as identify suitable candidates for entry into trials. Our data, in contrast, show that, in as few as 20 patients treated with the antiepileptic agent Topiramate, spontaneous nerve fiber regeneration can be quantified within 18 weeks (63). Our technique uses confocal microscopy, but it is not certain yet that the two approaches would yield very different results. Thus, it appears that, as this technique becomes more widespread, it will provide another means for examining the effects of various therapies on sensory fibers that are compromised in diabetic neuropathy.

Combined Measures of Nerve Function

The NIS-LL is a quantitative method of scoring the abnormalities of neurologic examination. This scale is quantitative, validated, and reproducible although not reaching the standards of other objective measures. The NIS-LL is a direct evaluation of the clinical deficits present in neuropathy, which lead to the severe end-stage complications of the diabetic foot such as recurrent foot ulceration, gangrene, and amputation. Dyck's scale has been utilized in small clinical trials (e.g., phase II nerve growth factor study) and has shown positive clinical change in response to treatment. A change in the scale is considered a significant alteration in polyneuropathy as the scale is designed to document relatively large changes.

The NIS-LL is a scoring system graduated from 0 points (the normal finding) to a maximum of 88 points (the absence of all motor, sensory, and reflex activity in the lower extremities). The scale is additive of all deficits (64 potential points for muscle strength, 8 points for reflexes, and 16 points for sensory function) in the lower extremities. Combining the scale with other measures ensures that other important features of neuropathy (which may predispose to other complications) are not overlooked. For example, autonomic dysfunction that causes early mortality in all patients and impotence in males should not be overlooked. Chronic painful symptoms can be disabling in a subset of diabetic neuropathy patients and need to be addressed as well. Patients' problems in diabetic polyneuropathy are not restricted to foot ulceration, gangrene, and amputation.

IDENTIFICATION OF CANDIDATES FOR PARTICIPATION IN RESEARCH STUDIES

Accurate diagnosis and staging of DPN and exclusion of conditions that mimic DPN are critical prerequisites of clinical trials designed to evaluate an intervention (72). However, what appears to be just as critical is the need to evaluate the level of impairment because "dead nerves" are unlikely to respond to any form of intervention. Patients with less severe impairment because of DPN may be the most responsive to a therapeutic intervention (73–75) designed to reverse or slow the progression (73–76). Thus, early identification of neuropathy disease-state impairment may help identify a population of patients who are most amenable to intervention with experimental therapies beyond glycemic control.

Traditionally, VDT has been recognized as a sensitive tool for the detection of neuropathy. Nonetheless, VDT for the prediction of responsiveness in clinical trials has not proven to be infallible. When vibration impairment is observed, other markers of less severe DPN need to be identified. The medial plantar SNAP has been suggested as a sensitive indicator of diabetic neuropathy; however, it is absent at a younger age in diabetes (mean 43.7 ± 1.2 years of age), and therefore, this nerve cannot be tested in many patients with diabetes and vibration loss (77). Reflexes are often used as an early marker of

DPN; however, changes in reflexes are not as sensitive as nerve-fiber function *(45)*. On the basis of several studies, what has emerged is that the presence or absence of a sural SNAP may serve as a valid marker of less severe DPN with vibratory impairment *(78–82)*.

Because the presence or absence of a sural SNAP had not been adequately evaluated as a marker of less severe DPN responsiveness to therapeutic intervention in large multinational clinical trials *(83–87)*, we assessed the presence of sural SNAPs as a marker of vibratory impairment in less severe DPN in patients enrolled in a multinational, placebo-controlled, randomized clinical trial, where the effects of ruboxistaurin (a specific inhibitor of the beta isoform of protein kinase C) were measured *(10–88)*. We have recently reported *(28)* that, in patients with impaired VDT of $\geq$ 97 percentile, preserved sural SNAPs identified a subset of patients with less severe DPN who were ideal candidates to select for clinical trials who could be predicted to respond to intervention. Identifying patients with DPN amenable to therapy is a challenge. To determine whether the amplitude of the sural SNAP reflects the severity of DPN, an analysis was performed in 205 patients with DPN, identified by an abnormal VDT, who were enrolled in a multinational clinical trial investigating ruboxistaurin mesylate *(28)*. Nerve conduction velocity and response amplitude and latency were measured and compared. VDT was significantly lower in those with preserved sural SNAPs ($n = 128$) than in those in whom they were absent ($n = 77$; 21.5 vs. 22.7 JND units, $p = 0.002$). Thus, preserved sural SNAP denoted less severe DPN. Logistic regression analyses evaluating baseline characteristics, HbA1c, and baseline symptom scores identified only DPN duration as a factor that might contribute to the presence of sural SNAP ($p = 0.004$; odds ratio = 0.896). We concluded that, in patients with abnormal VDT, preserved sural SNAP identifies a patient population with less severe DPN who may respond to therapeutic intervention in clinical trials.

The following summarizes our view of prospective endpoints in Diabetic Neuropathy Trials:

1. Symptoms: include Nerve Symptom Score, NSC, Total Symptom Score, Visual Analogue Scale for pain, Brief Pain Inventory, McGill pain questionnaire, Weekly Pain Inventories, Nerve Total Symptom Score 6, Clinical global Impression: *subjective but proven measures in clinical trials on pain relieving drugs.*
2. Quantitative neurologic exam focusing on distal sensorimotor function (sensation, strength, and reflexes): *semi-objective.*
3. Neurophysiology (velocity, amplitude, F-wave, multiple nerve, both sensory and motor): *objective.*
4. QST (vibration, thermal, and pain): *semi-objective.*
5. Morphology: (skin biopsy – density, branching pattern) – *objective.*

6. Neurovascular function: *objective*.
7. Autonomic testing: *objective*.
8. QOL: *subjective*.

CONCLUSIONS

There are now a large range of tools that have been developed for the evaluation of novel treatments for both the symptoms and the underlying disorders of diabetic neuropathies. Evaluation of pain and its relief appears to have come of age with the approval of two drugs specifically for diabetic neuropathic pain despite using different endpoints but nonetheless well-designed and executed trials. It has nonetheless become clear that using symptoms as an endpoint in longer-term studies with drugs that have the potential for changing the biology of the disease is fraught with danger because the natural history of diabetic neuropathy is changing for reasons that are not clear but may relate to improved general well-being, attention to the reduction of multiple risk factors for the development of neuropathy, healthier lifestyles and regular exercise and improved nutrition apart from the use of statins and ACEs and ARBs almost universally in the diabetic population that may impact neuropathy. Furthermore, the regression to the mean is also relevant to the evaluation of symptoms because the condition is self-liming, and there is a huge placebo effect. Indeed one of the best things one can do with patients in pain is to enter them into a trial, at least 30% will have a 30% improvement even if they only receive placebo.

Progression is being made with trials that are using harder endpoints for the evaluation of large fiber, small fiber, and autonomic nerve function. Recent trials of Aldose Reductase inhibitors have shown changes in electrophysiology and vibration perception; PKC inhibition has been associated with reduction symptoms and improved vibration and alpha lipoic acid with improved autonomic function. More recently, there is evidence that topiramate can induce small fiber regeneration of IENFs. It thus seems that advances are being made, so that it will not be the trials that fail but rather that the drugs that fail, and hopefully, we will have a new cadre of agents that address the underlying biological disturbance in diabetic neuropathy that can be shown to pass muster in clinical trials with appropriate endpoints.

REFERENCES

1. Young, M.J., Boulton, A.J.M., MacLeod, A.F., Williams, D.R.R., and Sonksen, P.H. 1993. A multicenter study of the prevalence of diabetic peripheral neuropathy in the United Kingdom hospital clinic population. *Diabetologia* 36:1–5.
2. Dyck, P.J. 1988. Detection, characterization and staging of polyneuropathy: assessed in diabetes. *Muscle Nerve* 11:21–32.

3. Vinik, A.I. and Mitchell, B. 1988. Clinical aspects of diabetic neuropathies. *Diabetes Metab Rev* 4:223–253.

4. Ziegler, D., Hanefeld, M., Ruhnau, K.J., Meissner, H.P., Lobisch, M., Schutte, K., and Gries, F.A. 1995. Treatment of symptomatic diabetic peripheral neuropathy with the anti-oxidant alpha-lipoic acid. A 3-week multicentre randomized controlled trial (ALADIN Study). *Diabetologia* 38:1425–1433.

5. Feldman, E.L., Stevens, M.J., Thomas, P.K., Brown, M.B., Canal, N., and Greene, D.A. 1994. A practical two-step quantitative clinical and electrophysiological assessment for the diagnosis and staging of diabetic neuropathy. *Diabetes Care* 17:1281–1289.

6. Apfel, S.C., Asbury, A., Bril, V., Burns, T., Campbell, J., Chalk, C., Dyck, P., Dyck, P.J., Feldman E, Fields, H. *et al.* 2001. Positive neuropathic sensory symptoms as endpoints in diabetic neuropathy trials. *J Neurol Sci* 189:3–5 (Abstract).

7. Dyck, P.J., Davies, J.L., Litchy, W.J., and O'Brien, P.C. 1997. Longitudinal assessment of diabetic polyneuropathy using a composite score in the Rochester Diabetic Neuropathy Study cohort. *Neurology* 49:229–239.

8. Melzack, R. 1999. Pain–an overview. *Acta Anaesthesiol Scand* 43:880–884.

9. Gracely, R.H. 1999. Pain measurement. *Acta Anaesthesiol Scand* 43:897–908.

10. Bastyr, E., Zhang, D., Bril, V., and The MBBQ Study Group. 2002. Neuropathy Total symptom Score-6 Questionnaire (NTSS-6) Is a valid instrument for assessing the positive symptoms of diabetic peripheral neuropathy (DPN). *Diabetes* 51:A199.

11. Vinik, A., Bril, V., Kempler, P., Litchy, W., Dyck, P., Tesfaye, S., Price, K., Bastyr, E., and for the MBBQ Study. 2005. Treatment of symptomatic diabetic peripheral neuropathy with protein kinase CB inhibitor ruboxistaurin mesylate during a 1-year randomized, placebo-controlled, double-blind clinical trial. *Clin Therap* 27:1164–1180.

12. Raskin, P., Donofrio, P., Rosenthal, N., Hewitt, D., Jordan, D., Xiang, J., and Vinik, A. 2004. Topiramate vs placebo in painful diabetic neuropathy: Analgesic and metabolic effects. *Neurology* 63:865–873.

13. Boulton, A.J., Vinik, A.I., Arezzo, J.C., Bril, V., Feldman, E.L., Freeman, R., Malik, R.A., Maser, R.E., Sosenko, J.M., and Ziegler, D. 2005. Diabetic neuropathies: a statement by the American Diabetes Association. *Diabetes Care* 28:956–962.

14. Vinik, A.I., Suwanwalaikorn, S., Stansberry, K.B., Holland, M.T., McNitt, P.M., and Colen, L.E. 1995. Quantitative measurement of cutaneous perception in diabetic neuropathy. *Muscle Nerve* 18:574–584.

15. Low, P.A., Caskey, P.E., Tuck, R.R., Fealey, R.D., and Dyck, P.J. 1983. Quantitative sudomotor axon reflex test in normal and neuropathic subjects. *Ann Neurol* 14:573–580.

16. Benbow, S. J., Wallmahmed, M. E., and MacFarlane, I. A. 1998. Diabetic peripheral neuropathy and quality of life. *Q J Med* 91:733–737.

17. Fryback, D.G. 2005. A US valuation of the EQ-5D. *Med Care* 43:199–200.

18. Ware, J.A. and Coller, B.S. 1995. Platelet morphology, biochemistry and function. In *Williams Hematology*. Beutler, E., Lichtman, M.A., Coller, B.S., and Kipps, T.J., editors. McGraw-Hill, New York, 1161–1201.

19. Grootenhuis, P.A., Snoek, F.J., Heine, R.J., and Bouter, L.M. 1994. Development of a type 2 diabetes symptom checklist: a measure of symptom severity. *Diabet Med* 11:253–261.

20. Vinik, E., Hayes, R., Oglesby, A., Bastyr, E., Barlow, P., Ford-Molvik, S., and Vinik, A. 2005. The Development and validation of the Norfolk QOL-DN a new measure of patients' perception of the effects of diabetes and diabetic neuropathy. *Diabetes Technol Ther* 7(3):497–508.

21. Vileikyte, L., Peyrot, M., Bundy, C., Rubin, R.R., Leventhal, H., Mora, P., Shaw, J.E., Baker, P., and Boulton, A.J. 2003. The development and validation of a neuropathy- and foot ulcer-specific quality of life instrument. *Diabetes Care* 26:2549–2555.

22. Vinik, E.J., Hayes, C., Oglesby, A., and Vinik, A.I. 2004. Identification of factors in the nerve fiber specific quality of life (QOL-DN) inventory that reflect QOL and health status. *Diabetes* 53:A295.

23. Vinik, E., Stansberry, K., Doviak, M., Ruck, S., and Vinik, A. 2003. Norfolk quality of life (QOL) tool: scoring and reproducibility in healthy people, diabetic controls and patients with neuropathy. *Diabetes* 52(Suppl 1):A198.

24. DCCT Research Group. 1993. The effect of intensive treatment of diabetes on the development and progression of long-term complications in insulin dependent diabetes mellitus. *N Engl J Med* 329:977–986.

25. Sima, A.A., Bril, V., Nathaniel, V., McEwen, T.A., Brown, M.B., Lattimer, S.A., and Greene, D.A. 1988. Regeneration and repair of myelinated fibers in sural-nerve biopsy specimens from patients with diabetic neuropathy treated with sorbinil. *N Engl J Med* 319:548–555.

26. Dyck, P.J. and O'Brien, P.C. 1989. Meaningful degrees of prevention or improvement of nerve conduction in controlled clinical trials of diabetic neuropathy. *Diabetes Care* 12:649–652.

27. Arezzo, J.C. 1997. The use of electrophysiology for the assessment of diabetic neuropathy. *Neurosci Res Comm* 21, 13–22.

28. Vinik, A.I., Bril, V., Litchy, W.J., Price, K.L., and Bastyr, E.J., III. 2005. Sural sensory action potential identifies diabetic peripheral neuropathy responders to therapy. *Muscle Nerve* 32:619–625.

29. Kohara, N., Kimura, J., Kaji, R., Goto, Y., Ishii, J., Takiguchi, M., and Nakai, M. 2000. F-wave latency serves as the most reproducible measure in nerve conduction studies of diabetic polyneuropathy: multicentre analysis in healthy subjects and patients with diabetic polyneuropathy. *Diabetologia* 43:915–921.

30. Vinik, A., Mehrabyan, A., Colen, L., and Boulton, A. 2004. Focal entrapment neuropathies in diabetes. *Diabetes Care* 27(7):1783–1788.

31. Sharma K., Cross J., Farronay O., Ayyar D., Sheber R., and Bradley W. 2002. Demyelinating neuropathy in diabetes mellitus. *Arch Neurol* 59:758–765.

32. Consensus Statement. 1988. Report and recommendations of the San Antonio conference on diabetic neuropathy. American Diabetes Association American Academy of Neurology. *Diabetes Care* 11:592–597.

33. Arezzo, J.C. and Zotova, E. 2002. Electrophysiologic measures of diabetic neuropathy: mechanism and meaning. *Int Rev Neurobiol* 50:229–255.

34. Shy, M.E., Frohman, E.M., So, Y.T., Arezzo, J.C., Cornblath, D.C., Giuliani, M.J., and the subcommittee of the American Academy of Neurology. 2003. Quantitative sensory testing. *Neurology* 602:898–906.

35. Bril, V., Kojic, J., Ngo, M., and Clark, K. 1997. Comparison of a neurothesiometer and vibration in measuring vibration perception thresholds and relationship to nerve conduction studies. *Diabetes Care* 20:1360–1362.

36. Dyck, P.J., Bushek, W., Spring, E.M., Karnes, J.L., Litchy, W.J., O'Brien, P.C., and Service, F.J. 1987. Vibratory and cooling detection thresholds compared with other tests in diagnosing and staging diabetic neuropathy. *Diabetes Care* 10:432–440.

37. Steiness, I. 1957. Vibratory perception in diabetics; a biothesiometric study. *Acta Med Scand* 158:327–335.

38. Steiness, I. 1957. Vibratory perception in normal subjects; a biothesiometric study. *Acta Med Scand* 158:315–325.

39. Malik, R.A., Newrick, P.G., Sharma, A.K., Jennings, A., Ah-See, A.K., and Mayhew, T.M. 1989. Microangiopathy in human diabetic neuropathy: relationship between capillary abnormalities and the severity of neuropathy. *Diabetologia* 32:92–102.

40. Giannini, C. and Dyck, P. 1995. Basement membrane reduplication and pericyte degeneration precede development of diabetic polyneuropathy and are associated with its severity. *Ann Neurol* 37:498–504.

41. Resnick, H.E., Vinik, A.I., Schwartz, A.V., Leveille, S.G., Brancati, F.L., Balfour, J., and Guralnik, J.M. 2000. Independent effects of peripheral nerve dysfunction on lower-extremity physical function in old age: the Women's Health and Aging Study. *Diabetes Care* 23:1642–1647.

42. Resnick, H.E., Stansberry, K.B., Harris, T.B., Tirivedi, M., Smith, K., Morgan, P., and Vinik, A.I. 2002. Diabetes, peripheral neuropathy, and old age disability. *Muscle Nerve* 25:43–50.

43. Young, M.J., Breddy, J.L., Veves, A., and Boulton, A.J. 1994. The prediction of diabetic neuropathic foot ulceration using vibration perception thresholds. A prospective study. *Diabetes Care* 17:557–560.

44. Coppini, D.V., Young, P.J., Weng, C., MacLeod, A.F., and Sonksen, P.H. 1998. Outcome on diabetic foot complications in relation to clinical examination and quantitative sensory testing: a case-control study. *Diabet.Med* 15:765–771.

45. Abbott, C.A., Vileikyte, L., Williamson, S., Carrington, A.L., and Boulton, A.J. 1998. Multicenter study of the incidence of and predictive risk factors for diabetic neuropathic foot ulceration. *Diabetes Care* 21:1071–1075.

46. Consensus Statement. 1992. Proceedings of a consensus development conference on standardized measures in diabetic neuropathy. *Muscle Nerve* 15:1143–1170.

47. Apfel, S.C., Schwartz, S., Adornato, B., Freeman, R., Biton, V., Rendell, M., Vinik, A., Giuliani, M., Stevens, J., Barbano, R., et al. 2000. Efficacy and safety of recombinant human nerve growth factor in patients with diabetic polyneuropathy. *JAMA* 284: 2215–2221.

48. Vinik, A.I., Maser, R.E., Mitchell, B.D., and Freeman, R. 2003. Diabetic autonomic neuropathy. *Diabetes Care* 26(5):1553–1579.

49. Suarez, G.A., Opfer-Gehrking, T.L., Offord, K.P., Atkinson, E.J., O'Brien, P.C., and Low, P.A. 1999. The Autonomic Symptom Profile: a new instrument to assess autonomic symptoms. *Neurology* 52:523–528.

50. Low, P.A., Benrud-Larson, L.M., Sletten, D.M., Opfer-Gehrking, T.L., Weigand, S.D., O'Brien, P.C., Suarez, G.A., and Dyck, P.J. 2004. Autonomic symptoms and diabetic neuropathy: a population-based study. *Diabetes Care* 27:2942–2947.

51. Vinik, E., Snoek, F., Hayes, R., Oglesby, A., Bastyr, E., and Vinik, A. Validation of the Norfolk QOL-DN, a new measure of patients' perception of the effects of diabetes and diabetic neuropathy. *Diabetic Med* (submitted).

52. Reaven, G.M., Lithell, H., and Lindsberg, L. 1996. Hypertension and associated metabolic abnormalities - the role of insulin resistance and the sympathoadrenal system. *N Engl J Med* 334:374–381.

53. DeFronzo, R.A. and Ferrannini, E. 1991. Insulin resistance: A multifaceted syndrome responsible for NIDDM, obesity, hypertension, dyslipidemia and atherosclerotic cardiovascular disease. *Diabetes Care* 14:173–194.

54. Ferrannini, E., Harrner, S.M., Nitchell, B.D., and Stern, M.P. 1991. Hyperinsulinemia: the key feature of a cardiovascular and metabolic syndrome. *Diabetologia* 34:416–422.

55. Zeng, G. and Quon, M.J. 1996. Insulin-stimulated production of nitric oxide is inhibited by wortmannin. Direct measurement in endothelial cells. *J Clin Invest* 98:894–898.
56. Baron, A.D., Laakso, M., Brechtel, G., and Edelman, S.V. 1991. Mechanism of insulin resistance in insulin-dependent diabetes mellitus: a major role for reduced skeletal muscle blood flow. *J Clin Endocrinol Metab* 73:637–643.
57. Baron, A.D. 1999. Vascular reactivity. *Am J Cardiol* 84:25J–27J.
58. Jaap, A.J., Hammersley, M.S., Shore, A.C., and Tooke, J.E. 1994. Reduced microvascular hyperaemia in subjects at risk of developing Type 2 (non-insulin-dependent) diabetes mellitus. *Diabetologia* 37:214–216.
59. Caballero, A.E., Arora, S., Saouaf, R., Lim, S.C., Smakowski, P., Park, J.Y., King, G.L., LoGerfo, F.W., Horton, E.S., and Veves, A. 1999. Microvascular and macrovascular reactivity is reduced in subjects at risk for type 2 diabetes. *Diabetes* 48:1856–1862.
60. Stansberry, K.B., Hill, M.A., Shapiro, S.A., McNitt, P.M., Bhatt, B.A., and Vinik, A.I. 1997. Impairment of peripheral blood flow responses in diabetes resembles an enhanced aging effect. *Diabetes Care* 20:1711–1716.
61. Vinik, A. I., Erbas, T., and Park, T. S. 2001. Methods for evaluation of peripheral neurovascular dysfunction. *Diabetes Technol Ther* 3:29–50.
62. Vinik, A., Erbas, T., Park, T., Stansberry, K., Scanelli, J., and Pittenger, G. 2001. Dermal neurovascular dysfunction in type 2 diabetes. *Diabetes Care* 24:1468–1475.
63. Pittenger, G., Simmons, K., Anandacoomaraswamy, D., Rice, A., Barlow, P., and Vinik, A. 2005. Topiramate improves intraepidermal nerve fiber morphology and quantitative neuropathy measures in diabetic neuropathy patients. *J Peripher Nerv Sys* 10(Suppl 1): (Abstract).
64. Vinik, A., Pittenger, G., Anderson, A., Stansberry, K., McNear, E., and Barlow, P. 2003. Topiramate improves C-fiber neuropathy and features of the dysmetabolic syndrome in type 2 diabetes. *Diabetes* 52(Suppl 1):A130.
65. Polydefkis, M., Griffin, J.W., and McArthur, J. 2003. New insights into diabetic polyneuropathy. JAMA 290:1371–1376.
66. Polydefkis, M., Hauer, P., Griffin, J.W., and McArthur, J.C. 2001. Skin biopsy as a tool to assess distal small fiber innervation in diabetic neuropathy. *Diabetes Technol Ther* 3:23–28.
67. Pittenger, G.L., Ray, M., Burcus, N.I., McNulty, P., Basta, B., and Vinik, A.I. 2004. Intraepidermal nerve fibers are indicators of small-fiber neuropathy in both diabetic and nondiabetic patients. *Diabetes Care* 27:1974–1979.
68. Pittenger, G., Mehrabyan, A., Simmons, K., Rice, A., Barlow, P., and Vinik, A. 2005. Small fiber neuropathy is associated with the metabolic syndrome. *Metab Syndr Relat Disord* 3(2):113–121.
69. Simone, D. A., Nolano, M., Johnson, T., Wendelschafer-Crabb, G., and Kennedy, W. R. 1998. Intradermal injection of capsaicin in humans produces degeneration and subsequent reinnervation of epidermal nerve fibers: correlation with sensory function. *J Neurosci* 18(21):8947–8959.
70. Nolano, M., Simone, D.A., Wendelschafer-Crabb, G., Johnson, T., Hazen, E., and Kennedy, W.R. 1999. Topical capsaicin in humans: parallel loss of epidermal nerve fibers and pain sensation. *Pain* 81:135–145.
71. Polydefkis, M., Hauer, P., Sheth, S., Sirdofsky, M., Griffin, J.W., and McArthur, J.C. 2004. The time course of epidermal nerve fibre regeneration: studies in normal controls and in people with diabetes, with and without neuropathy. *Brain* 127:1606–1615.

72. Vinik, A., Hewitt, D., and Xiang, J. 2003. Topiramate in the treatment of painful diabetic neuropathy: results from a multicenter, randomized, double-blind, placebo-controlled trial (abstract). *Neurology* 60(Suppl 1):A154–A155.
73. Albers, J.W., Brown, M.B., Sima, A.A., and Greene, D.A. 1996. Nerve conduction measures in mild diabetic neuropathy in the Early Diabetes Intervention Trial: the effects of age, sex, type of diabetes, disease duration, and anthropometric factors. Tolrestat Study Group for the Early Diabetes Intervention Trial. *Neurology* 46:85–91.
74. Sima, A.A. and Laudadio, C. 1996. Design of controlled clinical trials for diabetic polyneuropathy. *Semin Neurol* 16:187–191.
75. Sundkvist, G., Armstrong, F.M., Bradbury, J.E., Chaplin, C., Ellis, S.H., Owens, D.R., Rosen, I., and Sonksen, P. 1992. Peripheral and autonomic nerve function in 259 diabetic patients with peripheral neuropathy treated with ponalrestat (an aldose reductase inhibitor) or placebo for 18 months. United Kingdom/Scandinavian Ponalrestat Trial. *J Diabetes Complications* 6:123–130.
76. Arezzo, J.C. 1999. New developments in the diagnosis of diabetic neuropathy. *Am J Med* 107:9S–16S.
77. Abraham, R.M. and Abraham, R.R. 1987. Absence of the sensory action potential of the medial plantar nerve: a sensitive indicator of diabetic neuropathy. *Diabet Med* 4:469–474.
78. Behse, F. and Buchthal. 1978. Sensory action potentials and biopsy of the sural nerve in neuropathy. *Brain* 101:473–493.
79. Izzo, K.L., Sobel, E., Berney, S., and Demopoulos, J.T. 1985. Distal sensory nerves of the lower extremity in peripheral neuropathy: comparison of medial dorsal cutaneous and sural nerve abnormalities. *Arch Phys Med Rehabil* 66:7–10.
80. Izzo, K.L., Sobel, E., and Demopoulos, J.T. 1986. Diabetic neuropathy: electrophysiologic abnormalities of distal lower extremity sensory nerves. *Arch Phys Med Rehabil* 67:7–11.
81. Killian, J.M. and Foreman, P.J. 2001. Clinical utility of dorsal sural nerve conduction studies. *Muscle Nerve* 24:817–820.
82. Shin, J.B., Seong, Y.J., Lee, H.J., Kim, S.H., Suk, H., and Lee, Y.J. 2000. The usefulness of minimal F-wave latency and sural/radial amplitude ratio in diabetic polyneuropathy. *Yonsei Med J* 41:393–397.
83. Ekberg, K., Brismar, T., Johansson, B.L., Jonsson, B., Lindstrom, P., and Wahren, J. 2003. Amelioration of sensory nerve dysfunction by C-Peptide in patients with type 1 diabetes. *Diabetes* 52:536–541.
84. Greene, D.A., Arezzo, J.C., and Brown, M.B. 1999. Effect of aldose reductase inhibition on nerve conduction and morphometry in diabetic neuropathy. Zenarestat Study Group. *Neurology* 53:580–591.
85. Laudadio, C., Pfeifer, M., Sima, A., and Ponalrestat group. 1998. Progression rates of diabetic neuropathy endpoints in patients assigned to placebo in an 10 month Clinical Research Trial. *J Diabetes Complications* 3:121–127.
86. Ziegler, D., Mayer, P., Rathmann, W., and Gries, F.A. 1991. One-year treatment with the aldose reductase inhibitor, ponalrestat, in diabetic neuropathy. *Diabetes Res Clin Pract* 14:63–73.
87. Ziegler, D., Mayer, P., Muhlen, H., and Gries, F.A. 1991. The natural history of somatosensory and autonomic nerve dysfunction in relation to glycaemic control during the first 5 years after diagnosis of type 1 (insulin-dependent) diabetes mellitus. *Diabetologia* 34:822–829.
88. Vinik, A., Tesfaye, S., Zhang, D., and Bastyr, E. 2002. LY333531 treatment improves diabetic peripheral neuropathy (DPN) with symptoms. *Diabetes* 51(Suppl 2):A79.

9 Intensive Insulin Therapy for the Critically Ill Patient

Ilse Vanhorebeek, PhD
and Greet Van den Berghe, MD, PhD

CONTENTS

SUMMARY

More and more evidence argues against the concept that the characteristic dysregulation of glucose homeostasis in critical illness or "diabetes of injury" is an adaptive, benefical response in the modern intensive care era. Stress hyperglycemia has been linked to poor outcome of the patients in several studies. Proof of a causal relationship has been provided by a large, prospective, randomized, controlled study where strict blood glucose control to normoglycemia with intensive insulin therapy strongly reduced

From: *Contemporary Endocrinology: Controversies in Treating Diabetes:*
Clinical and Research Aspects
Edited by: D. LeRoith and A. I. Vinik © Humana Press, Totowa, NJ

mortality and morbidity of surgical intensive care patients. These results were recently confirmed in a medical intensive care patient population. Most of the clinical benefits of intensive insulin therapy appear to be related to the blood glucose control, but also non-glycemic metabolic and non-metabolic actions of insulin contribute. Although substantial progress has been made in the understanding of the pathways involved, more studies are needed to improve our knowledge on their relative importance and that of those yet to be unravelled.

Key Words: Critical illness, hyperglycemia, insulin, mortality, morbidity

INTRODUCTION

With the discovery of insulin in 1922, Banting and Best were the pioneers of a revolutionary break-through in medicine. Whereas type 1 diabetes used to be a lethal condition because of the development of ketoacidosis, patients with this disorder nowadays can be treated with insulin, and this approach has dramatically improved outcome. Already in the late nineteenth century, dysregulated glucose homeostasis also appeared to be a hallmark of critical illness (CI). Indeed, hyperglycemia commonly develops during several types of CI, irrespective of previously diagnosed diabetes, and has long been considered an adaptive and beneficial stress response. However, it is becoming increasingly clear that the development of hyperglycemia is detrimental to the critically ill patient. Moreover, a recent large prospective randomized trial clearly demonstrated a plethora of clinical benefits of strict blood glucose control with intensive insulin therapy with, most strikingly, an almost 50% reduction in mortality *(1)*. The importance of this observation is illustrated by the lack of any intervention with such a pronounced beneficial effect on overall intensive care survival since the introduction of mechanical ventilation in the 1950s.

CLINICAL COMPLICATIONS ASSOCIATED WITH CI

The progress in intensive care medicine starting with the introduction of mechanical ventilation in the 1950s has largely increased the chances of short-term survival of patients suffering from previously lethal, acute insults. Consequently, patients now frequently enter a chronic phase of CI, during which they remain dependent on vital organ support for a more or less extended time period. As this condition resulted from artificial interference by humans, with sophisticated mechanical devices, a wide array of drugs, and high-tech monitoring systems, nature has not been able to select survival mechanisms to overcome this challenge. As such, mortality has remained high among these prolonged critically ill patients, mostly because of non-resolving multiple organ failure and regardless of the initial disease requiring intensive care unit (ICU) admission.

Unlike in diabetic nephropathy, mainly affecting the glomerulus, CI-associated kidney failure mostly results from acute tubular necrosis. Extracorporeal hemofiltration or dialysis is the only therapeutic option that can be applied to bridge the time to spontaneous recovery (2). Taking measures to prevent deterioration of renal function in these patients, such as maintaining or optimizing renal perfusion and diligence with monitoring of nephrotoxic therapies, is therefore of crucial importance.

Prolonged critically ill patients often suffer from a diffuse axonal polyneuropathy (3). CI polyneuropathy clinically presents as a tetraparesis with muscle atrophy. However, confirmation by using electromyography is required. The course of this complication usually is self-limited and good recovery is expected once the underlying disease is overcome. Nevertheless, it severely delays weaning from the ventilator and mobilization of the patient (4). Specific prevention or treatment of CI polyneuropathy is hampered by the poor understanding of the exact pathogenesis (5), although several factors have been implicated in the etiology of this condition, such as sepsis and the accompanying release of cytokines, use of high-dose corticosteroids, and use of neuromuscular blocking agents.

Increased susceptibility to and insufficient control of severe infections because of suppressed innate immunity, referred to as "immunoparalysis," renders the patients vulnerable for infectious complications (6). Although at first sight paradoxical, the patients are also at high risk of excessive systemic inflammation, associated with cellular injury and coagulation abnormalities, thus contributing to multiple organ failure (7). The development of anemia is another common clinical problem in critically ill patients and is associated with substantial red blood cell transfusion requirements (8).

Within hours and during the first days following an acute severe insult, a hyperactive anterior pituitary gland evokes a hypercatabolic response (9–11). Clinical manifestations, including fever, tachypnea, and tachycardia, are accompanied by hyperglycemia, lipid abnormalities, and accelerated proteolysis. Its main purpose is the provision of endogenous substrates to wounded tissues and reparative cells, for healing at a time when caloric intake is limited. However, the sustained hypercatabolic response during prolonged CI induces profound erosion of lean body mass by ongoing proteolysis, despite artificial feeding and relative preservation of adipose tissue, referred to as the "wasting syndrome" of CI. Patients can lose 10% or even more of their muscle mass in a week (12,13), but also other organs are affected, including liver, kidney, and heart, leading to impaired function. Prolonged mechanical ventilatory support is often required because of extreme muscle weakness and fatigue. Prolonged CI is invariably associated with neuroendocrine changes, which are related to the hypercatabolism (9–11). More specifically, relatively suppressed function of the anterior pituitary gland is now responsible for suppressed function of its peripheral target organs.

All the described changes are thought to contribute to multiple organ failure, or the lack of recovery hereof, and to prolonged need of intensive care and high risk of death.

HYPERGLYCEMIA IN CI

In normal individuals, blood glucose levels are tightly regulated within the narrow range of 60–140 mg/dl. However, glucose levels usually rise during CI, labeled "stress diabetes" or "diabetes of injury" (14,15). Until recently, it was considered state of the art to tolerate blood glucose levels up to 220 mg/dl in fed critically ill patients (16), and only excessive hyperglycemia exceeding this value was treated. Reasons to treat hyperglycemia above this threshold included the occurrence of hyperglycemia-induced osmotic diuresis and fluid shifts at these high levels and the knowledge from the diabetes literature that uncontrolled and pronounced hyperglycemia predisposes to infectious complications (15,17). Arguments to tolerate glucose levels up to 220 mg/dl were the classic dogma that moderate hyperglycemia in critically ill patients is beneficial for organs that largely rely on glucose for their energy supply but do not require insulin for glucose uptake, such as the brain and blood cells, and the fear for occasional hypoglycemia and consequent brain injury with tight glucose management.

Development of Hyperglycemia in CI Patients

In the acute phase of CI, an upregulation of both gluconeogenesis and glycogenolysis enhances hepatic glucose production. After a transient fall in insulin levels hyperinsulinemia develops. Such high insulin levels normally suppress both pathways but in CI are unable to maintain normoglycemia. Increased levels of glucagon, cortisol, growth hormone, catecholamines, and cytokines all play a role (18–23). How the hyperglycemic response is maintained during prolonged CI remains relatively unclear. In comparison with the acute phase, cortisol, growth hormone, catecholamine, and cytokine levels usually decrease in the chronic phase of CI, whereas glucagon levels are not well documented. In addition to the stimulation of glucose production, impaired glucose uptake contributes to the development of hyperglycemia.

The important exercise-stimulated glucose uptake in skeletal muscle is likely abolished in view of the immobilization of the patient. Insulin-stimulated glucose uptake by glucose transporter-4 (GLUT-4) is compromised (24,25). Nevertheless, whole body glucose uptake is increased, accounted for by tissues that are not dependent on insulin for glucose uptake, such as brain and blood cells (15,26). The combined picture of higher levels of insulin, elevated hepatic glucose production and impaired peripheral glucose uptake, reflects the development of peripheral insulin resistance during CI.

Hyperglycemia and Outcome of CI Patients

Several recent studies clearly identify the development of hyperglycemia as an important risk factor for mortality and morbidity of critically ill patients. Elevated glucose levels predicted increased mortality and length of ICU and hospital stay of trauma patients and were associated with infectious morbidity and prolonged need of mechanical ventilation (27–30). Apart from the predictive value of hyperglycemia for worse survival of patients suffering from severe brain injury, a significant relationship was found between high blood glucose levels and worse neurologic status, impaired pupil reactivity, intracranial hypertension, and longer hospital length of stay (31,32). Similarly, hyperglycemia predicted a higher risk of death after stroke and a poor functional recovery in those patients who survived (33). In addition, a strong link has been described between increased blood glucose levels and the risk of CI polyneuropathy in sepsis and the systemic inflammatory response syndrome (34). A meta-analysis on myocardial infarction also revealed an association between stress hyperglycemia and increased risk of in-hospital mortality and congestive heart failure or cardiogenic shock (35) and even mild elevations in fasting glucose levels in patients with coronary artery disease undergoing percutaneous coronary intervention have been associated with a substantial mortality risk (36). Furthermore, the glucose level of patients undergoing coronary artery bypass grafting appeared to be an important predictor of delayed extubation (37). Retrospective analysis of a heterogeneous population of critically ill patients revealed that even a modest degree of hyperglycemia was associated with a substantially increased hospital mortality (38). A study on the occurrence of hyperglycemia among critically ill children with widely varying pathology showed a correlation with higher in-hospital mortality and longer length of stay (39). Peak blood glucose levels and duration of hyperglycemia appeared independently associated with mortality of critically ill children (40). In severely burned children, mortality, incidence of bacteremia and fungemia, and number of skin-grafting procedures were higher in hyperglycemic than in normoglycemic patients (41).

BLOOD GLUCOSE CONTROL WITH INTENSIVE INSULIN THERAPY IN CI

First strong evidence against the traditional concept of tolerating glucose levels up to as high as 200 mg/dl came from the landmark prospective, randomized, controlled study on intensive insulin therapy in surgical critically ill patients (1). This study of a large group of patients admitted to the ICU predominantly after extensive, complicated surgery or trauma indeed revealed major clinical benefits of strict glycemic control with insulin. In the conventional approach, patients received insulin only if glucose concentrations exceeded 215 mg/dl with the aim of keeping concentrations between 180 and 200 mg/dl, resulting in mean blood glucose levels of 150–160 mg/dl (hyperglycemia). Insulin was administered to the patients in the intensive insulin therapy group to maintain blood glucose levels between 80 and 110 mg/dl, which resulted in mean blood glucose levels of 90–100 mg/dl (normoglycemia). Tight blood glucose control with insulin strikingly lowered ICU mortality from 8.0 to 4.6% (43% reduction). The benefit was particularly attributed to the group of patients who required intensive care for more than 5 days with a 48% mortality reduction from 20.2 to 10.6%. Besides saving lives, intensive insulin therapy largely prevented several CI-associated complications. The incidence of CI polyneuropathy was reduced by 44%, the development of blood stream infections by 46%, and acute renal failure requiring dialysis or hemofiltration by 41%. The number of patients who acquired liver dysfunction with hyperbilirubinemia was lowered by 16%. Furthermore, anemia less frequently developed as illustrated by the 50% reduction in the median number of red blood cell transfusions needed. Finally, patients were also less dependent on prolonged mechanical ventilation and intensive care. A large number of patients were included in the study after complicated cardiac surgery. Nevertheless, the clinical benefits of this therapy were equally present in most other diagnostic subgroups. Particularly in the group of patients with isolated brain injury, intensive insulin therapy was able to protect the central and peripheral nervous system from secondary insults and improved long-term rehabilitation (42).

An important confirmation of the clinical benefits of intensive insulin therapy was recently obtained with the demonstration, by a large randomized controlled trial, that the Leuven protocol of glycemic control with insulin in adult surgical critically ill patients (1) was similarly effective in a strictly medical ICU patient population (43). Indeed, hospital mortality was reduced from 40.0 to 37.3% in the intention-to-treat population (not significant) and from 52.5 to 43.0% in the target group of long-stay patients needing at least a third day of intensive care, for which the study had been powered based on the results of the surgical study. Intensive insulin therapy significantly reduced morbidity in the intention-to-treat group, with lower occurence of new development of kidney injury and hyperbilirubinemia, earlier weaning from mechanical ventilation and earlier discharge from the ICU and from the hospital. The reduction in morbidity was even more striking in the target group of patients remaining in ICU for at least a third day. These patients were discharged from the hospital alive on average 10 days earlier than on conventional insulin therapy. The number of long-stay patients with hyper-inflammation was also reduced. In "real life" intensive care of a heterogeneous medical/surgical patient population, an observational study (44) had evaluated the impact of implementing a tight glucose management protocol by comparison with historical controls as a reference and also largely confirmed the clinical benefits (1). In this study, intravenous insulin was only administered if glucose levels exceeded 200 mg/dl on two successive measurements and aimed to lower glycemia below 140 mg/dl. Hence, blood glucose control was somewhat less strict and resulted in mean glucose levels of 131 mg/dl in the protocol period, compared with 152 mg/dl in the baseline period. In comparison with the historical control group, patients did clinically better after the implementation of the glucose control protocol, with a 29% decrease in hospital mortality, length of ICU stay decreased by 11%, 75% less patients developed new renal failure, and 19% less patients required red blood cell transfusion. No effect was seen with regard to prevention of severe infections, but the incidence of this complication was already low in the baseline period. In a predominantly general surgical patient population, however, another prospective, randomized, controlled study, albeit a small one, confirmed the findings of a decreased incidence of total nosocomial infections (including intravascular device, blood stream, intravascular device-related blood stream, and surgical site infections) with intensive insulin therapy targeting glucose levels between 80 and 120 mg/dl (45). This intervention resulted in mean daily glucose levels of 125 versus 179 mg/dl in the standard glycemic control group. In an observational study of patients with diabetes mellitus undergoing cardiac surgery, intravenous insulin infusion to eliminate hyperglycemia also lowered in-hospital mortality compared with the historical control group, with fewer deep sternal wound infections and shorter length of hospital stay (46).

INTENSIVE INSULIN THERAPY AND THE RISK
OF HYPOGLYCEMIA

The risk of hypoglycemia is a major concern when intensive insulin therapy is administered to critically ill patients. Severe hypoglycemia (<30 mg/dl) or prolonged hypoglycemia can lead to convulsions, coma, and irreversible brain damage and also cardiac arrhythmias can be induced (47). Patients who have an altered mental status, who are intubated, or who are severely ill may be unable to recognize or communicate hypoglycemic symptoms *(16)*. Moreover, clinical symptoms of the autonomic response (sweating, tachycardia, tremor) and central nervous symptoms such as dizziness, blurred vision, altered mental acuity, confusion, and eventually convulsions may be masked by concomitant diseases and by inherent intensive care treatments such as sedation, analgesia, and mechanical ventilation.

The hazard of hypoglycemia clearly warrants adequate training of the nursing and medical staff, at least initially making use of a strict and detailed insulin titration protocol. The best way to achieve blood glucose control during intensive care is by continuous insulin infusion, and the use of oral anti-diabetic agents in the patients with previously diagnosed diabetes should be discontinued *(16)*. This way of administration is quite obvious for several reasons. First, feeding of the ICU patients is usually a continuous process, whether this occurs by enteral or total parenteral nutrition or with a combination of both. Continuous intravenous administration of insulin is more reliable and consistent than subcutaneous injections. Furthermore, insulin need in this way can be more easily and precisely titrated in response to the actual blood glucose levels and, discontinuing or reducing the insulin infusion allows rapid cessation of insulin action in case the patient develops hypoglycemia, as intravenous insulin has a short half-life.

Specific measures to prevent hypoglycemia include the concomitant administration of insulin and carbohydrates (intravenous dextrose or tube feeds) and close monitoring of blood glucose levels *(16)*. Within the first 12–24 h after admission of the patients in the large surgical ICU study *(1)*, glucose levels were measured every 1–2 h. The frequency of the measurements was scaled down to every 4 h once the targeted blood glucose level was reached with a stable insulin dose. However, one has to remain alert after stable glucose levels are obtained. Indeed, although the incidence of hypoglycemia in the study was relatively low *(1)*, many of the cases where it did develop were attributed to inadequate insulin dose reduction during interruption of enteral feeding.

MECHANISM BY WHICH INTENSIVE INSULIN THERAPY ACHIEVES BLOOD GLUCOSE CONTROL

Data from the studies performed by our group suggest that mainly stimulation of glucose uptake by skeletal muscle explains how intensive insulin therapy lowers circulating glucose levels in critically ill patients, rather than an effect of insulin on hepatic glucose handling (Fig. 1) *(48,49)*. This is illustrated by improved responsiveness of insulin-regulated genes in skeletal muscle, whereas it appeared that insulin resistance in the liver is not overcome by

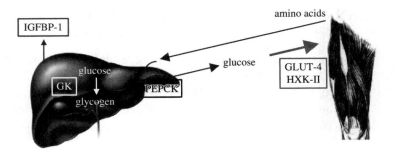

Fig. 1. Lowering of blood glucose levels by intensive insulin therapy in critical illness. Data from previous studies performed by our group suggest that insulin lowers blood glucose levels predominantly through increased skeletal muscle glucose uptake, rather than through an effect on hepatic glucose handling *(48,49)*. Improved responsiveness of insulin-regulated genes in patients from the intensive insulin therapy group is indicated in green, whereas refractoriness to insulin is indicated in red. GLUT-4: glucose transporter-4, HXK-II: hexokinase-II, GK: glucokinase, PEPCK: phosphoenolpyruvate carboxykinase, IGFBP-1: insulin-like growth factor-binding protein-1.

intensive insulin therapy. In muscle, GLUT-4 controls insulin-stimulated glucose uptake, whereas hexokinase-II is the rate-limiting enzyme in intracellular insulin-stimulated glucose metabolism. mRNA expression of both genes in postmortem skeletal muscle biopsies of critically ill patients was increased by intensive insulin therapy *(48)*. In contrast, mRNA expression of glucokinase, the rate-limiting enzyme for insulin-mediated glucose uptake and glycogen synthesis in liver, was not affected by insulin therapy in postmortem liver biopsies of the patients *(48)*. Repression of gluconeogenesis by insulin was not enhanced, as shown by comparable transcript levels of its rate-limiting enzyme phospho-enolpyruvate carboxy-kinase in both conventional and intensive insulin therapy groups *(49)*. Likewise, intensive insulin therapy was not able to counteract the increase in insulin-like growth factor-binding protein-1 (another protein transcriptionally regulated by insulin and shown to correlate with mortality), neither at the mRNA level nor at the protein level in the circulation *(49)*.

In contrast to our results for prolonged critically ill patients, whole-body glucose disposal was not affected in a small study on only 6 severely trauma-tized patients in the acute phase of illness, whereas endogenous glucose production appeared to be reduced *(50)*. It has to be emphasized, however, that acute and prolonged critically ill patients may have very different neuroen-docrine characteristics *(9–11)*. Furthermore, whole-body glucose disposal was studied without distinguishing between insulin-dependent and insulin-independent glucose uptake, which are oppositely affected by insulin and thus may explain the absence of an effect on this parameter.

MECHANISMS EXPLAINING THE IMPROVED OUTCOME WITH INTENSIVE INSULIN THERAPY

Both hyperglycemia and the administration of a high dose of insulin were associated with a high risk of death in surgical critically ill patients, as revealed by multivariate logistic regression analysis (1,51). This indicates that it was the blood glucose control and/or other metabolic effects of insulin that accompany tight blood glucose control, and not the insulin dose administered per se, that contributed to the improved survival with intensive insulin therapy. Other data also suggest that the mortality benefits can be attributed to glycemic control rather than the absolute insulin doses administered (38,52). The observed association between high insulin dose and mortality is likely explained by more severe insulin resistance in the sicker patients, who have a high risk of death. Glycemic control accounted for most morbidity effects, including the reduced incidence of CI polyneuropathy and bacteremia (51). Both glucose control and insulin dose contributed to the reduced inflammation, albeit with a superior effect of lowering glucose levels.

In this study, the risk of death appeared to be linearly correlated with the degree of hyperglycemia, with no clear cut-off level below which there was no further benefit (51). Indeed, the patients who received conventional insulin therapy and who developed only moderate hyperglycemia (110–150 mg/dl) had a lower risk of death than those with severe hyperglycemia (150–200 mg/dl), whereas they were at higher risk of death than patients whose blood glucose levels were controlled below 110 mg/dl with intensive insulin therapy (Fig. 2). Tight glycemic control below 110 mg/dl similarly appeared to be of crucial importance for the prevention of CI polyneuropathy, bacteremia, anemia, and acute renal failure (Fig. 2) (51). In particular, a positive linear correlation was observed between glycemia and the risk of developing CI polyneuropathy, where multivariate logistic regression analysis also confirmed the crucial role of preventing glucose toxicity to protect the neurons (42).

Mechanisms of Glucose Toxicity in CI and Effects of Intensive Insulin Therapy

If indeed avoiding even a moderate degree of hyperglycemia is crucial, it is striking that by doing so only during the relatively short period the patients needed intensive care, this strategy prevented the most feared complications of CI. Normal cells respond to moderate hyperglycemia by downregulation of glucose transporters to protect themselves from deleterious effects (53). In diabetic patients, chronic hyperglycemia also causes severe complications, but in a time frame which is several orders of magnitude longer than the time it took to prevent life-threatening complications with intensive insulin

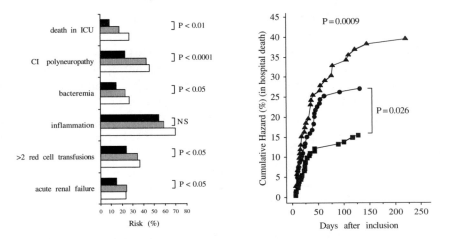

Fig. 2. Stratification of risk of death and morbidity factors for mean blood glucose levels. Left panel: Post-hoc analysis of the percentage of risk of death in intensive care unit (ICU), development of critical illness (CI), polyneuropathy, bacteremia, inflammation [C-reactive protein (CRP) higher than 150 mg/l for more than 3 days], need for more than two red cell transfusions, and acute renal failure requiring hemofiltration/dialysis among long-stay (more than 5 days) patients stratified for mean blood glucose levels. Filled bars represent patients with a mean blood glucose level lower than 110 mg/dl, shaded bars represent patients with a mean blood glucose level between 110 and 150 mg/dl, and unfilled bars represent patients with a mean blood glucose level higher than 150 mg/dl. The indicated p-values were obtained using the χ^2-test. Reproduced with permission from *(51)*. Right panel: Kaplan–Meier cumulative risk of in-hospital death among long-stay patients with a mean blood glucose level lower than 110 mg/dl (■), between 110 and 150 mg/dl (●) and higher than 150 mg/dl (▲). The p-value of 0.0009, obtained with Mantel–Cox log-rank test, indicates the significance level of the overall difference in risk of death among the groups, and the p-value of 0.026 indicates the significance level of the difference between the <110 mg/dl and 110–150 mg/dl groups. Reproduced with permission from *(51)*.

therapy in CI. Therefore, the obvious question is why hyperglycemia would be more acutely toxic in critically ill patients than in healthy individuals or diabetic patients.

Glucose uptake independent of insulin, mediated by the facilitative glucose transporters, GLUT-1, GLUT-2, or GLUT-3, may play a role. Indeed, several factors induced in CI have been shown to upregulate the expression and membrane localization of GLUT-1 and GLUT-3 in different cell types. These include cytokines, angiotensin II, endothelin-1, vascular endothelial growth factor, and transforming growth factor-β but also hypoxia appears to be a regulatory factor *(54–58)*. In this way, the normal downregulatory protective response against hyperglycemia may be overruled. Furthermore, GLUT-2 and GLUT-3 allow glucose to enter cells directly proportional to the extracellular glucose level over the range of glycemia present in CI (Km $\approx$ 9 mmol/l for GLUT-3 and much higher for GLUT-2) *(59)*. Hence, cellular glucose overload may develop in the central and peripheral nervous system, endothelial, epithelial and immune cells, as well as hepatocytes, renal tubules, pancreatic β cells and gastrointestinal mucosa. In contrast, cellular systems and tissues that predominantly rely on insulin-dependent glucose transport through GLUT-4, such as skeletal muscle and myocardium, may be relatively protected against hyperglycemia-induced cellular glucose overload and toxicity.

Recent data on mitochondrial ultrastructure and function in tissues from surgical critically ill patients are consistent with this concept *(60)*. We showed that prevention of hyperglycemia with intensive insulin therapy is protective to the hepatocytic mitochondrial compartment of critically ill patients *(60)*. In hepatocytes of patients in the conventional treatment group, hypertrophic mitochondria were observed with an increased number of abnormal and irregular cristae as well as reduced electron density of the matrix (Fig. 3). However, these severe ultrastructural abnormalities were virtually absent in patients with blood glucose levels tightly controlled to normoglycemia. At the functional level, this was associated with higher activities of respiratory chain complex I and complex IV in the patients who received intensive insulin therapy. In contrast to liver, no morphological abnormalities were detected in skeletal muscle, nor were any of the respiratory chain enzyme complexes affected by insulin therapy. This is in line with a direct effect of avoiding glucose toxicity on the hepatocytic mitochondrial compartment by strict blood glucose control rather than of insulinization. Mitochondrial dysfunction and the associated bioenergetic failure have been regarded as factors contributing to multiple organ failure, the most common cause of death in sepsis and prolonged CI, and have indeed been related to lethal outcome in patients and in a resuscitated long-term rat model of sepsis *(61,62)*. As such, prevention of hyperglycemia-induced mitochondrial damage to cellular systems with passive glucose uptake in addition to liver could theoretically explain some of the protective effects of intensive insulin therapy in severe illness.

There is substantial evidence that links diabetes and hyperglycemia to the development of increased oxidative stress. This is in part accounted for by enhanced mitochondrial superoxide production *(63)*, but also, transition metal-catalyzed glucose oxidation and activation of NADPH oxidase take part, amongst other mechanisms *(64,65)*. In turn, high levels of reactive oxygen radicals have been shown to inhibit the glycolytic enzyme glyceraldehyde-3-phosphate dehydrogenase. Consequently, glycolysis is blocked and glucose is shuttled into toxic pathways, contributing to vascular damage to tissues and organs *(63)*. Moreover, nitric oxide levels are increased in CI

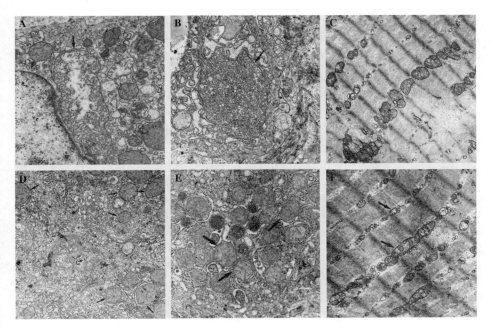

Fig. 3. Mitochondrial ultrastructure in liver and skeletal muscle of critically ill patients. Electron micrographs show greatly enlarged mitochondria with an increased number of disarrayed cristae and reduced electron density of the matrix in hepatocytes adjacent to normal mitochondria (A and B), contrasting with normal mitochondrial morphology in skeletal muscle (**C**) of conventionally treated patients. In most of the intensively treated patients, hepatocytic mitochondrial ultrastructure was normal [D (c: canaliculus), E], as in all muscle biopsy samples from these patients (**F**). Original magnification: ×23,000 [reprinted with permission from Elsevier *(60)*].

because of cytokine-induced activation of nitric oxide synthesis, whereas hypoxia-reperfusion in the patients aggravates superoxide production. In this way, the formation of the reactive nitrogen species peroxynitrite is promoted, able to induce tyrosine nitration of proteins, and thus affect their normal function *(66)*. Mitochondrial complex I is just one example of an activity suppressed by tyrosine nitration *(67)*.

High glucose levels also affect all major components of innate immunity *(68)*. Polymorphonuclear neutrophil function and intracellular bactericidal and opsonic activity are compromised by hyperglycemia *(69–72)*. This may play a role in the increased risk of infections observed for patients who are exposed to such high glucose levels *(17,73)*. Tight glycemic control has been shown to ameliorate the leukocyte oxidative burst and phagocytotic activity in patients with diabetes *(69,72)* . Importantly, intensive insulin therapy largely prevented severe nosocomial infections and lethal sepsis also in non-diabetic surgical

ICU patients *(1)*. In an animal model of prolonged CI *(74)*, glucose control with insulin beneficially affected innate immunity by preservation of phagocytosis and oxidative burst function of monocytes *(75)*.

Non-Glycemic Metabolic Effects of Intensive Insulin Therapy

The serum lipid profile is severely disturbed in critically ill patients. Most characteristically, levels of triglycerides are elevated (due to an increase in very-low-density lipoprotein), whereas levels of high-density lipoprotein (HDL)- and low-density lipoprotein (LDL)-cholesterol are very low *(76–78)*. Intensive insulin therapy prevented the rise in serum triglycerides during full nutritional support and substantially increased circulating HDL and LDL and the level of cholesterol associated with these lipoproteins *(48)*. Insulin treatment also decreased serum triglycerides and free fatty acids in burned children *(79)*. Given the important role of triglycerides in energy provision and of lipoproteins in transportation of lipid components (cholesterol, triglycerides, phospholipids, lipid-soluble vitamins) and endotoxin scavenging *(80–82)*, a contribution of the (partial) correction of the lipid profile to improved outcome may be expected. Multivariate logistic regression analysis indeed revealed that improvement of the dyslipidemia with insulin therapy explained a significant part of the reduced mortality and organ failure *(48)*. Surprisingly, these effects surpassed those of glycemic control. Furthermore, when the model was controlled for all metabolic effects of insulin, including the lipid effect, the risk associated with high-dose insulin administration disappeared *(48,52)*. As such, this important finding argues in favor of titrating insulin to doses required to achieve its metabolic effects.

Insulin has a well-recognized anabolic effect, which comprises both stimulation of muscle protein synthesis and attenuation of protein breakdown *(83–85)*. Therefore, its administration has been put forward as an intervention to attenuate the catabolic syndrome of prolonged CI *(86)*. In surgical critically ill patients who received intensive insulin therapy *(1)*, this anabolic effect of insulin was not obvious from clinical observation. However, intensive insulin therapy resulted in a higher protein content in postmortem skeletal muscle biopsies of the patients *(60)* and prevented weight loss in a rabbit model of prolonged CI *(75)*. Altered regulation at the level of the somatotropic axis appeared not to be involved in the anabolic effect of insulin, unlike expectations *(87)*.

Non-Metabolic Effects of Intensive Insulin Therapy

Independent of its preventive effect on infection, intensive insulin therapy was able to preclude excessive inflammation in critically ill patients, as illustrated by lower serum C-reactive protein (CRP) and mannose-binding lectin levels compared with conventional insulin therapy *(88)*. In multivariate analysis, the effect on CRP significantly contributed to the observed outcome benefit *(48)*. However, it was no longer independently related to the outcome benefit when the changes in lipid metabolism were taken into account *(48)*. In that way, a link may be put forward between the anti-inflammatory effect of intensive insulin therapy and its amelioration of the lipid profile, but a mechanistic explanation for the dominant effect of serum lipid correction still needs to be delineated. Attenuation of the CRP response by insulin therapy was also confirmed in a rabbit model of prolonged CI *(75)*. We recently investigated the effect of intensive insulin therapy on an extensive series of pro- and anti-inflammatory cytokines in surgical critically ill patients, but found no major effect *(89)*. In burned children, however, the administration of insulin resulted in lower pro-inflammatory cytokines and proteins, whereas the anti-inflammatory cascade was stimulated, although these effects were largely seen only late after the insult *(79)*. Similar results were obtained from endotoxemic rats and thermally injured rats *(90,91)*. Also, in an endotoxin-induced porcine model of CI, hyperinsulinemia was shown to lower pro-inflammatory cytokines *(92)*. Although anti-inflammatory effects of insulin therapy may be direct, prevention of hyperglycemia may be crucial as well.

Insulin has also shown to improve myocardial function and to protect the myocardium during acute myocardial infarction, open-heart surgery, endotoxic shock, and other critical conditions *(93,94)*. Direct anti-apoptotic properties of insulin independent of glucose uptake and involving insulin signaling play a role *(93,95,96)*. However, insulin's cardioprotective action may at least partly be due to lowering of glucose levels *(93)*, which likely explains the disappointing results in the absence of adequate glucose control obtained in the recent large, randomized CREATE-ECLA trial on glucose-insulin-potassium (GIK) infusion in patients with acute myocardial infarction *(97)* and the DIGAMI-2 trial in patients with diabetes and myocardial infarction *(98)*.

Finally, as in patients with diabetes, prevention of endothelial dysfunction and hypercoagulation may contribute to the protective effects of insulin therapy in CI *(99)*. We indeed demonstrated that maintenance of normoglycemia with intensive insulin therapy protected the endothelium, which contributed to prevention of organ failure and death with this intervention *(89)*. The therapy reduced endothelial activation, reflected in lower levels of adhesion molecules. The mechanism likely involves inhibition of excessive inducible nitric oxide synthase (iNOS)-induced NO release. Moreover, intensive insulin therapy reduced the levels of asymmetric dimethylarginine *(100)*, an endogenous inhibitor of nitric oxide synthase activity, which competes with cellular transport of its substrate arginine and thus interferes with nitric oxide production. The modulation of this arginine derivative by insulin was associated with a better outcome, most likely mediated by reducing the inhibition of the constitutively expressed endothelial nitric oxide synthase *(101)*, contributing to preservation of organ blood flow.

CONCLUSIONS

The development of hyperglycemia is detrimental for the outcome of critically ill patients. However, the simple metabolic intervention of maintaining normoglycemia with intensive insulin therapy to a large extent improves survival of critically ill patients and reduces morbidity. In the last few years, substantial progress has been made in the understanding of the mechanisms underlying these clinical benefits, and it appears that both strict glycemic control and other metabolic and non-metabolic effects of the insulin administered contribute. However, more studies are needed to further elucidate the exact pathways involved, as well as the relative contribution of prevention of glucose toxicity and direct non-glycemic effects of insulin. This knowledge will open new perspectives for developing strategies to further improve outcome of CI.

ACKNOWLEDGMENTS

The work was supported by research grants from the Catholic University of Leuven (OT/03/56) and the FWO Flanders Belgium (G.0278.03, G.0533.06). I. Vanhorebeek is a Post-doctoral Fellow of the FWO Flanders Belgium. G. Van den Berghe holds an unrestrictive Catholic University of Leuven Novo Nordisk Chair of Research.

REFERENCES

1. Van den Berghe G, Wouters P, Weekers F, et al. Intensive insulin therapy in critically ill patients. *N Engl J Med* 2001; 345:1359–1367.
2. Murray P, Hall J. Renal replacement therapy for acute renal failure. *Am J Respir Crit Care Med* 2000; 162:777–781.
3. Hund E. Neurological complications of sepsis: critical illness polyneuropathy and myopathy. *J Neurol* 2001; 248:929–934.
4. Leijten FS, De Weerd AW, Poortvliet DC, et al. Critical illness polyneuropathy in multiple organ dysfunction syndrome and weaning from the ventilator. *Intensive Care Med* 1996; 22:856–861.
5. Bolton CF, Young GB. Critical illness polyneuropathy. *Curr Treat Options Neurol* 2000; 2:489–498.
6. Docke WD, Randow F, Syrbe U, et al. Monocyte deactivation in septic patients: restoration by IFN-gamma treatment. *Nat Med* 1997; 3:678–681.
7. Parrillo JE. Pathogenetic mechanisms of septic shock. *N Engl J Med* 1993; 328: 1471–1477.
8. Corwin HL, Parsonnet KC, Gettinger A. RBC transfusion in the ICU. Is there a reason? *Chest* 1995; 108:767–771.

9. Van den Berghe G, de Zegher F, Bouillon R. Acute and prolonged critical illness as different neuroendocrine paradigms. *J Clin Endocrinol Metab* 1998; 83:1827–1834.
10. Van den Berghe G. Dynamic neuroendocrine responses to critical illness. *Front Neuroendocrinol* 2002; 23:370–391.
11. Vanhorebeek I, Langouche L, Van den Berghe G. Endocrine aspects of acute and prolonged critical illness. *Nat Clin Pract Endocrinol Metab* 2006; 2:20–31.
12. Gamrin L, Andersson K, Hultman E, et al. Longitudinal changes of biochemical parameters in muscle during critical illness. *Metabolism* 1997; 46:756–762.
13. Reid CL, Campbell IT, Little RA. Muscle wasting and energy balance in critical illness. *Clin Nutr* 2004; 23:273–280.
14. Thorell A, Nygren J, Ljungqvist O. Insulin resistance: a marker of surgical stress. *Curr Opin Clin Nutr Metab Care* 1999; 21:69–78.
15. McCowen KC, Malhotra A, Bistrian BR. Stress-induced hyperglycae mia. *Crit Care Clin* 2001; 17:107–124.
16. Boord JB, Graber AL, Christman JW, et al. Practical management of diabetes in critically ill patients. *Am J Respir Crit Care Med* 2001; 164:1763–1767.
17. Pozzilli P, Leslie RD. Infections and diabetes: mechanisms and prospects for prevention. *Diabet Med* 1994; 11:935–941.
18. Hill M, McCallum R. Altered transcriptional regulation of phosphoenolpyruvate carboxykinase in rats following endotoxin treatment. *J Clin Invest* 1991; 88:811–816.
19. Khani S, Tayek JA. Cortisol increases gluconeogenesis in humans: its role in the metabolic syndrome. *Clin Sci (Lond)* 2001; 101:739–747.
20. Watt MJ, Howlett KF, Febbraio MA, et al. Adrenalin increases skeletal muscle glycogenolysis, pyruvate dehydrogenase activation and carbohydrate oxidation during moderate exercise in humans. *J Physiol* 2001; 534:269–278.
21. Flores EA, Istfan N, Pomposelli JJ, et al. Effect of interleukin-1 and tumor necrosis factor/cachectin on glucose turnover in the rat. *Metabolism* 1990; 39:738–743.
22. Sakurai Y, Zhang XJ, Wolfe RR. TNF directly stimulates glucose uptake and leucine oxidation and inhibits FFA flux in conscious dogs. *Am J Physiol* 1996; 270:E864–E872.
23. Lang CH, Dobrescu C, Bagby GJ. Tumor necrosis factor impairs insulin action on peripheral glucose disposal and hepatic glucose output. *Endocrinology* 1992; 130:43–52.
24. Wolfe RR, Durkot MJ, Allsop JR, et al. Glucose metabolism in severely burned patients. *Metabolism* 1979; 28:1031–1039.
25. Wolfe RR, Herndon DN, Jahoor F, et al. Effect of severe burn injury on substrate cycling by glucose and fatty acids. *N Engl J Med* 1987; 317:403–408.
26. 26. Mizock BA. Alterations in carbohydrate metabolism during stress: a review of the literature. *Am J Med* 1995; 98:75–84.
27. Yendamuri S, Fulda GJ, Tinkoff GH. Admission hyperglycemia as a prognostic indicator in trauma. *J Trauma* 2003; 55:33–38.
28. Laird AM, Miller PR, Kilgo PD, et al. Relationship of early hyperglycemia to mortality in trauma patients. *J Trauma* 2004; 56:1058–1062.
29. Bochicchio GV, Sung J, Joshi M, et al. Persistent hyperglycemia is predictive of outcome of critically ill trauma patients. *J Trauma* 2005; 58:921–924.
30. Sung J, Bochicchio GV, Joshi M, et al. Admission hyperglycemia is predictive of outcome in critically ill trauma patients. *J Trauma* 2005; 59:80–83.
31. Rovlias A, Kotsou S. The influence of hyperglycemia on neurological outcome in patients with severe head injury. *Neurosurgery* 2000; 46:335–342.
32. Jeremitsky E, Omert LA, Dunham M, et al. The impact of hyperglycemia on patients with severe brain injury. *J Trauma* 2005; 58:47–50.

33. Capes SE, Hunt D, Malmberg K, et al. Stress hyperglycemia and prognosis of stroke in nondiabetic and diabetic patients: a systematic overview. *Stroke* 2001; 32:2426–2432.
34. Bolton CF. Sepsis and the systemic inflammatory response syndrome: neuromuscular manifestations. *Crit Care Med* 1996; 24:1408–16.
35. Capes SE, Hunt D, Malmberg K, et al. Stress hyperglycaemia and increased risk of death after myocardial infarction in patients with and without diabetes: a systematic overview. *Lancet* 2000; 355:773–778.
36. Muhlestein JB, Anderson JL, Horne BD, et al. Effect of fasting glucose levels on mortality rate in patients with and without diabetes mellitus and coronary artery disease undergoing percutaneous coronary intervention. *Am Heart J* 2003; 146:351–358.
37. Suematsu Y, Sato H, Ohtsuka T, et al. Predictive risk factors for delayed extubation in patients undergoing coronary artery bypass grafting. *Heart Vessels* 2000; 15:214–220.
38. Krinsley JS. Association between hyperglycemia and increased hospital mortality in a heterogeneous population of critically ill patients. *Mayo Clin Proc* 2003; 78:1471–1478.
39. Faustino EV, Apkon M. Persistent hyperglycemia in critically ill children. *J Pediatr* 2005; 146:30–34.
40. Srinivasan V, Spinella PC, Drott HR, et al. Association of timing, duration, and intensity of hyperglycemia with intensive care unit mortality in critically ill children. *Pediatr Crit Care Med* 2004; 5:329–336.
41. Gore DC, Chinkes D, Heggers J, et al. Association of hyperglycemia with increased mortality after severe burn injury. *J Trauma* 2001; 51:540–540.
42. Van den Berghe G, Schoonheydt K, Becx P, et al. Insulin therapy protects the central and peripheral nervous system of intensive care patients. *Neurology* 2005; 64:1348–1353.
43. Van den Berghe G, Wilmer A, Hermans G, et al. Intensive insulin therapy in the medical ICU. *N Engl J Med* 2006; 354:449–461.
44. Krinsley JS. Effect of an intensive glucose management protocol on the mortality of critically ill adult patients. *Mayo Clin Proc* 2004; 79:992–1000.
45. Grey NJ, Perdrizet GA. Reduction of nosocomial infections in the surgical intensive-care unit by strict glycemic control. *Endocr Pract* 2004; 10(Suppl 2):46–52.
46. Furnary AP, Wu Y, Bookin SO. Effect of hyperglycemia and continuous intravenous insulin infusions on outcomes of cardiac surgical procedures: the Portland Diabetic Project. *Endocr Pract* 2004; 10(Suppl 2):21–33.
47. Allen KV, Frier BM. Nocturnal hypoglycemia: clinical manifestations and therapeutic strategies toward prevention. *Endocr Pract* 2003; 9:530–543.
48. Mesotten D, Swinnen JV, Vanderhoydonc F, et al. Contribution of circulating lipids to the improved outcome of critical illness by glycemic control with intensive insulin therapy. *J Clin Endocrinol Metab* 2004; 89:219–226.
49. Mesotten D, Delhanty PJ, Vanderhoydonc F, et al. Regulation of insulin-like growth factor binding protein-1 during protracted critical illness. *J Clin Endocrinol Metab* 2002; 87:5516–5523.
50. Thorell A, Rooyackers O, Myrenfors P, et al. Intensive insulin treatment in critically ill trauma patients normalizes glucose by reducing endogenous glucose production. *J Clin Endocrinol Metab* 2004; 89:5382–5386.
51. Van den Berghe G, Wouters PJ, Bouillon R, et al. Outcome benefit of intensive insulin therapy in the critically ill: insulin dose versus glycemic control. *Crit Care Med* 2003; 31:359–366.
52. Finney SJ, Zekveld C, Elia A, et al. Glucose control and mortality in critically ill patients. JAMA 2003; 290:2041–2047.

53. Klip A, Tsakiridis T, Marette A, Ortiz PA. Regulation of expression of glucose transporters by glucose: a review of studies in vivo and in cell cultures. FASEB J 1994; 8:43–53.
54. Pekala P, Marlow M, Heuvelman D, Connolly D. Regulation of hexose transport in aortic endothelial cells by vascular permeability factor and tumor necrosis factor alfa, but not by insulin. J Biol Chem 1990; 265:18051–18054.
55. Shikhman AR, Brinson DC, Valbracht J, Lotz MK. Cytokine regulation of facilitated glucose transport in human articular chondrocytes. J Immunol 2001; 167:7001–7008.
56. Quinn LA, McCumbee WD. Regulation of glucose transport by angiotensin II and glucose in cultured vascular smooth muscle cells. J Cell Physiol 1998; 177:94–102.
57. Clerici C, Matthay MA. Hypoxia regulates gene expression of alveolar epithelial transport proteins. J Appl Physiol 2000; 88:1890–1896.
58. Sanchez-Alvarez R, Tabernero A, Medina JM. Endothelin-1 stimulates the translocation and upregulation of both glucose transporter and hexokinase in astrocytes: relationship with gap junctional communication. J Neurochem 2004; 89:703–714.
59. Tirone TA, Brunicardi C. Overview of glucose regulation. World J Surg 2001; 25: 461–467.
60. Vanhorebeek I, De Vos R, Mesotten D, et al. Strict blood glucose control with insulin in critically ill patients protects hepatocytic mitochondrial ultrastructure and function. Lancet 2005; 365:53–59.
61. Brealey D, Brand M, Hargreaves I, et al. Association between mitochondrial dysfunction and severity and outcome of septic shock. Lancet 2002; 360:219–223.
62. Brealey D, Karyampudi S, Jacques TS, et al. Mitochondrial dysfunction in a long-term rodent model of sepsis and organ failure. Am J Physiol Regul Integr Comp Physiol 2004; 286:R491–497.
63. Brownlee M. Biochemistry and molecular cell biology of diabetic complications. Nature 2001; 414:813–820.
64. Hunt JV, Dean RT, Wolff SP. Hydroxyl radical production and autoxidative glycosylation. Biochem J 1988; 256:205–212.
65. Bonnefont-Rousselot D. Glucose and reactive oxygen species. Curr Opin Clin Nutr Metab Care 2002; 5:561–568.
66. Aulak KS, Koeck T, Crabb JW, Stuehr DJ. Dynamics of protein nitration in cells and mitochondria. Am J Physiol Heart Circ Physiol 2004; 286:H30–H38.
67. Frost M, Wang Q, Moncada S, Singer M. Hypoxia accelerates nitric oxide-dependent inhibition of mitochondrial complex I in activated macrophages. Am J Physiol Regul Integr Comp Physiol 2005; 288:R394–R400.
68. Turina M, Fry DE, Polk HC Jr. Acute hyperglycemia and the innate immune system: clinical, cellular, and molecular aspects. Crit Care Med 2005; 33:1624–1633.
69. Rassias AJ, Marrin CA, Arruda J, et al. Insulin infusion improves neutrophil function in diabetic cardiac surgery patients. Anesth Analg 1999; 88:1011–1016.
70. Nielson CP, Hindson DA. Inhibition of polymorphonuclear leukocyte respiratory burst by elevated glucose concentrations in vitro. Diabetes 1989; 38:1031–1035.
71. Perner A, Nielsen SE, Rask-Madsen J. High glucose impairs superoxide production from isolated blood neutrophils. Intensive Care Med 2003; 29:642–645.
72. Rayfield EJ, Ault MJ, Keusch GT, et al. Infection and diabetes: the case for glucose control. Am J Med 1982; 72:439–450.
73. Furnary AP, Zerr KJ, Grunkemeier GL, Starr A. Continuous intravenous insulin infusion reduces the incidence of deep sternal wound infection in diabetic patients after cardiac surgical procedures. Ann Thorac Surg 1999; 67:352–360.

74. Weekers F, Van Herck E, Coopmans W, et al. A novel in vivo rabbit model of hyper-catabolic critical illness reveals a bi-phasic neuroendocrine stress response. *Endocrinology* 2002; 143:764–774.
75. Weekers F, Giuletti A-P, Michalaki M, et al. Endocrine and immune effects of stress hyperglycemia in a rabbit model of prolonged critical illness. *Endocrinology* 2003, 144:5329–5338.
76. Lanza-Jacoby S, Wong SH, Tabares A, et al. Disturbances in the composition of plasma lipoproteins during gram-negative sepsis in the rat. *Biochim Biophys Acta* 1992; 1124:233–240.
77. Khovidhunkit W, Memon RA, Feingold KR, Grunfeld C. Infection and inflammation-induced proatherogenic changes of lipoproteins. *J Infect Dis* 2000; 181:S462–S472.
78. Carpentier YA, Scruel O. Changes in the concentration and composition of plasma lipoproteins during the acute phase response. *Curr Opin Clin Nutr Metab Care* 2002; 5:153–158.
79. Jeschke MG, Klein D, Herndon DN. Insulin treatment improves the systemic inflammatory reaction to severe trauma. *Ann Surg* 2004; 239:553–560.
80. Tulenko TN, Sumner AE. The physiology of lipoproteins. *J Nucl Cardiol* 2002; 9:638–649.
81. Harris HW, Grunfeld C, Feingold KR, Rapp JH. Human very low density lipoproteins and chylomicrons can protect against endotoxin-induced death in mice. *J Clin Invest* 1990; 86:696–702.
82. Harris HW, Grunfeld C, Feingold KR, et al. Chylomicrons alter the fate of endotoxin, decreasing tumor necrosis factor release and preventing death. *J Clin Invest* 1993; 91:1028–1034.
83. Gore DC, Wolf SE, Sanford AP, et al. Extremity hyperinsulinemia stimulates muscle protein synthesis in severely injured patients. *Am J Physiol Endocrinol Metab* 2004; 286:E529–E534.
84. Agus MSD, Javid PJ, Ryan DP, Jaksic T. Intravenous insulin decreases protein breakdown in infants on extracorporeal membrane oxygenation. *J Pediatr Surg* 2004; 39:839–844.
85. Zhang XJ, Chinkes DL, Irtun O, Wolfe RR. Anabolic action of insulin on skin wound protein is augmented by exogenous amino acids. *Am J Physiol Endocrinol Metab* 2002; 282:E1308–E1315.
86. Vanhorebeek I, Van den Berghe G. Hormonal and metabolic strategies to attenuate catabolism in critically ill patients. *Curr Opin Pharmacol* 2004; 4:621–628.
87. Mesotten D, Wouters PJ, Peeters RP, et al. Regulation of the somatotropic axis by intensive insulin therapy during protracted critical illness. *J Clin Endocrinol Metab* 2004; 89:3105–3113.
88. Hansen TK, Thiel S, Wouters PJ, et al. Intensive insulin therapy exerts anti-inflammatory effects in critically ill patients, as indicated by circulating mannose-binding lectin and C-reactive protein levels. *J Clin Endocrinol Metab* 2003; 88:1082–1088.
89. Langouche L, Vanhorebeek I, Vlasselaers D, et al. Intensive insulin therapy protects the endothelium of critically ill patients. *J Clin Invest* 2005; 115:2277–2286.
90. Jeschke MG, Klein D, Bolder U, Einspanier R. Insulin attenuates the systemic inflammatory response in endotoxemic rats. *Endocrinology* 2004; 145:4084–4093.
91. Klein D, Schubert T, Horch RE, et al. Insulin treatment improves hepatic morphology and function through modulation of hepatic signals after severe trauma. *Ann Surg* 2004; 240:340–349.
92. Brix-Christensen V, Andersen SK, Andersen R, et al. Acute hyperinsulinemia restrains endotoxin-induced systemic inflammatory response: an experimental study in a porcine model. *Anesthesiology* 2004; 100:861–870.

93. Das UN. Insulin: an endogenous cardioprotector. *Curr Opin Crit Care* 2003; 9:375–383.
94. Jonassen A, Aasum E, Riemersma R, et al. Glucose-insulin-potassium reduces infarct size when administered during reperfusion. *Cardiovasc Drugs Ther* 2000; 14:615–623.
95. Gao F, Gao E, Yue T, et al. Nitric oxide mediates the antiapoptotic effect of insulin in myocardial ischemia-reperfusion: the role of PI3-kinase, Akt and eNOS phosphorylation. *Circulation* 2002; 105:1497–1502.
96. Jonassen A, Sack M, Mjos O, Yellon D. Myocardial protection by insulin at reperfusion requires early administration and is mediated via Akt and p70s6 kinase cell-survival signalling. *Circ Res* 2001; 89:1191–1198.
97. The CREATE-ECLA Trial Group Investigators. Effect of glucose-insulin-potassium infusion on mortality in patients with acute ST-segment elevation myocardial infarction. The CREATE-ECLA randomized controlled trial. *JAMA* 2005; 293:437–446.
98. Malmberg K, Ryden L, Wedel H, et al. Intense metabolic control by means of insulin in patients with diabetes mellitus and acute myocardial infarction (DIGAMI-2): effects on mortality and morbidity. *Eur Heart J* 2005; 26:650–661.
99. Van den Berghe G. How does blood glucose control with insulin save lives in intensive care? *J Clin Invest* 2004; 114:1187–1195.
100. Siroen MPC, van Leeuwen PAM, Nijveldt RJ, et al. Modulation of asymmetric dimethylarginine in critically ill patients receiving intensive insulin treatment: a possible explanation of reduced morbidity and mortality? *Crit Care Med* 2005; 33:504–510.
101. Nijveldt RJ, Teerlink T, van Leeuwen PA. The asymmetric dimethylarginine (ADMA)-multiple organ failure hypothesis. *Clin Nutr* 2003; 22:99–104.

10 Childhood Diabetes Explosion

Michael S. Stalvey, MD, and Desmond A. Schatz, MD

CONTENTS

INTRODUCTION
WHAT HAS LED TO BOTH CHILDHOOD TYPE 1
    AND TYPE 2 DIABETES REACHING EPIDEMIC
    LEVELS?
TACKLING THE PROBLEMS
CONCLUSION
ACKNOWLEDGMENTS
REFERENCES

SUMMARY

A century ago, the incidence of both Type 1 (T1D) and Type 2 (T2D) was very low. Worldwide epidemics of both T1D and T2D have placed tremendous burdens on both affected individuals and society. Disproportionate resources are spent on complications of the diseases. Although multiple etiologies have been promulgated, for T1D, causative factors and the precise mechanisms leading to the disease remain elusive. In contrast, the rising incidence of T2D in children is closely associated with the obesity explosion which is strongly linked to an increased food supply and decreased physical activity. The rising incidence of obesity has reached pandemic proportions with more than a billion people affected worldwide. Focus needs to be directed to understanding the complex interaction between genes, the environment, and the immune system culminating in T1D and tackling the obesity epidemic. This chapter will discuss the emergence of the diabetes explosion, the proposed pathogenic mechanisms, and potential interventions.

From: *Contemporary Endocrinology: Controversies in Treating Diabetes:*
Clinical and Research Aspects
Edited by: D. LeRoith and A. I. Vinik © Humana Press, Totowa, NJ

Key Words: Type 1 diabetes, type 2 diabetes, autoimmunity, obesity, insulin resistance

INTRODUCTION

An explosion inevitably conjures images of destruction, chaos, anxiety, fear, and panic. The twenty-first century confronts the world with new health challenges, if not explosions, at least alarming epidemics not only of childhood type 2 diabetes (T2D) but also, and perhaps less well recognized, of type 1 diabetes (T1D) (Table 1; Figs 1 and 2). At the beginning of the twentieth century, when hunger was rampant even in industrialized nations, no one would have envisioned that both childhood and adult obesities and its comorbidities including T2D would become one of our greatest healthcare problems.

A hundred years ago, the worldwide incidence of both T1D and T2D was very low. Because insulin had yet to be discovered, children or adults who developed T1D had a short life expectancy. With the advent of insulin therapy

Table 1
Comparison of Type 1 and Type 2 Diabetes

	T1D	*T2D*
Usual clinical course	Insulin-dependent	Non-insulin-dependent (initially)
Usual age of onset	<18 y LADA recognized in 5-15% of adults with T2D	>40 y but increasing, especially among obese teen minorities
Body weight	Lean	Obesity 80-90%
Clinical presentation	Acute-onset	Subtle
Ketosis-prone	Yes	No
Family history	≤15% with affected first-degree relative	Common
Ethnicity	Predominantly Caucasian	More common in people of Asian, African, Latino, Native American origin
Islet autoantibodies (GADA, ICA, IA-2A, IAA)	Present at onset	Absent
HLA-DR3,DR4, DQB1*0201, *0302	Increased frequency	No increased frequency

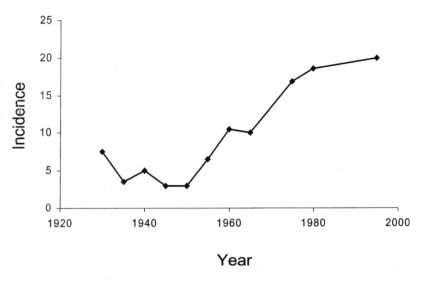

Fig. 1. Increasing incidence of type 1 diabetes in children in Norway from 1950 to present. Reproduced from Gale, EA *(1)* with permission.

and the subsequent refinements in insulin synthesis and delivery, the survival of individuals with T1D has permitted normal reproductive lives. The "explosion" of T1D cannot, however, be attributed to increased numbers of genetically susceptible offspring of people with T1D. The dramatic increase in T1D around

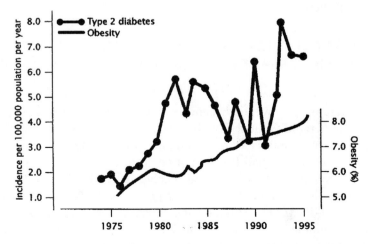

Fig. 2. Annual incidence of type 2 diabetes and prevalence of obesity among Japanese school children. Reproduced from Alberti et al *(2)* with permission.

the mid-twentieth century can only be explained by environmental factors. Although the dramatic rise in T1D slowed in the late twentieth century and the beginning of the twenty-first century, the incidence continues to increase.

The contemporary availability of high caloric density, low cost, convenient, and heavily promoted foods, together with environmental impediments to physical activity, has led to accelerating rates of obesity and rapidly rising numbers of T2D in both the adult and more recently the adolescent populations. The frequency of T2D has far exceeded T1D for many decades and targets all population groups. Edwin Gale *(3)* aptly describes T2D as "targeting the rich in poor countries and the poor in rich countries." T2DM, which 20–25 years ago, accounted for less than 3% of all cases of new-onset diabetes in children and adolescents, today accounts for up to 45% of new-onset cases among adolescents *(4)*.

In 1987, the Center for Disease Control and Prevention estimated that diabetes affected 6.8 million individuals in the USA *(5)*. By 2002, reports indicated that diabetes affected over 18 million individuals, with T2D accounting for approximately 90–95% of all cases *(6)*. The number of persons worldwide with diabetes is predicted to reach 300 million by the year 2025. King et al. *(7)* predict a 42% increase in developed countries and a 170% increase in developing countries.

The burden of diabetes is great on both the individual and the society. Despite improvements in therapy, a disproportionate amount of resources is spent on patients with macro- and microvascular complications of diabetes. In the USA alone, the direct cost of diabetes more than doubled from 1997 to 2002 ($44 billion to $92 billion). The projected direct costs for diabetes healthcare in the USA are $138 billion in the year 2020 *(8)*.

WHAT HAS LED TO BOTH CHILDHOOD TYPE 1 AND TYPE 2 DIABETES REACHING EPIDEMIC LEVELS?

Type 1 Diabetes

At the start of the twentieth century, childhood diabetes was considered to be rare and rapidly fatal. By the end of the century, 3–4 children per 1000 in Western countries were developing T1D by age of 20 years, and a steady rise in incidence had been reported from other parts of the world *(7)*. In 1890, the reported death rate from diabetes of children less than 15 years of age in the USA was 1.3/100,000/year *(1)* rising to 2–7/100,000/year over the years 1900–1920 *(1)*. Although the reliability of these data is uncertain because of variable access to medical care and absence of validation of diagnosis, physician surveys and other clinical/hospital records do not suggest a substantial increase in incidence during the era of 1920–1950 *(1)*. In the second half of the twentieth century, multiple studies from Europe (Norway, Denmark, Sardinia, and UK) and the USA reported a dramatic increase in the incidence of T1D. The incidence appears to be increasing in linear fashion *(1)*. These findings are most prominent in countries known for high prevalence rates of diabetes. In Finland, in the 1950s, incidence rates were 10–12/100,000/year and are now (45–50/100,000/year. Almost 1 of 160 Finnish children develop T1D by age 16 years. Although increases in T1D frequency have been observed in almost every country where it has been monitored, the rates are still smaller than those noted for T2D. Extrapolation of current trends suggests that the global incidence of T1D will increase by 40% over the period 1998–2010 *(9)*.

Worldwide, Finland and Sardinia have the highest T1D incidence (45–50/100,000/year) *(10,11)*. The USA has an annual incidence of approximately 15/100,000 children or more than 12,000 new cases per year. The peak incidence occurs at adolescence, however a more modest peak is noted in preschool age children. There is evidence that the increasing worldwide incidence of T1D is especially noted in young children *(9,12–14)*. Not included in these incidence data are the increasing number of adult patients initially diagnosed with T2D who have latent autoimmune diabetes of adults (LADA), a slowly progressive form of T1D *(15–23)*. Between 4 and 17% of T2D patients have LADA based on the presence of islet autoantibodies, with the highest percentages being in young patients. Among 25- to 34-year-old T2D patients in the United Kingdom Prospective Diabetes Study, 34% had one or more diabetes-specific autoantibodies and 47% of Swedish 15–34 year-old T2D patients were positive. LADA could affect as many individuals as classic, acute-onset T1D. The etiology of the increase in incidence is not well understood. The change in incidence within genetically stable populations indicates an effect of changes in the environment. The presence of disparate geographic differences in addition to the rising worldwide incidence as well as an approximate 50–66% discordance rate in identical twins further indicates that environmental agents must be operative *(24)*. Islet-specific autoantibodies can frequently be detected within the first few years of life *(25–27)*, implying environmental encounters affecting islet cells very early in development. As there is invariably a latent period between the appearance of autoantibodies and onset of disease, additional environmental factors—interacting with genetic predisposition further appear to modulate the rate of disease *(28)*. Many attempts have been made to explain the rising incidence of diabetes over the past 30 years. Early nutrition and infection have been the most frequently advanced hypotheses with exposure to cow's milk *(29)* or to rubella or enterovirus infection *(30)* most often proposed. There is, however, no direct evidence that either plays a major role in causation.

There is indirect evidence that in utero exposure may account for at least a portion of cases. Congenital rubella infection can cause ß-cell autoimmunity in 70% and diabetes in up to 40% of children infected in utero, but not in those infected postnatally (31–36). The incubation period of T1D in congenital rubella patients is 5–20 years, and persistent rubella virus infection of the pancreas has been demonstrated. The infection can also trigger autoimmune thyroiditis. Development of T1D in these patients is associated with the HLA-DR3 and four alleles (32). A molecular mimicry has been reported between a rubella virus protein and a 52-kDa pancreatic islet ß-cell autoantigen (36).Disappearance of the syndrome and the small but associated number of T1D cases following universal rubella vaccination have proven that T1D can be prevented by modification of environmental factors.

A relationship between islet autoimmunity and enteroviral infection exposure in utero has also been proposed (37–39). Studies from both Finland and Sweden indicate that maternal enterovirus infection increases the likelihood of subsequent diabetes in the offspring (37,38). In the Finnish study, significant increases in IgM antibodies to CBV5 and CBV5 procapsid enterovirus antigens were noted in the sera of pregnant mothers whose offspring subsequently developed T1D. In the Swedish studies, case mothers had significantly greater frequency of insulin CBV3 IgM antibodies than those whose offspring did not develop T1D. Molecular mimicry between the P2-C protein of Coxsackie virus and the glutamic acid decarboxylase (GAD) protein (40) has been proposed to account for the ß-cell autoimmunity. The presence of antibodies against enteroviruses in people with autoimmunity does not, however, prove a causal relationship. It should also be noted that the number of women not exposed during pregnancy is increasing and that infection in early childhood has become less common in the course of the century (41). These considerations do not exclude arguments based on changing antigenicity of viruses (or other environmental toxins or foods) or timing of exposure to them. People with autoimmunity may also be more prone to enteroviral infection, may have a stronger humoral response to infection because of their particular HLA genetic susceptibility, or may be in a non-specific hyperimmune state following exposure to various exogenous antigens (41). Islet-related autoantibodies have also been detected after mumps, rubella, measles, chickenpox, Coxsackie, and ECHO4 and rotavirus infections (42–45).

The hypothesis that there is an association between a protective effect of breastfeeding and early exposure to cow's milk on the incidence of autoimmunity and T1D is controversial (15–17, 46–48). Gerson's extensive meta-analysis demonstrated a weak but significant association between T1D and both a shortened period of breast-feeding and cow's milk exposure before 3–4 months of age *(18)*. In both the Bio Breeding (BB) rat and Non-Obese Diabetic (NOD) mouse (animal models of T1D), diet plays an important role in the development of T1D. Casein is the major protein fraction of cow's milk. Feeding semi-purified diets with simple sugars replacing complex carbohydrates and hydrolyzed casein as the protein source routinely retards the development of diabetes *(19,20)*. Karjalainen et al. *(48)* showed that antibodies to bovine serum albumin (BSA) (immunologically distinct from human serum albumin) were present in 100% of Finnish children with new-onset T1D, but were absent in controls. The majority of these antibodies were directed against a 17 amino acid fragment of BSA (ABBOS), to which peripheral blood lymphocytes from T1D patients were subsequently shown to respond by proliferation. Structural similarities between this ABBOS peptide and an islet autoantigen protein (ICA$_{69}$) invoked the appealing pathogenic concept of molecular mimicry, by which the early introduction of cow's milk would allow absorption of the intact protein before gut maturation, thus immunizing the infant and directing an immune response to the islets through its ICA$_{69}$ mimic *(21)*. There is evidence countervailing each argument for the cow's milk hypothesis *(17)*. The Diabetes Autoimmunity Study in the Young (DAISY) has found no association between early exposure to cow's milk and β-cell autoimmunity in young siblings and offspring of diabetes patients or when the analyses were restricted to those with the highest risk HLA genotypes *(16)*. The accuracy and relevance of the dietary recall information from the higher risk population may reflect bias *(22)*.

Breast-feeding patterns do not reflect changes in the incidence of childhood diabetes *(23)*. There is little to suggest that this is, in any way, related to changes in the incidence of childhood diabetes. Cow's milk consumption (per person per year) has been shown to be correlated with T1D incidence in some countries but not in others. In Sardinia, with the second highest incidence rate in Europe (after Finland), and where the incidence of T1D continues to rise, cow's milk consumption is less than half that in Finland *(49)*. Most studies examining infant feeding practices have looked at the first 3–6 months of life and not at other later nutritional practices. Other studies have suggested an association between an increased risk of diabetes and weaning foods, as well as milk and dairy product consumption, and the ingestion of foods containing nitrosamine in the 12 months before diagnosis. Atkinson et al. *(15)* were unable to show any link between the presence of antibodies to BSA and disease. Other studies in both childhood and adult-onset T1D patients have not supported the utility of measuring BSA antibodies as a marker of the disease either at diagnosis or in disease prediction *(50)*. ICA$_{69}$ are found in several other organs besides pancreatic cells and are seemingly not exclusive to T1D. The anticipated cross-reactivity of these antibodies with BSA has not been confirmed. In the animal models, there is little or no effect of the feeding of increased quantities of BSA or skim milk powder on diabetes frequencies.

That ingestion of nutrient-containing elements of plants such as soy and wheat may have an effect on the development of diabetes is suggested by studies of non-obese diabetic mice *(51)*. In humans, two recent studies—DAISY and the German study of offspring of T1D parents—provided evidence that susceptibility to T1D is associated with the timing of exposure to cereal and gluten *(52,53)*. In DAISY, initial exposure to cereal between birth and 3 months of age and after 7 months of age imparted risk of autoimmunity. In the German study of offspring of T1D parents, Zeigler and colleagues *(53)* demonstrated an increased risk for autoimmunity in infants initially exposed to gluten before 3 months of age and found no increased risk in infants whose initial exposure was after 6 months of age. Although both studies provided interesting findings, their conclusions are in some ways contradictory and demonstrate the need for larger collaborative investigations to determine appropriately how early dietary exposures affect risk for autoimmunity.

As previously noted, the highest incidence of T1D worldwide occurs in Finland (now almost 50/100,000/year), which is more than three times that in the USA. The incidence of the disease is related to distance north of the equator. Sun exposure in northern Finland is extremely limited, and low serum concentrations of vitamin D are common. Hypponen et al. *(54)* suggest that ensuring adequate vitamin D supplementation for infants could help to reverse the trend of increasing incidence of T1D. The investigators conducted a birth cohort study of almost 11,000 infants in northern Finland who were followed to age 1 year and concluded that dietary vitamin D supplementation (2000 IU daily) was associated with a subsequent reduced risk of T1D when adjusted for neonatal, anthropometric, and social characteristics. It has been proposed that vitamin D compounds act as selective immunosuppressants as exemplified by their ability to either prevent or markedly suppress development of autoimmune disease in animal models. Vitamin D given to mice genetically at risk to develop diabetes is also associated with a reduced risk of T1D *(55)*. Vitamin D has been shown to stimulate transforming growth factor (TGF)-$\beta 1$ and interleukin (IL)-4, which may suppress inflammatory T-cell ($T_H 1$) activity *(56)*. As T1D in the NOD mouse appears to be a $T_H 1$-mediated disease, altering the balance toward $T_H 2$ production may be protective. In addition, there is evidence for a genetic link between Vitamin D and diabetes risk. A recent study showed that a vitamin D receptor initiation codon polymorphism in exon 2 influences genetic susceptibility to T1D among the Japanese *(57)*. The number of incident cases, however, was small and, therefore, the absolute magnitude of the effect needs to be further assessed. Although a Norwegian study demonstrated that children born to women who took cod liver oil during pregnancy had a reduced risk of T1D, infants taking cod liver oil or other vitamin D supplements in the first year of life did not have an altered risk of diabetes (58). The results of this study are difficult to interpret, because vitamin D levels were not measured nor was there accurate quantification of intake.

Toxic doses of nitrosamine compounds can also cause diabetes because of the generation of free radicals (59,60). The effect of dietary nitrate, nitrite, or nitrosamine exposure on human T1D risk is less clear (61,62). Several perinatal risk factors for childhood diabetes are also associated with the development of T1D (63). The effect of maternal–child blood group incompatibility is fairly strong (both ABO and Rh factor with ABO > Rh) and needs to be further explored. Other perinatal factors conferring increased risk include preeclampsia, neonatal respiratory distress, neonatal infections, caesarian section, birth weight, gestational age, birth order, and maternal age (64–68). It will be important to determine whether these factors contribute and how they may act or be confounded by other unknown risk factors. Rodent studies indicated that administration of diphtheria–tetanus–pertussis vaccine at 2 months of age increased the incidence of diabetes compared with those unvaccinated or vaccinated at birth. Prospective studies in children, however, show no association between early childhood immunizations and ß-cell autoimmunity (69,70).

Recently, it has been argued that the rising incidence of T1D could be accounted for by protective factors in the environment that have been lost (71). There has been a parallel rise of asthma and allergy. The hygiene hypothesis proposes that early exposure to infective agents in early childhood is necessary for maturation of the immune response. In the absence of such exposure, there would be a failure of early immune regulation that might permit, depending on genetic susceptibility, the development of autoimmunity (T_H1) or allergy (T_H2) (71,72). This view is consistent with the fact that the NOD mouse is less likely to develop diabetes in the presence of pinworms and other infections (72).

Type 2 Diabetes

The first cases of childhood T2D were reported in Native Americans and Canadian First Nation People in 1979 and 1984 (4). Before 1994, the percentage of children in the USA and in other parts of the world diagnosed with T2D comprised less than 5% of all cases. (4,73). Over a period of 20 years, the prevalence of T2D increased sixfold for Pima Indian adolescents from a prevalence of 9/1000 in the 15- to 24-year age group in the 1970s to 51/1000 in the 15- to 19-year age group in the 1990s. In addition, a prevalence of 22/1000 was demonstrated in the 10- to 14-year age group in the 1990s, whereas this age group had no T2D (4). Similar trends have been reported among other populations in the USA. In a Cincinnati-based pediatric diabetes clinic, 2–4%

of newly diagnosed diabetes patients had T2D between 1982 and 1992, with a sharp increase to 16% by 1994. During the period of 1990–2000 at the Montifiore Medical Center in Bronx, NY, the number of patients <18 years diagnosed with T2D increased 10-fold (74). In 1990, T2D accounted for 12% of the newly diagnosed diabetes patients. By 2000, almost 50% of the newly diagnosed patients had T2D (4). In the USA, T2D now accounts for 8–45% of all pediatric diabetes, and its prevalence appears to be increasing (2,73).

Outside of the USA, similar trends in children and adults have been noted in both the developed and the developing worlds, based on reports which vary from public health surveys to clinic series and which include varying definitions of T2D. In Japan, 80% of all new instances of diabetes in children and adolescents are T2D (75), with a female predominance of 2:1 (4), and the increasing incidence over the past 20 years has paralleled the increase in obesity (76). This shift has occurred as the traditional Japanese diet has been replaced by one in which more calories as animal fat and protein are being consumed (77).

There appears to be a close relation between rates of T2D in adults and the appearance of the disorder in adolescents. This pattern has been noted in most geographic regions and ethnic and cultural groups that have been studied. Adolescents from minority groups in the USA (Pima Indians, African Americans, and Hispanic Americans), Canada (First Nations people), Australia (Aboriginal), and New Zealand (Maori) have a disproportionately high prevalence of T2D (4,78–80). For example, in the Maori population between 1997 and 1999, T2D accounted for 12% of new cases of diabetes. This percentage rose to almost 36% in 2001 (81). Similar trends are seen in both immigrants and their offspring where analyses of social trends suggest that adoption of a Western lifestyle is strongly associated with T2D in these populations (79). These studies suggest that minority populations and immigrants have increased rates of obesity. Asian-American and Hispanic adolescents born and raised in the USA are more than twice as likely to be obese as those in their native lands.

The rising incidence of T2D in children is closely linked to the obesity explosion in the general population and, specifically, among children (Fig. 1). Over the past 10 years especially, there has been an obesity explosion in the Asia-Pacific region, Europe, and the USA in both adults and children, paralleling the increasing incidence of T2D (82). Obesity is now the most common nutritional disease of children and adolescents in the USA (83). In 2002, the US prevalence of overweight [body mass index (BMI) >25 in 2002] was a staggering 66%. Obesity defined as BMI > 30% occurred in 30.5% and extreme obesity (BMI > 40.0) in 5.1%. (84). Overweight children were over four times more likely to be overweight adults than were normal weight children *(85)*. Obese adults beget obese children. If a child has two non-obese parents, there is an 8% chance of adult obesity, whereas a 10- to 14-year-old child has a 79% chance of obesity if at least one parent is obese *(86)*.

Worldwide, the incidence of obesity continues to increase, reaching pandemic proportions with more than a billion people affected *(87–90)*. As previously discussed, developing countries have not been spared. The Asia-Pacific subcontinent includes perhaps the largest populations of diabetes in the world. Greater than 12% of Indians have diabetes and another approximately 14% demonstrate glucose intolerance *(91)*. The incidence of diabetes in adults continues to grow at an alarming rate, and by 2025, China is expected to show an increase in incidence of up to 68%, followed closely by India with 59%, and the other Asian countries and the Pacific Islands (41%). These data have implications for screening programs among youngsters and for public obesity prevention programs. The thrifty genotype hypothesis, i.e. evolutionary selection of individuals able to survive through periods of famine by enhanced energy storage capabilities when food was obtainable, coupled with continuous availability of food, explains this observed rising incidence of T2D in developing countries.

In the industrialized world, urbanization, easy access to motor vehicles, and availability of school busing, have led to most children and adolescents walking or cycling less than a few blocks to school or work after school. The discontinuation of physical education (PE) in schools and the lack of time spent in outside play by children have produced a generation of children accustomed to a more sedentary lifestyle. Concerns for safety have resulted in reduced neighborhood play, which has been replaced by television, video games, and other computer activity. Nesmith noted that participation in school-based PE decreased from 41.6% of students in 1991 to 24.5% in 1995. In addition, only 50% of the US children and adolescents aged 12–21 years reported regular vigorous physical activity and 25% reported no physical activity at all *(92)*. Proctor et al. have shown that time spent watching television is an independent predictor of childhood BMI and skinfold thickness. BMI of early adolescent children watching >3 h of television averaged 20.9 versus 18.6 kg/m^2 for those watching <1.75 h/day. The sum of five skinfolds for children who watch >3.0 h of television was 106 mm compared with 88 mm for children watching less than 1.75 h/day *(93)*. Gortmaker et al. *(94)* reported that children who watched more than 5 h of television per day were five times more likely to be overweight. In addition, the availability and low cost of fast foods contributes to obesity. Pereira et al. *(95)* have shown on a positive association of body weight and insulin resistance in individuals who consume fast food in excess of two times per week. Children who buy school lunches have an increased risk of being overweight *(96)*.

TACKLING THE PROBLEMS

Type 1 Diabetes

To prevent T1D, we must enhance our understanding of the mechanisms leading to autoimmune-mediated β-cell failure. These include the identification of potential environmental triggers and a better understanding of the deviant interaction of genes, the environment, and the immune system, which culminates in clinical disease. The ongoing NIH-funded The Environmental Determinants of Type 1 Diabetes in Youth (TEDDY) study seeks to identify infectious, dietary, or other environmental exposures and psychological factors that trigger or prevent T1D in genetically susceptible individuals. From birth, high-risk children from the general population and relatives of people with T1D will be tested for exposures to candidate environmental factors. Over 200,000 newborn babies will be screened by six centers in the USA (Florida/Georgia, Colorado, Washington state), Finland, Sweden, and Germany.

The unraveling of the natural history of pre-T1D, which has allowed for the identification of at-risk individuals both by genetic and by islet autoantibody testing of both high- and low-risk general populations, affords opportunities to intervene at varying time points in the prediabetic period (Fig. 3)

Over the past decade, well-designed, randomized, controlled clinical trials aimed at preventing T1D have been implemented. Although major transcontinental efforts (Diabetes Prevention Trial conducted in the USA and Canada) and the European Nicotinamide Diabetes Intervention Trial were unsuccessful in preventing T1D, both studies added significantly to our understanding of the natural history of pre-T1D and generated collaborative interactions across and

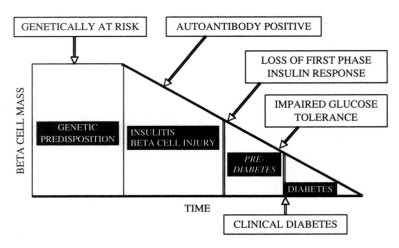

Fig. 3. Natural history of Type 1 diabetes and opportunities for prevention.

between continents. The creation of multicenter cooperative groups (akin to the childhood cancer collaborative centers) is vital to enable the simultaneous testing of primary and secondary prevention strategies in different population groups at different stages of the disease process. Studies are ongoing as part of the NIH-funded TrialNet and Immune Tolerance Networks.

Type 2 Diabetes

Opportunities in preventing the occurrence of T2D are shown in Fig. 4. Although there have been few metabolic studies in pre- and early T2D in youth, it is likely that a similar disease process occurs as in adults with both impaired insulin resistance and β-cell failure occurring early *(97)*.

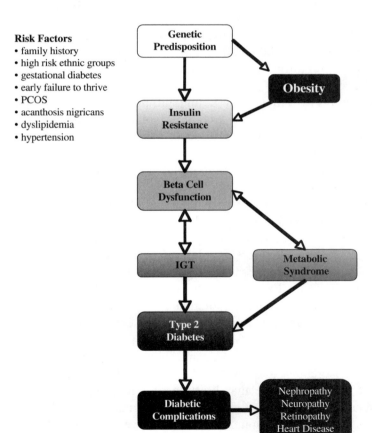

Fig. 4. Natural history of Type 2 diabetes in children and adolescents. Enhanced knowledge of the natural history of the disease in children and adolescents affords multiple opportunities to potentially intervene prior to onset.

Identifying and eliminating, or at least modifying, risk factors will be necessary to reduce the disease frequency. Curbing the obesity epidemic is essential to decreasing the T2D explosion as well as preventing early hyperlipidemia, hypertension, and cardiovascular disease. Obesity and increased waist circumference in prepubertal children is associated with subsequent hyperlipidemia and hypertension, impaired glucose tolerance, and T2D *(98)*. Up to a third of youth with T2D also have hypertension and hypertriglyceridemia *(99)*, and mico-albuminuria has been reported in 14–22% of cases *(80,100)*.

Substantial resources must be directed globally to effect lifestyle changes. Communities, schools, and individuals must all be targeted. The challenges are enormous in contemporary society where daily physical activity opportunities are limited for our youth, entertainment is more sedentary than physically challenging, labor-saving devices abound and high-fat, high-energy calorie dense foods are cheap, ubiquitous, and heavily promoted.

Efforts at treating childhood obesity have been generally disappointing. Other risk factors for T2D in youth include a strong family history of T2D, visceral adiposity (an independent risk factor), acanthosis nigricans, ethnicity (minority ethnic and immigrant populations), polycystic ovarian disease, offspring of mothers with gestational pregnancy, and intrauterine growth retardation. Because early identification and treatment of the disease and comorbidities have been shown to prevent the development or progression of complications, criteria for testing children and youth at risk for developing T2D have been developed (Table 2) *(101)*.

Individuals with IGT (defined as a fasting glucose >100, but <126 mg/dL, and/or a 2-h postprandial glucose >140, but <200 mg/dL) should be targeted for intervention. A recent report by Duncan *(102)* estimated the frequency of impaired fasting glucose (IFG defined as BG > 100 mg/dl) to be about 11% in a tested subsample of 4370 youth aged 12–19 years in the National Health and Nutrition Examination Survey (NHANES). This is a substantial percentage of such a young population to have IFG, especially considering that the fasting serum glucose concentration rises later than does postprandial glycemia in the evolution of T2D. Importantly, as in adults, IFG correlates with subsequent progression to T2D and should trigger close attention to blood pressure measurement and testing of lipids. Studies in adults with impaired glucose tolerance indicate that lifestyle change (weight loss and increased physical activity) is effective in decreasing progression to T2D over periods of 5–6 years *(103–105)*. Although these studies were conducted in self-selected volunteers who were likely motivated to make lifestyle changes, there is reason to anticipate that motivated youth might have a similar positive outcome to a comprehensive intervention combining diet and physical activity changes. The goal of the multicenter National Institute of Diabetes and Digestive and Kidney

Table 2
ADA Recommendations for Testing for Type 2 Diabetes in Children

---

Criteria*
  Overweight (Body Mass Index of 85th percentile for age and sex, weight for height 85th percentile, or weight 120% of ideal for height)
Plus any two of the following risk factors:
- Family history of T2D in first- or second-degree relative
- Race/ethnicity (American Indian, African-American, Hispanic, Asian/Pacific Islander)
- Signs of insulin resistance or conditions associated with insulin resistance (acanthosis nigricans, hypertension, dyslipidemia, PCOS)

  Initiation of screening: age 10 years or at onset of puberty if puberty occurs at a younger age
Frequency of screening: every 2 years
Screening Method: fasting plasma glucose preferred

---

  *Clinical judgment should be used to test for diabetes in high-risk patients who do not meet these criteria.
  Adapted from American Diabetes Association, Diabetes Care 2000, published with permission *(101)*.

Diseases (NIDDK) -funded Studies to Treat or Prevent Pediatric (STOPP) T2D primary prevention protocol is to implement a population-based intervention in middle school children to prevent or decrease the development of risk factors for T2D. The primary objective is to moderate risk factors of adiposity and glycemic dysregulation, specifically decreasing BMI (>85th percentile), IFG, and fasting insulin (≥ 30 μU/ml). The study will involve changes in the nutritional quality of food and beverage offerings throughout the school, changes in the PE program, classroom activities designed to increase knowledge and decision making skills, individual and group behavior change initiatives aimed at enhancing healthier behaviors, family outreach activities to involve parents/guardians, and school-wide communications to enhance and promote changes in nutrition, activity, and behavior. The small Bienestar population-based lifestyle intervention study suggested that risk factors for T2D in children could be ameliorated. Twenty-seven elementary schools in San Antonio, Texas, were provided with a multi-faceted health program to Mexican American fourth graders *(106)*. Mean fasting blood glucose was statistically lower for children in the intervention schools compared with those in the control schools. Other school-based programs in the USA and Singapore have been shown to be effective *(74)*. Rocchini et al. *(107)*, in a study of 50 obese adolescents, demonstrated weight loss, blood pressure, and improved insulin sensitivity with lifestyle modification. Robinson studied 192 children who were randomized to reduce television viewing and video game play from 12 h per week to 8 h per week. A decrease in both BMI and waist circumference was observed over the 6 months of the study *(108)*.

The avoidance of smoking in adolescents should not be forgotten because smoking at any age, independently of obesity, is associated with greatly increased risks of atherosclerosis, even in modest amounts *(109)*.

CONCLUSION

Epidemics of both T1D and T2D in children and adolescents, beginning about mid-twentieth century and in the last decade of the twentieth century, respectively, are now evident. We must continue the pursuit of the epidemiologic and pathogenetic factors contributing to the increasing numbers of T1D, while also turning our focus to altering the recognized environmental factors predisposing to T2D. The obstacles to the latter effort are enormous in contemporary society. We must also continue to pursue the molecular understanding of both T1D and T2D. It is to be hoped that the recognition of this public health explosion will lead to an all-encompassing effort involving greatly augmented government, research, community, and individual commitments to prevent these disorders. The costs will be insignificant compared with the potential for prevention.

ACKNOWLEDGMENTS

We thank Dr. Arlan Rosenbloom for his critical comments and editorial assistance. Supported in part by grants U01 DK 60987-01, UO1DK60987-03, and 2MO1RR0082 from the National Institute of Health.

REFERENCES

1. Gale EA: Is there really an epidemic of type 2 diabetes? *Lancet* 362:503–504, 2003
2. Pinhas-Hamiel O, Zeitler P: The global spread of type 2 diabetes mellitus in children and adolescents. *J Pediatr* 146:693–700, 2005
3. Wetterhall SF, Olson DR, DeStefano F, Stevenson JM, Ford ES, German RR, Will JC, Newman JM, Sepe SJ, Vinicor F: Trends in diabetes and diabetic complications, 1980–1987. *Diabetes Care* 15:960–967, 1992
4. Centers for Disease Control and Prevention: National diabetes fact sheet: general information and national estimates on diabetes in the United States, 2005. Atlanta, GA: U.S. Department of Health and Human Services, Centers for Disease Control and Prevention, 2005
5. King H, Aubert RE, Herman WH: Global burden of diabetes, 1995–2025: prevalence, numerical estimates, and projections. *Diabetes Care* 21:1414–1431, 1998
6. Hogan P, Dall T, Nikolov P: Economic costs of diabetes in the US in 2002. *Diabetes Care* 26:917–932, 2003

7. Gale EA: The rise of childhood type 1 diabetes in the 20th century. *Diabetes* 51:3353–3361, 2002

8. Onkamo P, Vaananen S, Karvonen M, Tuomilehto J: Worldwide increase in incidence of Type I diabetes–the analysis of the data on published incidence trends. *Diabetologia* 42:1395–1403, 1999

9. Tuomilehto J, Lounamaa R, Tuomilehto-Wolf E, Reunanen A, Virtala E, Kaprio EA, Akerblom HK: Epidemiology of childhood diabetes mellitus in Finland–background of a nationwide study of type 1 (insulin-dependent) diabetes mellitus. The Childhood Diabetes in Finland (DiMe) Study Group. *Diabetologia* 35:70–76, 1992

10. Muntoni S, Stabilini L, Stabilini M, Mancosu G, Muntoni S: Steadily high IDDM incidence over 4 years in Sardinia. *Diabetes Care* 18:1600–1601, 1995

11. Karvonen M, Viik-Kajander M, Moltchanova E, Libman I, LaPorte R, Tuomilehto J: Incidence of childhood type 1 diabetes worldwide. Diabetes Mondiale (DiaMond) Project Group. *Diabetes Care* 23:1516–1526, 2000

12. Green A, Patterson CC: Trends in the incidence of childhood-onset diabetes in Europe 1989–1998. *Diabetologia* 44 Suppl 3:B3-8, 2001

13. Karvonen M, Pitkaniemi J, Tuomilehto J: The onset age of type 1 diabetes in Finnish children has become younger. The Finnish Childhood Diabetes Registry Group. *Diabetes Care* 22:1066–1070, 1999

14. Turner R, Stratton I, Horton V, Manley S, Zimmet P, Mackay IR, Shattock M, Bottazzo GF, Holman R: UKPDS 25: autoantibodies to islet-cell cytoplasm and glutamic acid decarboxylase for prediction of insulin requirement in type 2 diabetes. UK Prospective Diabetes Study Group. *Lancet* 350:1288–1293, 1997

15. Schranz DB, Bekris L, Landin-Olsson M, Torn C, Nilang A, Toll A, Sjostrom J, Gronlund H, Lernmark A: Newly diagnosed latent autoimmune diabetes in adults (LADA) is associated with low level glutamate decarboxylase (GAD65) and IA-2 autoantibodies. Diabetes Incidence Study in Sweden (DISS). *Horm Metab Res* 32:133–138, 2000

16. Olmos P, A'Hern R, Heaton DA, Millward BA, Risley D, Pyke DA, Leslie RD: The significance of the concordance rate for type 1 (insulin-dependent) diabetes in identical twins. *Diabetologia* 31:747–750, 1988

17. Ziegler AG, Hummel M, Schenker M, Bonifacio E: Autoantibody appearance and risk for development of childhood diabetes in offspring of parents with type 1 diabetes: the 2-year analysis of the German BABYDIAB Study. *Diabetes* 48:460–468, 1999

18. Rewers M, Bugawan TL, Norris JM, Blair A, Beaty B, Hoffman M, McDuffie RS, Jr., Hamman RF, Klingensmith G, Eisenbarth GS, Erlich HA: Newborn screening for HLA markers associated with IDDM: diabetes autoimmunity study in the young (DAISY). *Diabetologia* 39:807–812, 1996

19. Akerblom HK, Knip M, Simell O: From pathomechanisms to prediction, prevention and improved care of insulin-dependent diabetes mellitus in children. *Ann Med* 29:383–385, 1997

20. Leslie RD, Elliott RB: Early environmental events as a cause of IDDM. Evidence and implications. *Diabetes* 43:843–850, 1994

21. Harrison LC, Honeyman MC: Cow's milk and type 1 diabetes: the real debate is about mucosal immune function. *Diabetes* 48:1501–1507, 1999

22. Graves PM, Norris JM, Pallansch MA, Gerling IC, Rewers M: The role of enteroviral infections in the development of IDDM: limitations of current approaches. *Diabetes* 46:161–168, 1997

23. Menser MA, Forrest JM, Bransby RD: Rubella infection and diabetes mellitus. *Lancet* 1:57–60, 1978

24. Ginsberg-Fellner F, Witt ME, Yagihashi S, Dobersen MJ, Taub F, Fedun B, McEvoy RC, Roman SH, Davies RG, Cooper LZ, et al.: Congenital rubella syndrome as a model for type 1 (insulin-dependent) diabetes mellitus: increased prevalence of islet cell surface antibodies. *Diabetologia* 27 Suppl:87–89, 1984

25. Bodansky HJ, Grant PJ, Dean BM, McNally J, Bottazzo GF, Hambling MH, Wales JK: Islet-cell antibodies and insulin autoantibodies in association with common viral infections. *Lancet* 2:1351–1353, 1986

26. Blom L, Nystrom L, Dahlquist G: The Swedish childhood diabetes study. Vaccinations and infections as risk determinants for diabetes in childhood. *Diabetologia* 34:176–181, 1991

27. Clarke WL, Shaver KA, Bright GM, Rogol AD, Nance WE: Autoimmunity in congenital rubella syndrome. *J Pediatr* 104:370–373, 1984

28. Karounos DG, Wolinsky JS, Thomas JW: Monoclonal antibody to rubella virus capsid protein recognizes a beta-cell antigen. *J Immunol* 150:3080–3085, 1993

29. Hyoty H, Hiltunen M, Knip M, Laakkonen M, Vahasalo P, Karjalainen J, Koskela P, Roivainen M, Leinikki P, Hovi T, et al.: A prospective study of the role of coxsackie B and other enterovirus infections in the pathogenesis of IDDM. Childhood Diabetes in Finland (DiMe) Study Group. *Diabetes* 44:652–657, 1995

30. Dahlquist GG, Ivarsson S, Lindberg B, Forsgren M: Maternal enteroviral infection during pregnancy as a risk factor for childhood IDDM. A population-based case-control study. *Diabetes* 44:408–413, 1995

31. Clements GB, Galbraith DN, Taylor KW: Coxsackie B virus infection and onset of childhood diabetes. *Lancet* 346:221–223, 1995

32. Kaufman DL, Erlander MG, Clare-Salzler M, Atkinson MA, Maclaren NK, Tobin AJ: Autoimmunity to two forms of glutamate decarboxylase in insulin-dependent diabetes mellitus. *J Clin Invest* 89:283–292, 1992

33. Viskari HR, Koskela P, Lonnrot M, Luonuansuu S, Reunanen A, Baer M, Hyoty H: Can enterovirus infections explain the increasing incidence of type 1 diabetes? *Diabetes Care* 23:414–416, 2000

34. Helmke K, Otten A, Willems WR, Brockhaus R, Mueller-Eckhardt G, Stief T, Bertrams J, Wolf H, Federlin K: Islet cell antibodies and the development of diabetes mellitus in relation to mumps infection and mumps vaccination. *Diabetologia* 29:30–33, 1986

35. Champsaur HF, Bottazzo GF, Bertrams J, Assan R, Bach C: Virologic, immunologic, and genetic factors in insulin-dependent diabetes mellitus. *J Pediatr* 100:15–20, 1982

36. Honeyman MC, Coulson BS, Stone NL, Gellert SA, Goldwater PN, Steele CE, Couper JJ, Tait BD, Colman PG, Harrison LC: Association between rotavirus infection and pancreatic islet autoimmunity in children at risk of developing type 1 diabetes. *Diabetes* 49:1319–1324, 2000

37. Yoon JW, Austin M, Onodera T, Notkins AL: Isolation of a virus from the pancreas of a child with diabetic ketoacidosis. *N Engl J Med* 300:1173–1179, 1979

38. Borch-Johnsen K, Joner G, Mandrup-Poulsen T, Christy M, Zachau-Christiansen B, Kastrup K, Nerup J: Relation between breast-feeding and incidence rates of insulin-dependent diabetes mellitus. A hypothesis. *Lancet* 2:1083–1086, 1984

39. Martin JM, Trink B, Daneman D, Dosch HM, Robinson B: Milk proteins in the etiology of insulin-dependent diabetes mellitus (IDDM). *Ann Med* 23:447–452, 1991

40. Karjalainen J, Martin JM, Knip M, Ilonen J, Robinson BH, Savilahti E, Akerblom HK, Dosch HM: A bovine albumin peptide as a possible trigger of insulin-dependent diabetes mellitus. *N Engl J Med* 327:302–307, 1992

41. Atkinson MA, Bowman MA, Kao KJ, Campbell L, Dush PJ, Shah SC, Simell O, Maclaren NK: Lack of immune responsiveness to bovine serum albumin in insulin-dependent diabetes. *N Engl J Med* 329:1853–1858, 1993

42. Norris JM, Beaty B, Klingensmith G, Yu L, Hoffman M, Chase HP, Erlich HA, Hamman RF, Eisenbarth GS, Rewers M: Lack of association between early exposure to cow's milk protein and beta-cell autoimmunity. Diabetes Autoimmunity Study in the Young (DAISY). *Jama* 276:609–614, 1996

43. Schatz DA, Maclaren NK: Cow's milk and insulin-dependent diabetes mellitus. Innocent until proven guilty. *Jama* 276:647–648, 1996

44. Gerstein HC: Cow's milk exposure and type I diabetes mellitus. A critical overview of the clinical literature. *Diabetes Care* 17:13–19, 1994

45. Coleman DL, Kuzava JE, Leiter EH: Effect of diet on incidence of diabetes in nonobese diabetic mice. *Diabetes* 39:432–436, 1990

46. Elliott RB, Martin JM: Dietary protein: a trigger of insulin-dependent diabetes in the BB rat? *Diabetologia* 26:297–299, 1984

47. Pietropaolo M, Castano L, Babu S, Buelow R, Kuo YL, Martin S, Martin A, Powers AC, Prochazka M, Naggert J, et al.: Islet cell autoantigen 69 kD (ICA69). Molecular cloning and characterization of a novel diabetes-associated autoantigen. *J Clin Invest* 92:359–371, 1993

48. Vobecky JS, Vobecky J, Froda S: The reliability of the maternal memory in a retrospective assessment of nutritional status. *J Clin Epidemiol* 41:261–265, 1988

49. Wright AL: The rise of breastfeeding in the United States. *Pediatr Clin North Am* 48:1–12, 2001

50. Fava D, Leslie RD, Pozzilli P: Relationship between dairy product consumption and incidence of IDDM in childhood in Italy. *Diabetes Care* 17:1488–1490, 1994

51. Ivarsson SA, Mansson MU, Jakobsson IL: IgG antibodies to bovine serum albumin are not increased in children with IDDM. *Diabetes* 44:1349–1350, 1995

52. Scott FW, Marliss EB: Conference summary: diet as an environmental factor in development of insulin-dependent diabetes mellitus. *Can J Physiol Pharmacol* 69:311–319, 1991

53. Norris JM, Barriga K, Klingensmith G, Hoffman M, Eisenbarth GS, Erlich HA, Rewers M: Timing of initial cereal exposure in infancy and risk of islet autoimmunity. *Jama* 290:1713–1720, 2003

54. Ziegler AG, Schmid S, Huber D, Hummel M, Bonifacio E: Early infant feeding and risk of developing type 1 diabetes-associated autoantibodies. *Jama* 290:1721–1728, 2003

55. Hypponen E, Laara E, Reunanen A, Jarvelin MR, Virtanen SM: Intake of vitamin D and risk of type 1 diabetes: a birth-cohort study. *Lancet* 358:1500–1503, 2001

56. Saggese G, Federico G, Balestri M, Toniolo A: Calcitriol inhibits the PHA-induced production of IL-2 and IFN-gamma and the proliferation of human peripheral blood leukocytes while enhancing the surface expression of HLA class II molecules. *J Endocrinol Invest* 12:329–335, 1989

57. Mathieu C, Waer M, Laureys J, Rutgeerts O, Bouillon R: Prevention of autoimmune diabetes in NOD mice by 1,25 dihydroxyvitamin D3. *Diabetologia* 37:552–558, 1994

58. Pani MA, Knapp M, Donner H, Braun J, Baur MP, Usadel KH, Badenhoop K: Vitamin D receptor allele combinations influence genetic susceptibility to type 1 diabetes in Germans. *Diabetes* 49:504–507, 2000

59. Stene LC, Ulriksen J, Magnus P, Joner G: Use of cod liver oil during pregnancy associated with lower risk of Type I diabetes in the offspring. *Diabetologia* 43:1093–1098, 2000

60. Schein PS, Alberti KG, Williamson DH: Effects of streptozotocin on carbohydrate and lipid metabolism in the rat. *Endocrinology* 89:827–834, 1971

61. Pont A, Rubino JM, Bishop D, Peal R: Diabetes mellitus and neuropathy following Vacor ingestion in man. *Arch Intern Med* 139:185–187, 1979

62. Kostraba JN, Gay EC, Rewers M, Hamman RF: Nitrate levels in community drinking waters and risk of IDDM. An ecological analysis. *Diabetes Care* 15:1505–1508, 1992

63. Dahlquist GG, Blom LG, Persson LA, Sandstrom AI, Wall SG: Dietary factors and the risk of developing insulin dependent diabetes in childhood. *Bmj* 300:1302–1306, 1990

64. Dahlquist GG, Patterson C, Soltesz G: Perinatal risk factors for childhood type 1 diabetes in Europe. The EURODIAB Substudy 2 Study Group. *Diabetes Care* 22:1698–1702, 1999

65. Dahlquist G, Kallen B: Maternal-child blood group incompatibility and other perinatal events increase the risk for early-onset type 1 (insulin-dependent) diabetes mellitus. *Diabetologia* 35:671–675, 1992

66. Blom L, Dahlquist G, Nystrom L, Sandstrom A, Wall S: The Swedish childhood diabetes study–social and perinatal determinants for diabetes in childhood. *Diabetologia* 32:7–13, 1989

67. Flood TM, Brink SJ, Gleason RE: Increased incidence of type I diabetes in children of older mothers. *Diabetes Care* 5:571–573, 1982

68. Patterson CC, Carson DJ, Hadden DR, Waugh NR, Cole SK: A case-control investigation of perinatal risk factors for childhood IDDM in Northern Ireland and Scotland. *Diabetes Care* 17:376–381, 1994

69. McKinney PA, Parslow R, Gurney K, Law G, Bodansky HJ, Williams DR: Antenatal risk factors for childhood diabetes mellitus; a case-control study of medical record data in Yorkshire, UK. *Diabetologia* 40:933–939, 1997

70. Classen JB: The timing of immunization affects the development of diabetes in rodents. *Autoimmunity* 24:137–145, 1996

71. Hummel M, Ziegler AG: Vaccines and the appearance of islet cell antibodies in offspring of diabetic parents. Results from the BABY-DIAB Study. *Diabetes Care* 19:1456–1457, 1996

72. Todd JA: A protective role of the environment in the development of type 1 diabetes? *Diabet Med* 8:906–910, 1991

73. Singh B: Stimulation of the developing immune system can prevent autoimmunity. *J Autoimmun* 14:15–22, 2000

74. Bobo N, Evert A, Gallivan J, Imperatore G, Kelly J, Linder B, Lorenz R, Malozowski S, Marschilok C, Minners R, Moore K, Perez Comas A, Satterfield D, Silverstein J, Vaughn GG, Warren-Boulton E: An update on type 2 diabetes in youth from the National Diabetes Education Program. *Pediatrics* 114:259–263, 2004

75. Grinstein G, Muzumdar R, Aponte L, Vuguin P, Saenger P, DiMartino-Nardi J: Presentation and 5-year follow-up of type 2 diabetes mellitus in African-American and Caribbean-Hispanic adolescents. *Horm Res* 60:121–126, 2003

76. Alberti G, Zimmet P, Shaw J, Bloomgarden Z, Kaufman F, Silink M: Type 2 diabetes in the young: the evolving epidemic: the international diabetes federation consensus workshop. *Diabetes Care* 27:1798–1811, 2004

77. Cockram CS: The epidemiology of diabetes mellitus in the Asia-Pacific region. *Hong Kong Med J* 6:43–52, 2000

78. Kitagawa T, Owada M, Urakami T, Tajima N: Epidemiology of type 1 (insulin-dependent) and type 2 (non-insulin-dependent) diabetes mellitus in Japanese children. *Diabetes Res Clin Pract* 24 Suppl:S7–13, 1994

79. Kitagawa T, Owada M, Urakami T, Yamauchi K: Increased incidence of non-insulin dependent diabetes mellitus among Japanese schoolchildren correlates with an increased intake of animal protein and fat. *Clin Pediatr (Phila)* 37:111–115, 1998

80. Popkin BM, Udry JR: Adolescent obesity increases significantly in second and third generation U.S. immigrants: the National Longitudinal Study of Adolescent Health. *J Nutr* 128:701–706, 1998

81. Hara H, Egusa G, Yamakido M, Kawate R: The high prevalence of diabetes mellitus and hyperinsulinemia among the Japanese-Americans living in Hawaii and Los Angeles. *Diabetes Res Clin Pract* 24 Suppl:S37–42, 1994

82. McGrath NM, Parker GN, Dawson P: Early presentation of type 2 diabetes mellitus in young New Zealand Maori. *Diabetes Res Clin Pract* 43:205–209, 1999

83. Hotu S, Carter B, Watson PD, Cutfield WS, Cundy T: Increasing prevalence of type 2 diabetes in adolescents. *J Paediatr Child Health* 40:201–204, 2004

84. Ebbeling CB, Pawlak DB, Ludwig DS: Childhood obesity: public-health crisis, common sense cure. *Lancet* 360:473–482, 2002

85. Silink M, Kaichi K, Rosenbloom A: *Type 2 Diabetes in Childhood and Adolescence: A global perspective*. London, Martin Dunitz, Taylor & Francis Group, 2003

86. Hedley AA, Ogden CL, Johnson CL, Carroll MD, Curtin LR, Flegal KM: Prevalence of overweight and obesity among US children, adolescents, and adults, 1999–2002. *Jama* 291:2847–2850, 2004

87. Freedman DS, Khan LK, Serdula MK, Dietz WH, Srinivasan SR, Berenson GS: The relation of childhood BMI to adult adiposity: the Bogalusa Heart Study. *Pediatrics* 115:22–27, 2005

88. Whitaker RC, Wright JA, Pepe MS, Seidel KD, Dietz WH: Predicting obesity in young adulthood from childhood and parental obesity. *N Engl J Med* 337:869–873, 1997

89. Miller J, Rosenbloom A, Silverstein J: Childhood obesity. *J Clin Endocrinol Metab* 89:4211–4218, 2004

90. Thorburn AW: Prevalence of obesity in Australia. *Obes Rev* 6:187–189, 2005

91. Frye C, Heinrich J: Trends and predictors of overweight and obesity in East German children. *Int J Obes Relat Metab Disord* 27:963–969, 2003

92. Yajnik CS: Early life origins of insulin resistance and type 2 diabetes in India and other Asian countries. *J Nutr* 134:205–210, 2004

93. Ramachandran A, Snehalatha C, Kapur A, Vijay V, Mohan V, Das AK, Rao PV, Yajnik CS, Prasanna Kumar KM, Nair JD: High prevalence of diabetes and impaired glucose tolerance in India: National Urban Diabetes Survey. *Diabetologia* 44:1094–1101, 2001

94. Nesmith JD: Type 2 diabetes mellitus in children and adolescents. *Pediatr Rev* 22:147–152, 2001

95. Proctor MH, Moore LL, Gao D, Cupples LA, Bradlee ML, Hood MY, Ellison RC: Television viewing and change in body fat from preschool to early adolescence: The Framingham Children's Study. *Int J Obes Relat Metab Disord* 27:827–833, 2003

96. Gortmaker SL, Must A, Sobol AM, Peterson K, Colditz GA, Dietz WH: Television viewing as a cause of increasing obesity among children in the United States, 1986–1990. *Arch Pediatr Adolesc Med* 150:356–362, 1996

97. Pereira MA, Kartashov AI, Ebbeling CB, Van Horn L, Slattery ML, Jacobs DR, Jr., Ludwig DS: Fast-food habits, weight gain, and insulin resistance (the CARDIA study): 15-year prospective analysis. *Lancet* 365:36–42, 2005

98. Veugelers PJ, Fitzgerald AL: Prevalence of and risk factors for childhood overweight and obesity. *Cmaj* 173:607–613, 2005

99. Gungor N, Thompson T, Sutton-Tyrrell K, Janosky J, Arslanian S: Early signs of cardio-vascular disease in youth with obesity and type 2 diabetes. *Diabetes Care* 28:1219–1221, 2005

100. Maffeis C, Pietrobelli A, Grezzani A, Provera S, Tato L: Waist circumference and cardiovascular risk factors in prepubertal children. *Obes Res* 9:179–187, 2001

101. Pinhas-Hamiel O, Dolan LM, Daniels SR, Standiford D, Khoury PR, Zeitler P: Increased incidence of non-insulin-dependent diabetes mellitus among adolescents. *J Pediatr* 128:608–615, 1996

102. Fagot-Campagna A, Nelson RG, Knowler WC, Pettitt DJ, Robbins DC, Go O, Welty TK, Lee ET, Howard BV: Plasma lipoproteins and the incidence of abnormal excretion of albumin in diabetic American Indians: the Strong Heart Study. *Diabetologia* 41: 1002–1009, 1998

103. Type 2 diabetes in children and adolescents. American Diabetes Association. *Diabetes Care* 23:381–389, 2000

104. Duncan G: Prevalence of diabetes and impaired fasting glucose levels among US adoles-cents: National Health and Nutrition Examination Survey, 1999–2002. *Arch Pediatr Adolesc Med* 2006 May; 160(5):523–8.

105. Tuomilehto J, Lindstrom J, Eriksson JG, Valle TT, Hamalainen H, Ilanne-Parikka P, Keinanen-Kiukaanniemi S, Laakso M, Louheranta A, Rastas M, Salminen V, Uusitupa M: Prevention of type 2 diabetes mellitus by changes in lifestyle among subjects with impaired glucose tolerance. *N Engl J Med* 344:1343–1350, 2001

106. Swinburn BA, Metcalf PA, Ley SJ: Long-term (5-year) effects of a reduced-fat diet intervention in individuals with glucose intolerance. *Diabetes Care* 24:619–624, 2001

107. Knowler WC, Barrett-Connor E, Fowler SE, Hamman RF, Lachin JM, Walker EA, Nathan DM: Reduction in the incidence of type 2 diabetes with lifestyle intervention or metformin. *N Engl J Med* 346:393–403, 2002

108. Trevino RP, Yin Z, Hernandez A, Hale DE, Garcia OA, Mobley C: Impact of the Bienestar school-based diabetes mellitus prevention program on fasting capillary glucose levels: a randomized controlled trial. *Arch Pediatr Adolesc Med* 158:911–917, 2004

109. Rocchini AP, Katch V, Schork A, Kelch RP: Insulin and blood pressure during weight loss in obese adolescents. *Hypertension* 10:267–273, 1987

110. Robinson TN: Reducing children's television viewing to prevent obesity: a randomized controlled trial. *Jama* 282:1561–1567, 1999

111. Calle EE, Thun MJ, Petrelli JM, Rodriguez C, Heath CW, Jr.: Body-mass index and mortality in a prospective cohort of U.S. adults. *N Engl J Med* 341:1097–1105, 1999

11 Weight Loss in Type 2 Diabetic Patients

Is it Worth the Effort?

Rena R. Wing, PhD,
Heather M. Niemeier, PhD,
and Angela Marinilli Pinto, PhD

Contents

Summary

This chapter reviews the evidence regarding the role of weight loss in the prevention and treatment of type 2 diabetes. Strategies to improve adherence to diet and physical activity interventions that have been shown to be most effective for individuals with type 2 diabetes are also reviewed. Evidence

From: *Contemporary Endocrinology: Controversies in Treating Diabetes:*
Clinical and Research Aspects
Edited by: D. LeRoith and A. I. Vinik © Humana Press, Totowa, NJ

for the role of lifestyle changes in successful long-term weight loss maintenance is provided. Lastly, recent efforts to disseminate successful weight loss interventions are described.

Key Words: weight loss, weight loss maintenance, dietary intervention, physical activity, type 2 diabetes

LIFESTYLE INTERVENTION

It is well accepted that obesity and a sedentary lifestyle are related to the development of type 2 diabetes. With the rapid increase in obesity over the last few decades, a consequent increase in the rates of diabetes has already been noted and is expected to worsen. The epidemic rates of obesity have heightened interest in efforts to prevent obesity through interventions in young children and public health approaches, such as development of walking paths and taxation of junk foods. Although such efforts are important, they are fueled in part by the belief that once a person becomes overweight, there is no chance of recovery. The purpose of this chapter is to present evidence to the contrary—showing that successful weight loss is indeed possible and that lifestyle intervention can play an important role in the prevention and treatment of diabetes. In addition, the chapter will address specific issues being debated in the field, related to the type of diet and the level of physical activity that should be prescribed for weight loss, whether behavioral weight loss programs have adverse effects, and current efforts to effectively disseminate lifestyle interventions to increase their accessibility.

IS WEIGHT LOSS WORTH THE EFFORT?

Weight Loss and the Prevention of Diabetes

Probably the strongest evidence for the benefits of lifestyle intervention come from several large randomized controlled trials demonstrating convincingly that lifestyle intervention reduces the risk of developing type 2 diabetes. Of particular note is the Diabetes Prevention Program *(1)* conducted in 27 clinical centers in the USA. This study involved 3234 overweight individuals (BMI > 24 kg/m^2; BMI >22 kg/m^2 in Asian Americans) with impaired glucose tolerance. Participants averaged 51 years of age: 68% were women and 45% were members of minority groups. These participants were randomly assigned to receive either intensive lifestyle intervention or standard lifestyle intervention combined with Metformin (850 mg twice daily) or placebo. The intensive lifestyle intervention involved 16 individual sessions over 24 weeks followed by a contact at least every 2 months (typically once a month) throughout the trial. The goals of the lifestyle intervention were to lose 7%

of initial body weight, maintain this weight loss, and achieve at least 150 min/week of physical activity using activities that were similar in intensity to brisk walking. Physical activity was considered important for preventing diabetes in its own right and also for improving weight loss and maintenance.

The findings from Diabetes Prevention Program (DPP) were very dramatic, and thus the trial was stopped early, after an average follow-up of 2.8 years. The lifestyle intervention used in DPP was effective in producing weight loss and increased physical activity, both short and long term. Fifty percent of lifestyle participants achieved the 7% weight loss goal at week 24, and 38% achieved this goal at study end. Using self-reported diary data, 74% met the physical activity goal at 24 weeks and 58% at the final visit.

The intervention was extremely effective in reducing the risk of diabetes. The crude incidence of diabetes was 11.0, 7.8, and 4.8 cases per 100-person year for placebo, metformin, and lifestyle, respectively. Thus, lifestyle intervention reduced the risk of diabetes by 58% compared with placebo, and metformin reduced the risk by 31%. Moreover, lifestyle intervention was effective in all age, gender, and ethnic subgroups.

Similar results were obtained in two other large trials. In the Finnish Diabetes Prevention Study (2), lifestyle intervention also reduced risk of diabetes by 58% compared with the control group. The Da Quing Study (3) demonstrated that diet, exercise, and the combination reduced the risk of diabetes by 31–36%, with no significant difference among these behavioral approaches.

With the exception of the Da Quing Study, the lifestyle intervention used in these studies combined weight loss and physical activity, and thus it is difficult to reach conclusions about the independent effects of each of these behavior changes on diabetes risk. In a re-analysis of the DPP lifestyle intervention, it has been shown that weight loss was the dominant determinant of the reduction in disease risk (4). Although changes in diet and physical activity predicted weight loss, these behavior changes had no independent effect on diabetes risk in the entire DPP lifestyle cohort. For the lifestyle cohort as a whole, for each kilogram of weight loss, there was a 16% reduction in diabetes risk. However, in those who did not meet the weight loss goal, physical activity did have a beneficial effect.

Thus, one effect of weight loss that suggests that it is indeed worth the effort is the reduction of the risk of diabetes. However, this immediately raises the question of the cost of providing such an intensive intervention. In the DPP, investigators conducted an economic evaluation of the lifestyle and metformin intervention from perspectives of the payer and society (5). From a societal perspective, the lifestyle intervention implemented in DPP costs $24,000 per case of the disease prevented and the metformin intervention costs $34,500. From a payer perspective, the costs were $15,700 and $31,300 for lifestyle and metformin, respectively. Thus, the lifestyle intervention was more cost effective than metformin. Ways of further reducing the costs of the lifestyle intervention, for example, by using group treatment rather than individual case management deserve further attention.

Weight Loss and Glycemic Control and Cardiovascular Disease Risk Factors

In a chapter on evidence-based diabetes care, Wing (6) reviewed research testing the effects of different types of weight loss intervention on glycemic control. The conclusion was that with larger weight losses, achieved by behavioral programs, medication, or surgery, there was a clear long-term benefit of weight loss on glycemic control; more modest weight loss produced more variable outcomes.

The strongest evidence of a long-term benefit for individuals with type 2 diabetes comes from studies using gastrointestinal surgery. In the Swedish Obesity Study (SOS), for example, diabetic patients who underwent surgery for their obesity (typically vertical banded gastroplasty) had a relative risk of recovery from diabetes (reducing glucose to <120 mg/dl with no drugs) of 3.7 compared with control subjects (7). The effect of weight loss on recovery from diabetes was stronger than the effect on recovery from hypertension, hypertriglyceridemia, or hypercholesterolemia.

Weight loss medications have also been shown to be beneficial for individuals with diabetes. Orlistat (Xenical), a lipase inhibitor, was tested in yearlong trials with type 2 diabetic patients on metformin, sulfonylureas, and insulin (8–10). In each trial, Orlistat produced better weight losses than placebo and consequently greater improvements in glycemic control. The effect of Orlistat on glycemic control was directly related to improved weight loss. However, Orlistat also improved serum lipid levels; at any given level of weight loss, the improvements in lipids were greater on Orlistat than on placebo.

Likewise, Sibutramine (Meridia), which is a serotonin and norepinephrine reuptake inhibitor, improves weight loss relative to placebo in diabetic and non-diabetic individuals. For example, in a 1-year trial of 195 subjects with type 2 diabetes treated with metformin, weight losses were 5.5, 8.0, and 0.2 kg for patients treated with 15 mg Sibutramine, 20 mg Sibutramine, and placebo, respectively (11). Glycemic control improved with this weight loss; subjects who lost ≥10% of their body weight (which occurred in 15% of patients on 15 mg of Sibutramine and 27% of those on 20 mg of Sibutramine, but 0% on placebo) had a 1.2% decrease in HbA1c. Again, the improvement in glycemic control was directly related to the weight loss achieved. In contrast to these positive changes, Sibutramine has been associated with increased pulse rate and blood pressure.

Finally, there are many lifestyle intervention studies showing that dietary changes, physical activity, and their combination can result in improved glycemic control and cardiovascular disease (CVD)-risk factors in individuals with diabetes. Wing and colleagues *(6)* have conducted a large number of studies on this topic. Based on 114 overweight type 2 diabetic patients followed for 1 year, they concluded that modest weight losses (>6.9 kg) resulted in long-term improvements in HbA1, fasting glucose, insulin, high-density lipoprotein (HDL)-cholesterol, and triglycerides *(12)*. A dose–response relationship was observed between the magnitude of weight loss and the improvements in these risk factors. In addition, the short-term effects of weight loss were more dramatic than the long-term effects. However, the fact that even modest weight losses can be beneficial for at least 1 year is an important positive message to convey to patients attempting to lose weight.

Does Weight Loss Reduce CVD or All-Cause Mortality in Individuals with Type 2 Diabetes?

As described above, there are a large number of clinical studies suggesting that weight loss improves CVD risk factors and glycemic control. However, most of these studies are short term. To date, no long-term trials have been conducted evaluating the effects of weight loss on hard end points, notably CVD or death. Several observational studies have raised concerns about possible adverse effects of weight loss on cardiovascular and all-cause mortality. In these studies, individuals with or without diabetes are followed over time, and those who lose weight are compared with those who remain weight stable (or gain) on the subsequent risk of mortality over an extended follow-up. In a review of six observational studies of the effect of weight loss in type 2 diabetic individuals *(13)*, two studies found that weight loss was associated with decreased mortality, one with increased mortality, one showed no association, and in two the results differed by subgroup. A major concern in these studies is that intentional weight loss cannot be distinguished from unintentional weight loss. More recent studies have tried to distinguish intentional and unintentional weight loss. In a recent study *(14)*, intentional weight loss in individuals with diabetes was associated with 23% lower mortality rate compared with those not reporting trying to lose weight, whereas unintentional weight loss was associated with a 58% higher mortality rate. Another study *(15)* of over 4000 men aged 56–75 years suggested that even intentional weight loss carried out because of a physician's advice or ill health (including the diagnosis of diabetes) was associated with increased mortality; in this study, only intentional weight loss for personal reasons was beneficial.

In contrast, an historical prospective study of intentional weight loss in 336 overweight individuals with at least one CVD-risk factor *(16)* found that those who underwent at least 6 months of dietary counseling and lost at least 4.5 kg had a risk factor adjusted odds ratio for coronary heart disease (CHD) incidence, over 4 years of follow-up, of only 0.57 (CI = 0.39–0.84). In the group of individuals with diabetes ($n = 282$), the odds ratio for CHD in those losing 4.5 kg was also 0.57 (CI = 0.29–1.14).

Unfortunately, none of these studies can provide a definitive answer to the question of the long-term health effects of weight loss, as none utilized a randomized clinical trial design in which some participants are randomized to lose weight and others (of comparable baseline characteristics) are not provided with weight loss intervention. Such a randomized controlled trial is currently underway. This study, entitled Look AHEAD (Action for Health in Diabetes), is assessing the long-term effects (up to 11.5 years) of an intensive weight loss program in over 5000 overweight and obese individuals with type 2 diabetes (17). Participants are randomly assigned to the lifestyle intervention or to a control condition that is given diabetic education and support. The primary outcome measure is time to incidence of a major CVD event. Other outcomes, including CVD risk, cost and cost effectiveness, diabetes control and complications, and hospitalizations, are also being assessed.

In answer to the question of whether weight loss is worth the effort, the answer is YES. Weight loss has been found to improve several health parameters including decreasing the risk of diabetes, improving glycemic control, and improving CVD risk factors. Its effect on CVD and mortality needs further study; however, evidence to date suggests that weight loss should definitely be recommended for overweight individuals.

ARE THERE ADVERSE PSYCHOLOGICAL EFFECTS OF WEIGHT LOSS?

Questions have been raised regarding whether behavioral weight loss treatments, with their focus on regular weighing and dietary restriction, may lead to or exacerbate eating disorders in participants. This concern is largely based on the cognitive behavioral theory of the development of bulimia nervosa and binge eating disorder (BED) which theorizes that strict dietary restriction leads to binge eating. A recent study by Wadden et al. (18) addressed this question. These investigators recruited 123 overweight women who did not display disordered eating and randomly assigned them to a weight loss program using 1000 kcal/day diet with meal replacement products (MRs), a 1200–1500 kcal/day conventional food diet, or a non-dieting approach. They found no differences among the groups in the number of women who reported binge eating episodes, and no participant in the study met criteria for BED at any time during the study. There were also no differences among the groups on their reported level of hunger or disinhibition (a measure of thoughts, feelings, and behaviors associated with loss of control and binge eating). Thus, the authors concluded that behavioral weight loss does not contribute to the development of binge eating in participants who do not display it before entering treatment.

Another approach to this question is to examine whether individuals with eating disorders who undergo behavioral weight loss treatment experience an exacerbation of their symptoms. BED, characterized by episodes of overeating and feelings of loss of control without compensatory behaviors (such as vomiting or laxative use), is prevalent among individuals seeking behavioral weight loss; rates of BED range from 5–10% in such treatment-seeking populations (19). Several studies have shown that behavioral weight loss treatment actually ameliorates binge eating in participants meeting criteria for BED before treatment (20,21). Porzelius et al. (21)compared a standard behavioral weight loss program to a program modified to specifically address binge eating problems and found that both treatments significantly reduced binge eating at both posttreatment and follow-up with no differences between the groups. Not only do participants with BED experience a decrease in binge eating following behavioral weight loss, but they also have been shown to lose as much weight as non-BED participants in such programs (22–24).

Therefore, from available evidence to date, a focus on weight loss through dietary restriction in the context of behavioral weight loss programs does not appear to create or exacerbate eating disorders in obese populations. Conversely, such programs have been found to actively decrease binge eating and also produce weight loss in participants with a diagnosis of BED. These findings led the National Task Force on the Prevention and Treatment of Obesity to recommend moderate caloric restriction and increased physical activity for overweight and obese individuals regardless of binge status (25).

DOES ANYONE SUCCEED AT LONG-TERM WEIGHT LOSS?

Prevalence of Successful Weight Loss Maintenance

Another controversy facing the weight loss field is whether long-term weight loss maintenance is even possible. There is tremendous pessimism regarding the issue of successful long-term weight loss, but this belief does not appear to be justified. Data showing the lack of success typically come from weight loss treatment studies, where a group of participants are followed through one weight loss effort. Such data may underestimate the prevalence of success, because it may require several attempts before success is achieved. In addition, individuals who join such weight loss programs may have more difficulty with weight loss and maintenance than the general population of overweight individuals.

Population-based studies suggest that approximately 20% of overweight individuals will succeed in losing weight and maintaining it. McGuire surveyed 500 US adults regarding their lifelong weight history *(26)*. Of those who were overweight (BMI $\geq$ 27) at some point in their life (*n* = 228), 20.6% had lost at least 10% of their weight and maintained it at least 1 year. In a re-analysis of data reported by Moore *(27)*, Phelan and Wing *(28)* found that 57% of healthy overweight individuals who lost at least 1.8 kg over a 4-year period sustained a 1.8 kg loss over the next 4 years. Thus, there may be greater levels of success than often recognized.

Another point to consider is that weight loss, even if followed by regain, may help ameliorate the development of obesity observed during middle age. Using data from the Nurses' Health Study, Field et al. *(29)* found that women who lost >10% of their body weight between 1989 and 1991 subsequently gained more weight between 1991 and 1995 than those who had initially remained weight stable. Despite their greater regain, however, these women were far more successful overall (1989–1995). Thus, for example, women with a BMI of 25–29.9 (*n* = 9229) who initially lost >10% had a median weight reduction of 10.0 kg in 1989–1991, followed by a median weight regain of 10.9 kg and overall experienced no weight change. In contrast, those who did not lose >10% experienced a 2.3 kg gain from 1989–1991, a further 4.5 kg gain from 1991–1995, and overall a 6.8 kg gain. This weight gain would increase these women's risk of developing diabetes and CVD *(30,31)*.

The National Weight Control Registry

In an effort to learn more about successful weight loss maintenance, Hill and Wing established the National Weight Control Registry (NWCR) in 1994. The registry enrolls individuals who are over 18 years of age and who report having lost at least 30 pounds and kept it off at least 1 year *(32)*. The NWCR has received extensive media coverage, and individuals who read about the registry are invited to enroll. Thus, the NWCR is a self-selected population of successful weight losers; findings from the registry cannot be assumed to generalize to the broader population of successful weight losers. However, the self-reported weights of NWCR members have been shown to be very accurate *(33)*, and a population-based study of successful weight losers confirmed that the behaviors reported by registry members are also observed in the general population of successful weight losers *(34)*.

Participants in the registry complete a variety of questionnaires when they enroll and are then followed annually. At present, there are approximately 5000 individuals in the registry. The NWCR members are 77% women, 82% are college educated, 95% are Caucasian, and 64% are married; average age is 46.8 years. These participants report having lost an average of 33 kg, reducing from a BMI of 36.7 kg/m^2 to 25.1 kg/m^2. They have maintained a weight loss of at least 30 lbs for an average of 5.7 years; 13% have maintained the weight loss for at least 10 years. Thus by any criterion one would use, these individuals are clearly successful.

Participants in the registry report that they lost their weight in different ways. About one-third of the participants report that they lost weight on their own—without help from a commercial program, dietician, or physician. Others did it through commercial programs or working with a dietician or physician. The common theme in how they lost their weight was that over 90% used both diet and exercise to accomplish their weight reduction.

Registry members report that their successful weight loss came after many previous unsuccessful attempts (35). This is an important message for clinicians and for those attempting weight loss; it is reminiscent of the smoking cessation literature, which suggests that many attempts are needed before a person is successful. The fact that an individual is initially unsuccessful and later becomes successful suggests that the difference between success and lack of success is not due to differences in metabolism or psychological factors. Rather, the same person is at one point unsuccessful and then subsequently becomes successful. When asked what distinguished this successful weight loss from prior unsuccessful attempts, registry members note that this time they were more committed, they dieted more strictly, and exercise was a greater part of their approach.

Although there is great variety in how registry members lost weight, there appears to be certain common themes regarding the strategies used for mainte-nance. These include following a low-calorie, low-fat diet, maintaining high levels of physical activity, and remaining vigilant about their weight (32). As a whole, findings from population-based studies of successful weight loss among overweight individuals and the registry suggest that it is indeed possible for people to maintain weight loss long term.

Successful Weight Loss in Individuals with Diabetes

Data from the NWCR indicate that individuals with diabetes can indeed be successful weight losers. Approximately 7.5% of members of the NWCR report that prior to their weight loss they had been diagnosed with diabetes. Of these, 93% report that their diabetes has improved, and 73% report that they do not currently need medication to control their blood glucose.

However, it appears that it may be more difficult for individuals with type 2 diabetes to lose weight than those without diabetes, and individuals with diabetes may be more likely to regain their weight. In one study, 12 diabetic patients and their non-diabetic spouses were enrolled together in a behavioral weight loss program. Although patients and spouses were of similar age and weight, those with diabetes lost only 7.5 kg over 20 weeks, whereas their non-diabetic spouses lost 13.4 kg (36). In another comparison of 20 women with type 2 diabetes and 23 non-diabetic women treated together in a 16-week behavioral weight loss program, initial weight losses were comparable (7.4 and 6.4 kg for diabetic and non-diabetic subjects, respectively), but at 1-year follow-up, those with diabetes maintained a weight loss of 2 kg, whereas the non-diabetics retained a weight loss of 5.4 kg (37).

The same phenomenon has been observed in studies with weight loss medications. In both within and between study comparisons, individuals with diabetes have smaller weight losses than those without diabetes, and this difference occurs in participants treated with the weight loss medication and in those on placebo (38,39).

There are several reasons why individuals with diabetes may be less successful at weight loss. As glycemic control improves with weight loss, individuals with diabetes may have decreased excretion of calories in their urine, thereby reducing their weight loss. As diabetics in poor glycemic control have more elevated energy expenditure, this too may normalize with weight loss and improved glycemic control. Physical problems associated with diabetes, including neuropathy, may limit physical activity. There may also be psychological reasons for poorer weight loss, including a longer history of failure to lose weight, and perhaps more frequent occurrence of depressive symptomatology. Finally, many of the medications used to improve glycemic control, including sulfonylureas, thiazolidinediones, and insulin, enhance anabolism and promote weight gain. As all of these factors may make weight loss more difficult, more intensive approaches may be needed to produce weight loss in individuals with diabetes. However, even individuals with diabetes can indeed lose weight successfully.

WHAT DIET STRATEGIES OPTIMIZE WEIGHT LOSS AND WEIGHT LOSS MAINTENANCE?

Evidence regarding the optimal dietary and physical activity prescriptions for weight loss and weight loss maintenance comes from both the strategies successfully used by registry members and randomized clinical trials testing different approaches.

Dietary Intake in Registry Members

Registry members complete the Block Food Frequency Questionnaire (40) indicating their dietary intake at the time of entering the registry when they are maintaining their successful weight loss. The majority of participants report a low-calorie, low-fat eating style. However, there has been some change in the diet over the 10 years of the registry. In 1994, when the diet of the first 784 members of the registry was assessed, the mean caloric intake was 1381 kcal/day, with 24% of calories coming from fat *(35)*. As dietary reports typically underestimate actual intake by 20–30%, we assume that registry members were eating closer to 1800 kcal/day. We have recently looked again at the dietary intake of successful weight losers recruited in 2003. The average caloric intake has remained fairly constant over time. However, the percent of calories from fat has increased to 29.4%. This change may be due to the popularity of the Atkins diet and other low-carbohydrate diets during recent years.

Regular consumption of breakfast appears to be another characteristic of successful weight losers *(41)*. Only 4% of registry members indicate that they never eat breakfast, whereas 78% state that they eat breakfast every day of the week. The typical breakfast seems to be a meal of cereal and fruit.

Raynor et al. *(42)* recently reported on dietary variety in registry members. Prior studies have suggested that the degree of variety in the diet is correlated with BMI; those with lower BMI report less dietary variety, especially in high-fat-dense foods (sweets and snacks) and greater variety in low-fat-dense foods (vegetables). Moreover, during a behavioral weight loss program, participants report a decrease in the amount of variety in high-fat-dense food categories and an increase in the variety of fruits and vegetables. Thus, we expected this pattern to be seen in registry members. Interestingly, however, registry members reported low variety in all categories of foods including both high-fat and low-fat-dense foods. As overall dietary variety was correlated with caloric intake, it appears that registry members may reduce the variety in all categories of their diet as a means to reduce overall intake.

Low-Fat Versus Low-Carbohydrate Diets for Individuals with Diabetes

The diet consumed by members of the NWCR is quite similar to the diet typically recommended for weight loss, namely a high-carbohydrate, low-fat, energy-restricted diet *(43)*. Such diets usually recommend that no more than 20–30% of calories come from fat. These diets are consistent with governmental recommendations described in the Food Guide Pyramid *(44)* as well as recommendations of many research and medical societies, including the American Heart Association *(45)* and the American Diabetes Association *(46)*. A low-fat diet is the most commonly used in behavioral weight loss interventions *(47)*, and therefore several randomized controlled trials have evaluated outcomes of this approach. Low-fat, energy-restricted diets, when prescribed in combination with standard behavioral interventions, achieve an average of 10.4 kg of weight loss at 6 months with an 8.1 kg weight loss being maintained by 18 months *(43)*. In studies with individuals with type 2 diabetes, average weight losses tend to be slightly lower. For example, Pascale et al. *(48)* reported an average weight loss of 7.7 kg at 16 weeks in women with type 2 diabetes following a calorie-restricted and fat-restricted diet, and at 1-year follow-up, participants had maintained an average of 5.2 kg of weight loss. As noted above, low-fat, energy-restricted diets combined with lifestyle intervention have been shown to lead not only to weight loss but also to decreased risk of the development of diabetes in those at risk *(49)* and improved glycemic control in those with diabetes *(48)*.

Although a low-fat, energy-restricted diet is recommended for those with diabetes, low-carbohydrate, high-protein diets such as that promoted by Atkins *(50)* have recently become popular weight loss approaches. Although popular among the public, questions have been raised as to the safety of this type of diet. Concerns include the effect of low-carbohydrate diets on metabolic functioning, particularly in individuals with CVD, type 2 diabetes, dyslipidemia, and hypertension *(51)*. Specifically, there are concerns that such a diet may cause abnormal metabolism of insulin, promote hyperlipidemia, and impair renal function among other potential negative consequences.

Several clinical trials have compared low-fat, hypocaloric diets with low-carbohydrate diets *(52–56.)* In both treatment conditions, participants received education combined with minimal professional support. With the exception of Samaha et al. *(54)* and their 12-month follow-up *(55)*, in each study, the low-carbohydrate diet prescribed a restriction of carbohydrate intake to <20 g per day for the first 2 weeks followed by a gradual increase in the grams of carbohydrates consumed as weight loss is achieved, consistent with the Atkins diet *(50)*. Samaha et al. *(54)* prescribed a diet containing fewer than 30 g of carbohydrate per day without the increase after 2 weeks. In each of these studies, this ad libitum low-carbohydrate diet was compared with a low-fat, energy-restricted diet. At 6 months, all studies showed greater weight losses in the low-carbohydrate condition than the low-fat condition. For the low-carbohydrate diet, 6-month weight losses ranged from 5.8 to 12.0 kg, and for the low-fat diet conditions, 6-month losses ranged from 1.9 to 6.5 kg. However, in the two studies that reported 12-month follow-up data, there were no significant differences found in weight loss between the two diets *(53,55)*. Importantly, of the four studies, only Samaha et al. included individuals with type 2 diabetes, and weight losses were not reported separately by diabetes diagnosis. In addition, it is important to note that these studies achieved weight losses that are less than those seen with more intensive behavioral weight loss interventions that include regular professional contact *(43)*.

Superior weight losses found in the low-carbohydrate diets at 6 months suggest that although calories are not targeted by such approaches, participants reduce their caloric intake to a greater degree than do those in the low-fat, energy-restricted conditions, at least for a period of time. There are several potential explanations for the greater energy deficit achieved by the low-carbohydrate diets, including decreased variety in the diet leading to reduced intake *(57)*, increased satiation due to increased protein intake *(58)*, or the relative simplicity of the diet (e.g., no calorie or fat gram counting). However, as no differences in weight loss have been found with longer follow-up, long-term adherence to the low-carbohydrate approach does not appear to be superior to adherence to the low-fat approach.

Interestingly, several differences were found between these dietary prescriptions in their effects on health parameters. Three studies found that the low-carbohydrate diet was associated with greater decreases in triglycerides *(53,55,56)* and greater increases (or less decrease) in HDL cholesterol levels *(53,55,56)*. With regards to total cholesterol and low-density lipoprotein (LDL) cholesterol, there were no differences between the groups in any of the studies *(52,53,55,56)*. These findings contradict the hypothesized effect of low-carbohydrate diets on lipid levels given the increased intake of saturated fat. This may be because of the weight losses achieved by the low-carbohydrate group counteracting the adverse effect of increased saturated fat intake on LDL cholesterol concentrations *(53)*.

Three of the studies included glucose and insulin testing *(52–55)*. In the only study that included individuals with diabetes, Samaha et al. *(54)* found greater reductions in glucose levels among diabetic participants in the low-carbohydrate condition than in the low-fat condition; this difference was no longer significant at the 12-month follow-up *(55)*. However, at 12 months, diabetic participants in the low-carbohydrate condition demonstrated greater decreases in hemoglobin A1c than those in the low-fat condition. Samaha et al. *(55)* also found greater increases in insulin sensitivity among non-diabetics in the low-carbohydrate condition, but these differences were not significant at the 1-year follow-up. Foster et al. *(53)* and Brehm et al. *(52)* did not find significant differences between groups on insulin or glucose levels.

Reviewing these studies, it appears that the optimal macronutrient composition of weight loss diets for individuals with diabetes is still unclear. Unfortunately, with one exception, the randomized controlled trials comparing the low-carbohydrate and low-fat, energy-restricted approaches conducted to date have excluded participants with type 2 diabetes. In addition, studies with more extensive follow-up are needed to investigate the long-term health consequences of low-carbohydrate diets, particularly in those with diabetes and other health conditions. Preliminary findings with the low-carbohydrate diet suggest that this approach warrants further research as it produces greater initial weight losses and does not appear to negatively impact key health parameters.

Improving Dietary Adherence in Weight Loss Programs

In order for weight loss to be attained and maintained long term, adherence to a reduced-calorie diet has to be achieved. Improving adherence is particularly important in individuals with type 2 diabetes because they tend to have a more difficult time achieving and maintaining weight loss. Several approaches to improving adherence have been attempted. One of the most successful approaches has been to increase the structure and simplicity of the diet through the provision of portion-sized foods, the use of structured meal plans and shopping lists, or the use of MRs (59–61). When combined with standard behavioral treatment (SBT), each of these techniques has been shown to improve weight losses as compared with SBT alone. Jeffery et al. (59) found that providing prepackaged, portion-controlled meals for 10 meals per week significantly improved weight losses as compared with SBT throughout the full 18 months of the study (6.4 vs. 4.1 kg of weight loss at 18 months). Wing et al. (60) found that either the provision of prepackaged foods or the provision of a structured meal plan and grocery list detailing the foods that should be consumed improved weight losses after 6 months of treatment as compared with SBT; this difference remained significant a full year after treatment (and the end of provision of food or meal plans).

More recently, MRs have been utilized as a means of increasing structure and simplicity of the diet in behavioral weight loss programs (61–64). MRs are nutritionally balanced drinks or bars typically prescribed as part of a hypocaloric (1200–1500 kcal/day), low-fat (<30% kcals from fat) diet and are used to replace two meals per day with the third meal being composed of conventional foods. The use of MRs is compared with a self-selected, conventional diet with identical calorie and fat gram goals. The use of MRs has been consistently shown to improve both initial weight loss and maintenance of weight loss over the long term (62–64). Weight losses following the initial weight loss period (ranging from 8–12 weeks) ranged from 6.4–7.8% with the use of MRs compared with 1.5–4.9% in the conventional diet groups (62–64). Ditchuneit and Flechtner-Mors (62) found that significant differences between weight losses were maintained a full 4 years later when 75% of their original sample was reevaluated. The MR group maintained an average weight loss of 8.4%, whereas the conventional diet group maintained an average weight loss of 3.3%.

The use of MRs has been shown to lead to significant improvements in blood pressure, glucose, insulin, triacylglycerol, total cholesterol, and LDL cholesterol (61–64). These effects are likely due to the greater weight losses achieved.

The use of MRs in patients with type 2 diabetes has been questioned by some health care providers due to the concerns that the simple sugars in such products may lead to hyperglycemia. Yip et al. *(64)* conducted a 12-week randomized controlled trial comparing the use of two different types of MRs (one containing lactose, fructose, and sucrose and the other in which fructose and sucrose were replaced with oligosaccharides) with the use of the Exchange Diet Plan in a group of obese patients with type 2 diabetes. Those groups using MRs lost significantly more weight than the group using the Exchange Diet (6.4 and 6.7% vs. 4.9%). There were no significant differences between the two groups using MRs. Those using either MR products showed significantly lower serum glucose concentrations than those using the Exchange Diet and significant decreases over time in insulin levels and HbA1c; no serious adverse events were reported with the use of MRs in this diabetic sample.

In a recent study with obese individuals with type 2 diabetes, Redmon et al. *(65,66)* combined the use of 10 mg of Sibutramine, MRs to replace one meal and one snack per day, and the use of exclusively MRs (totaling 900–1300 kcal/day) for 7 consecutive days every 2 months. They compared this combination group to a control condition receiving standard dietary counseling recommending a reduced-calorie conventional food diet. Those in the combination therapy lost significantly more weight (6.4 vs. 0.8%) and displayed a greater decrease in HbA1c (–0.6 vs. –0.2%) than those in the standard condition at the 1-year follow-up *(65)*. After the first year, the standard group received the combination therapy for 1 year, and the combination group remained on the same regimen. At 2-year follow-up, despite continuation of the diet and medications in the combination group, significant weight regain occurred such that by the end of year 2, the combination group maintained a total of 4.6 kg; the decrease in HbA1c was marginally significant at –0.5%. However, because the standard condition received the same treatment in year 2, it is unclear whether these improvements would have been superior to standard treatment alone. In combination with Yip et al. *(64)*, this study does support the safety and efficacy of the use of MRs in individuals with type 2 diabetes.

Achieving long-term adherence to a reduced calorie diet is a major challenge in behavioral weight loss. There is consistent evidence that the use of food provision, structured meal plans, and MRs improves weight loss outcomes in both short and long term. This is likely due to the increased structure and simplicity of the diet making reduction of calories and fat easier. With such structure, there is a decreased need for measurement and planning as well as increased ease of self-monitoring. In addition, such approaches reduce the variety in the diet, which has been shown to be associated with decreased intake and body weight *(57)*. Recent work with participants with diabetes suggests that such an approach is not only safe and effective in this population but also produces greater improvements in diabetes regulation than conventional approaches.

WHAT PHYSICAL ACTIVITY STRATEGIES OPTIMIZE WEIGHT LOSS AND MAINTENANCE?

The types of physical activity recommended for overweight and obese patients with type 2 diabetes include moderate-intensity aerobic exercise such as brisk walking, swimming, bicycling, and/or circuit-type resistance training (with proper supervision) targeting major muscle groups (67,68). Regular exercise (at least 150 min per week) offers significant benefits for patients with type 2 diabetes, including improved insulin sensitivity and glycemic control, and overall reductions in mortality (69–72). In addition, frequent moderate-intensity physical activity is an important element of any weight management program and is one of the best predictors of successful weight loss maintenance (73). Given the benefits of weight management for patients with type 2 diabetes, this section will address a number of questions that have been raised regarding the role of physical activity for successful weight loss.

Is Physical Activity Alone Effective for Weight Loss?

Current recommendations indicate that physical activity should be combined with dietary change for most effective weight loss. Studies have shown that while physical activity is an important part of weight loss *maintenance*, exercise alone produces only minimal weight *loss* among overweight and obese individuals (74). This conclusion was supported by a review conducted by the Expert Panel on the Identification, Evaluation, and Treatment of Overweight and Obesity convened by the National Heart, Lung, and Blood Institute in combination with the National Institute of Diabetes and Digestive and Kidney Disease (74). The Expert Panel identified randomized controlled trials with varying sample sizes that involved at least 3–4 months of treatment examining dietary interventions, exercise interventions, and their combination. Twelve studies compared the weight loss effect of exercise alone (primarily aerobic activity) to no treatment (74). Of these studies, two revealed no weight loss benefit of exercise, whereas the other 10 showed a mean weight loss of 2.4 kg in the exercise condition compared with controls (about 2.4% of body weight). Therefore, the Expert Panel concluded that aerobic physical activity produces modest weight loss among overweight and obese adults. This conclusion is supported by several meta-analyses as well. For example, Ballor and Keesey (75) reviewed 53 studies and revealed that interventions involving aerobic activity alone (e.g., walking and running) produced a significant but modest weight loss of 1.2 kg compared with no treatment over an average of 17 weeks of treatment (0.1 kg per week). Garrow and Summerbell *(76)* showed that compared with controls, aerobic exercise alone achieved weight losses of 3.0 kg and 1.4 kg for men and women, respectively, whereas resistance training had little effect on weight loss but increased fat-free mass by approximately 2 kg in men and 1 kg in women. Similar findings have been reported for exercise-only interventions with diabetic patients. In a meta-analysis examining the effect of exercise on body mass and glycemic control in patients with type 2 diabetes, Boule and colleagues *(69)* demonstrated that while exercise-only interventions improved HbA1c, there was no significant weight loss benefit compared with controls.

Is Physical Activity Combined with Diet More Effective than Diet Alone for Weight Loss?

In an effort to answer this question, the Expert Panel reviewed 15 randomized controlled trials that compared diet plus exercise to diet alone *(74)*. Of these studies, 12 showed that combined diet and physical activity interventions produce greater mean weight loss (1.9 kg) and greater mean reduction in BMI (0.3–0.5) compared with diet-only interventions. A review by Wing *(77)* reevaluated some of the studies identified by the Expert Panel as well as several others and reported that while most studies report greater weight losses for interventions that involve diet plus exercise, only two of the 13 studies reviewed showed *statistically significant* differences in weight loss *(78,79)*. Therefore, the conclusion of Wing *(77)* is that although a majority of studies show somewhat greater weight loss in the diet plus exercise condition compared with diet alone, in most studies, the addition of exercise does not significantly increase initial weight loss above and beyond that achieved through dietary change. A meta-analysis conducted by Miller and colleagues *(80)* that compared interventions focusing on diet, exercise, and diet plus exercise supports this conclusion. This analysis showed that on average, during 16 weeks of treatment, diet and diet plus exercise interventions produced comparable weight losses (10.7 vs. 11.0 kg, respectively), and both were significantly greater than exercise-only interventions (3 kg). Studies of diabetic patients have found similar results. For example, Giannopoulou et al. *(81)* compared a 14-week program of hypocaloric high-monounsaturated diet alone, exercise alone, or diet plus exercise in postmenopausal women with type 2 diabetes and showed significant weight losses in the diet-alone and diet plus exercise groups (−4.5 kg vs. −1.7 for exercise only). Although all groups reduced waist circumference, visceral adipose tissue decreased significantly only in the exercise and diet plus exercise conditions, suggesting a unique benefit of including exercise in the treatment of women with type 2 diabetes.

Although diet plus exercise does not appear to improve short-term weight loss compared with diet alone, this combination is of benefit for longer term weight loss maintenance. For example, the Expert Panel *(74)* identified three long-term randomized controlled trials examining diet plus exercise versus diet alone and revealed that all studies obtained a 1.5–3.0 kg greater weight loss in the combined treatment over a period of 9–24 months *(78,82,83)*. In Wing's *(77)* review, two of the six long-term studies evaluated demonstrated significantly greater weight losses at 1 year or more among patients in the diet plus exercise condition compared with diet only *(78,84)*. In the meta-analysis by Miller and colleagues *(80)*, the difference in weight loss maintenance at 1-year follow-up between patients receiving diet plus exercise (8.6 kg) compared with diet alone (6.6 kg) was not significant; however, the authors concluded that combined treatment was superior, because those patients maintained 77% of initial weight loss compared with 56% for patients in diet only programs.

Although many of the studies referenced above have been conducted with non-diabetic overweight individuals, the same findings regarding the benefits of activity are seen in studies with type 2 diabetic participants. Wing et al *(78)* compared a diet-only program to diet plus exercise in overweight patients with diabetes. Both groups attended three meetings per week for the first 10 weeks and then once a week for the next 10 weeks and monthly for 1 year. All participants were given an individualized calorie goal designed to produce a 1–2 lb/week weight loss. In addition, both groups received training in behavioral weight control techniques. The diet plus exercise group walked a 3-mile route at each of their meetings and were instructed to complete a fourth exercise session each week on their own. The diet group was instructed not to change their physical activity. As expected, participants in the two conditions reported comparable changes in diet, but the diet plus exercise group reported far greater increases in caloric expenditure from exercise (619 kcal/week at baseline, 1522 kcal/week at week 10, and 1561/week kcal at 1 year) than the diet-only condition (668, 816, and 853 kcal/week at the three time periods, respectively). The differences in physical activity produced significant differences in weight loss. At the end of the 10 weeks of intensive intervention, the diet-only group had lost 5.6 kg compared with 9.3 kg in diet plus exercise; at 1-year follow-up, overall weight losses were 3.8 and 7.9 kg for diet-only and diet plus exercise, respectively. Both groups experienced improved HbA1c (–1.9 and –2.4% for diet-only and diet plus exercise at week 10 and –0.8 and –1.4% at 1-year in the two groups, respectively) demonstrating the benefit of weight loss for glycemic control. Decreases in hypoglycemic medication were more frequent and larger in the diet plus exercise group. Moreover, both changes in weight and physical activity were independently related to improvements in glycemic control.

An important consideration in evaluating long-term randomized controlled trials is exercise adherence, as adherence declines over time *(85,86)*. Data indicate that patients who report continued adherence to exercise in combination with dietary change achieve greater weight losses than those who are non-adherent. For example, Wadden et al. *(87)* showed that patients who reported exercising regularly at 1-year follow-up had maintained significantly greater weight losses (12.1 kg) than their peers who were not exercising (6.1 kg).

Additional support for the benefit of diet plus exercise for long-term maintenance of weight loss is provided by correlational studies that indicate that individuals who continue to perform the most physical activity are the ones who achieve the largest long-term weight losses *(73)*. Research comparing weight loss maintainers with regainers has shown that 90% of individuals who maintained their weight loss for at least 2 years reported exercising regularly (3 or more days/week for 30 min or more), whereas only 34% of regainers report this level of physical activity *(88)*.

How Much Exercise is Needed for Weight Loss?

There has been recent interest in determining the optimal amount of physical activity for weight loss and improved health. In the short term, there appear to be no differences in weight loss between exercising 30 min per day versus 60 min per day in addition to dietary change *(89)*. However, several studies have provided evidence for a dose–response relationship between amount of physical activity and *long-term* weight loss *(35,90,91)*. In a study comparing the impact of intermittent versus continuous exercise on weight loss among women enrolled in an 18-month behavioral weight loss program, Jakicic and colleagues *(90)* found that participants with the greatest amount of physical activity achieved the greatest weight losses. Specifically, women who exercised more than 200 min per week throughout the 18-month intervention lost more weight than those exercising 150–200 min per week and those exercising less than 150 min per week.

Similarly, data from the NWCR suggest that successful weight loss maintainers do high levels of physical activity. Over 90% of registry members report using both diet and physical activity to lose weight and to maintain their weight loss. Registry members complete the Paffenbarger Physical Activity questionnaire *(92)* that assesses the amount of walking, stair climbing, and sports activities over the prior week. Women in the registry report expending 2545 calories/week in their leisure-time activities and men report expending 3293 calories/week *(35)*. These levels have remained very consistent over the 10 years of the registry. The most frequent type of activity is walking. Over 70% of participants report walking as part of their activity, but most (50%)

report some other type of activity in addition to walking. It is estimated that registry members are exercising at least 1 h a day to achieve their high level of caloric expenditure from exercise.

The benefit of higher doses of physical activity for weight loss maintenance has also been shown in a randomized clinical trial. Jeffery and colleagues *(91)* randomly assigned overweight men and women to standard behavioral weight loss treatment that included a physical activity goal of 1000 kcal/week in energy expenditure (~30 min of physical activity per day) or standard behavioral weight loss with a high physical activity goal of 2500 kcal/week of energy expenditure (~75 min of physical activity per day). Findings showed that high levels of physical activity in the context of a behavioral weight loss program produced significantly greater weight losses at 18 months (M = 6.7 kg) compared with a standard weight loss program with conventional physical activity goals (M = 4.1 kg). Findings from all of the above studies have led to changes in the recommendations for the dose of activity for weight loss maintenance. Currently, it is recommended that individuals attempting to maintain their weight loss try to achieve at least 60 min of activity each day.

Does Physical Activity have to be Done all at Once to be Effective for Weight Loss?

One of the primary reasons provided for non-adherence to an exercise program is lack of time. In an effort to improve adherence and to develop exercise prescriptions that may be more convenient for patients, researchers have investigated the effects of dividing exercise into multiple short bouts (e.g., 4 bouts of 10 min each) compared to exercising in one longer bout (e.g., 40 min). Research suggests that exercise completed in several short bouts is at least as effective as one longer bout of exercise in terms of weight loss and in some cases may be even more effective because of its positive effect on exercise adherence. For example, Jakicic and colleagues *(93)* randomly assigned obese sedentary females enrolled in a 20-week behavioral weight loss program to either a short bout or long bout exercise regimen. Both groups had the same exercise goal, which was to gradually increase exercise to 200 min per week. The long bout group was instructed to complete their exercise in one session each day (beginning with 20 min and building up to 40 min), whereas the short bout group was instructed to engage in several 10-min exercise sessions throughout the day (beginning with 2 sessions per day and building up to 4). Participants exercising in multiple short bouts had significantly better adherence to exercise and a trend toward greater weight loss compared with the long bout group (–8.9 ± 5.3 vs. –6.4 ± 4.5 kg).

In a long-term study, Jakicic et al. *(90)* compared three different exercise formats among overweight and obese women enrolled in an 18-month behavioral weight loss program. Participants were randomly assigned to long bout exercise, multiple short bout exercise, or multiple short bout exercise plus home treadmills for the course of the study. As in the earlier study, all groups had the same goal of reaching 40 min per day of exercise on 5 days a week. Results at 18 months showed similar weight losses and improvements in cardiorespiratory fitness between the multiple short-bout and long-bout groups. Participants who received home exercise equipment maintained a higher level of exercise than the long- and multiple short-bout groups not receiving home treadmills, suggesting that access to exercise facilitates long-term adherence.

In summary, the data indicate significant benefits of physical activity for patients with type 2 diabetes, including improved insulin sensitivity, glycemic control, and weight management. Although dietary restriction appears to be the most effective for short-term weight loss, the combination of dietary change and frequent moderate-intense physical activity, such as brisk walking, is important for successful weight loss maintenance. Findings from the registry and randomized controlled trials suggest that high levels of physical activity (e.g., 200 min or more per week) are most effective. This can be done in one long bout or multiple shorter bouts throughout the day.

HOW CAN EFFECTIVE STRATEGIES BE DISSEMINATED TO MORE PEOPLE?

As this chapter has demonstrated, weight loss is highly beneficial in improving health parameters for overweight and obese individuals with diabetes. Currently, the gold standard approach to weight loss treatment is professional, face-to-face delivery of standard behavioral weight loss programs. However, this approach is time consuming and has limited accessibility to many individuals seeking weight loss. In addition, although continued treatment contact results in improved weight loss outcomes *(94–96)*, long-term studies show that participant attendance at treatment sessions decreases sharply over time *(97)*. Concern about the accessibility of gold-standard programs has led obesity researchers to develop lifestyle interventions that can be more easily disseminated by replacing face-to-face therapist contact with weight loss counseling through telephone, mail, or Internet *(98–101)*.

In a large-scale randomized trial implementing a low-cost non-clinic-based intervention, Jeffery et al. *(101)* randomly assigned 1801 overweight members of a managed care organization to usual care, telephone, or mail intervention. The two active treatment groups received 10 behaviorally based lessons on nutrition, physical activity, and behavior management. Participants in the telephone intervention received a series of phone calls from a therapist to provide guidance about each lesson and those in the mail intervention received written guidance. At 6 months, weight losses in the telephone condition (2.4 kg) were greater than usual care (1.5 kg) but not different from participants in the mail intervention (1.9 kg). No group differences were found at 12 months. Wing and colleagues *(100)* evaluated the efficacy of a telephone-assisted intervention for weight loss maintenance among 53 women who had completed a 6-month weight loss program and had lost at least 4.5 kg. Participants were randomly assigned to a no-contact control group or to receive weekly phone calls for 12 months from a research assistant who collected data about self-monitoring of weight and eating. Results at 1 year posttreatment showed that although the telephone maintenance intervention was implemented relatively easily and was successful in inducing behavioral skills such as self-monitoring, average weight *regain* in this condition (3.9 kg) was not significantly different from that in the control group (5.6 kg). The authors propose that failure to find an effect of the telephone intervention may have been because of the lack of statistical power or the fact that telephone calls were made by trained staff rather than study therapists. In another study, Kirkman et al. *(102)* used a minimal intervention designed to improve glycemic control in a sample of primary care patients with type 2 diabetes. Patients were randomly assigned to receive usual care or usual care plus monthly telephone contacts by a nurse to review their medical regimen, which included diet, exercise, medication, and glucose monitoring. At 12 months, patients receiving telephone contacts had better glycemic control and were more likely to have seen a dietitian. However, there were no group differences in weight loss, lipid profiles, or self-reported adherence to diet and exercise recommendations. Taken together, these studies suggest that while phone interventions are feasible and may have some behavioral impact, their effect on weight loss and prevention of weight regain are minimal.

Another promising area of research has involved using computer technology to disseminate standard behavioral weight loss treatment. Tate et al. *(99)* randomly assigned 92 overweight and obese participants at risk for type 2 diabetes to one of two Internet treatments: a basic Internet weight loss program in which participants received a web-based weight loss tutorial, and weekly resource links and e-mail reminders to submit weight, or a basic Internet weight loss program plus individualized e-counseling. At 12 months, patients receiving basic Internet plus individualized e-counseling achieved greater weight losses (4.4 kg) than those receiving basic Internet alone (2.0 kg). These weight losses, although less than those achieved in face-to-face behavioral programs, are comparable to clinic-based commercial programs such as Weight Watchers

(*103–105*) and are more than four times those of Internet-based commercial programs like eDiets.com *(106)*.

Researchers have also examined the utility of using the Internet to facilitate weight loss *maintenance*. For instance, Harvey-Berino and colleagues *(98)* randomized 122 overweight adults who had completed a 6-month face-to-face standard behavioral weight loss program to one of three 12-month maintenance conditions: frequent in-person support, Internet support, or minimal in-person support. At 18-month follow-up, participants receiving Internet support had sustained significantly smaller weight losses (5.7 kg) than both frequent and minimal in-person support groups (10.4 kg). These results may reflect the fact that participants found it difficult to transition from a face-to-face approach used during treatment to an Internet maintenance program, a possibility supported by a second study by Harvey-Berino et al. *(107)*. In this study, 255 overweight adults who had completed a 6-month behavioral weight loss program delivered over interactive television were randomly assigned to one of three 12-month maintenance conditions: frequent in-person support, Internet support, or minimal in-person support. At 18 months, intent to treat analyses revealed no differences in weight losses sustained across the three maintenance conditions (3.9, 4.7, and 4.2 kg) for frequent in-person, Internet support, and minimal in-person, respectively. Thus, Internet approaches may be helpful for treatment and maintenance of weight loss, but they are currently less effective than conventional face-to-face approaches.

The research discussed above demonstrates that disseminating standard face-to-face behavioral weight loss treatment through media-based alternatives is feasible and can be implemented in different settings and various modalities. Such alternative approaches eliminate the need for travel and scheduling for specific meeting times and may be more convenient for certain patients than conventional programs. The data on telephone interventions suggest that they may be beneficial for increasing certain behavioral skills such as self-monitoring but appear to have little impact on weight loss or prevention of weight regain. Internet-based standard behavioral programs appear to be more promising, but further research is needed to refine these approaches and identify individuals who are best suited to this mode of intervention.

CONCLUSION

Rapidly rising rates of obesity have been accompanied by increased prevalence of type 2 diabetes. This chapter presents evidence that lifestyle interventions that promote weight loss through diet and exercise are effective in the prevention and treatment of diabetes. The literature reviewed demonstrates that hypocaloric low-fat diets typically recommended in behavioral weight loss programs produce successful weight loss among diabetic individuals. However, preliminary studies using low-carbohydrate diets have demonstrated positive results in the short-term and warrant further investigation. Physical activity plays an important role in long-term weight management and has additional health benefits for diabetic patients including improved insulin sensitivity and glycemic control. Although there is some evidence to suggest that diabetic patients may have more difficulty achieving weight loss and may need more intensive approaches, studies show that successful weight loss is indeed possible for individuals with diabetes and results in significant health benefits.

REFERENCES

1. Diabetes Prevention Program Research Group, Reduction in the incidence of type 2 diabetes with lifestyle intervention or metformin. *New England Journal of Medicine*, 2002. 346(6): p. 393–403.
2. Tuomilehto, J., J. Lindstrom, J. Eriksson, T. Valle, H. Hamalainen, P. Ilanne-Parikka, S. Keinanen-Kiukaanniemi, M. Laakso, A. Louheranta, M. Rasta, V. Salminen, M. Uusitupa, and for the Finnish Diabetes Prevention Study Group, Prevention of type 2 diabetes mellitus by changes in lifestyle among subjects with impaired glucose tolerence. *New England Journal of Medicine*, 2001. 344: p. 1343–1350.
3. Pan, X.R., G.W. Li, Y.H. Hu, J.X. Wang, W.Y. Yang, Z.X. An, Z.X. Hu, J. Lin, J.Z. Xiao, H.B. Cao, P.A. Liu, X.G. Jiang, Y.Y. Jiang, J.P. Wang, H. Zheng, H. Zhang, P.H. Bennett, and B.V. Howard, Effects of diet and exercise in preventing NIDDM in people with impaired glucose tolerance. *Diabetes Care*, 1997. 20(4): p. 537–544.
4. Hamman, R.F., R.R. Wing, S.L. Edelstein, J.M. Lachin, G.A. Bray, L. Delahanty, M. Hoskin, A.M. Kriska, E.J. Mayer-Davis, X. Pi-Sunyer, J. Regensteiner, B. Venditti, & J. Wylie-Rosett, Effect of weight loss with lifestyle intervention on risk of diabetes. *Diabetes Care*, 2006. 29(9): p. 2102–2107.
5. Diabetes Prevention Program Research Group, Within-trial cost-effectiveness of lifestyle intervention or metformin for the primary prevention of type 2 diabetes. *Diabetes Care*, 2003. 26(9): p. 2518–2523.
6. Wing, R.R., Weight loss in the management of type 2 diabetes, in *Evidence Based Diabetes Care*, H.C. Gerstein and R.B. Haynes, Editors. 2001, BC Decker Inc.: Ontario, Canada: p. 252–276.
7. Sjostrom, C., L. Lissner, H. Wedel, and L. Sjostrom, Reduction in incidence of diabetes, hypertension and lipid distrurbances after intentional weight loss induced by bariatric surgery: the SOS intervention study. *Obesity Research*, 1999. 7(5): p. 477–484.
8. Miles, J.M., L. Leiter, P. Hollander, T.A. Wadden, J.W. Anderson, M. Doyle, J. Foreyt, L. Aronne, and S. Klein, Effect of orlistat in overweight and obese patients with type 2 diabetes treated with metformin. *Diabetes Care*, 2002. 25(7): p. 1123–1128.
9. Hollander, P.A., S.C. Elbein, I.B. Hirsch, D. Kelley, J. McGill, T. Taylor, S.R. Weiss, S.E. Crockett, R.A. Kaplan, J. Comstock, C.P. Lucas, P.A. Lodewick, W. Canovatchel, J. Chung, and J. Hauptman, Role of orlistat in the treatment of obese patients with type 2 diabetes: A 1-year randomized double-blind study. *Diabetes Care*, 1998. 21(8): p. 1288–1294.

10. Kelley, D.E., G.A. Bray, F.X. Pi-Sunyer, S. Klein, J. Hill, J. Miles, and P. Hollander, Clinical efficacy of orlistat therapy in overweight and obese patients with insulin-treated type 2 diabetes: A 1-year randomized controlled trial. *Diabetes Care*, 2002. 25(6): p. 1033–1041.

11. McNulty, S.J., E. Ur, and G. Williams, A randomized trial of sibutramine in the management of obese type 2 diabetic patients treated with metformin. *Diabetes Care*, 2003. 26(1): p. 125–131.

12. Wing, R.R., R. Koeske, L.H. Epstein, M.P. Nowalk, W. Gooding, and D. Becker, Long-term effects of modest weight loss in type II diabetic patients. *Archives of Internal Medicine*, 1987. 147: p. 1749–1753.

13. Williamson, D.F., Weight loss and mortality in persons with type-2 diabetes mellitus: A review of the epidemiological evidence. *Experimental and Clinical Endocrinology and Diabetes*, 1998. 106(Suppl 2): p. 14–21.

14. Gregg, E.W., R.B. Gerzoff, T.J. Thompson, and D.F. Williamson, Trying to lose weight, losing weight, and 9-year mortality in overweight U.S. adults with diabetes. *Diabetes Care*, 2004. 27(3): p. 657–662.

15. Wannamethee, S.G., A.G. Shaper, and L. Lennon, Reasons for intentional weight loss, unintentional weight loss, and mortality in older men. *Archives of Internal Medicine*, 2005. 165(9): p. 1035–1040.

16. Eilat-Adar, S., M. Eldar, and U. Goldbourt, Association of intentional changes in body weight with coronary heart disease event rates in overweight subjects who have an additional coronary risk factor. *American Journal of Epidemiology*, 2005. 161(4): p. 352–358.

17. Look AHEAD Research Group, Look AHEAD: Action for Health in Diabetes Design and Methods for a Clinical trial of Weight Loss for the Prevention of Cardiovascular Disease in Type 2 Diabetes. *Controlled Clinical Trials*, 2003. 24: p. 610–628.

18. Wadden, T., G.D. Foster, D.B. Sarwer, D.A. Anderson, M. Gladis, R.S. Sanderson, R.V. Letchak, R. Berkowitz, and S. Phelan, Dieting and the development of eating disorders in obese women: results of a ramdomized controlled trial. *American Journal of Clinical Nutrition*, 2004. 80(3): p. 560–568.

19. Stunkard, A.J., Binge eating disorder and the night eating syndrome, in *Handbook of Obesity Treatment*, T.A. Wadden & A.J. Stunkard, Editors. 2001, Guilford press: Newyork, p. 107–124.

20. Agras, W., C. Telch, B. Arnow, K. Eldredge, D. Wilfley, S. Raeburn, J. Henderson, and M. Marnell, Weight loss, cognitive-behavioral and desipramine treatments in binge eating disorder: *An additive design. Behavioral Therapy*, 1994. 25: p. 209–238.

21. Porzelius, L.K., C. Houston, M. Smith, C. Arfkin, and E. Fisher, Comparison of a standard behavioral weight loss treatment and a binge eating weight loss treatment. *Behavior Therapy*, 1995. 26: p. 119–134.

22. Gladis, N.M., T.A. Wadden, R. Vogt, G. Foster, R.H. Kuehnel, and S.J. Bartlett, Behavioral treatment of obese binge eaters: Do they need different care? *Journal of Psychosomatic Research*, 1998. 44: p. 375–384.

23. Wadden, T.A., G.D. Foster, and K.A. Letizia, Response of obese binge eaters to treatment by behavior therapy combined with very low calorie diet. *Journal of Consulting and Clinical Psychology*, 1992. 60(5): p. 808–811.

24. Wadden, T.A., G.D. Foster, and K.A. Letizia, One-year behavioral treatment of obesity: Comparison of moderate and severe caloric restriction and the effects of weight maintenance therapy. *Journal of Consulting and Clinical Psychology*, 1994. 62: p. 165–171.

25. National Task Force on the Prevention and Treatment of Obesity, Dieting and the development of eating disorders in overweight and obese adults. *Archive of Internal Medicine*, 2000. 160: p. 2581–2589.

26. McGuire, M., R. Wing, and J. Hill, The prevalence of weight loss maintenance among American adults. *International Journal of Obesity*, 1999. 23: p. 1314–1319.

27. Moore, L.L., A.J. Visioni, M.M. Qureshi, M.L. Bradlee, R.C. Ellison, and R. D'Agostino, Weight loss in overweight adults and the long-term risk of hypertension: The Framingham study. *Archives of Internal Medicine*, 2005. 165(11): p. 1298–1303.

28. Phelan, S. and R.R. Wing, Prevalence of successful weight loss. *Archives of Internal Medicine*, 2005. 165(20): p. 2430.

29. Field, A.E., R.R. Wing, J.E. Manson, D.L. Spiegelman, and W.C. Willett, Relationship of a large weight loss to long-term weight change among young and middle-aged US women. *International Journal of Obesity*, 2001. 25: p. 1113–1121.

30. Ford, E.S., D.F. Williamson, and S. Liu, Weight change and diabetes incidence: Findings from a national cohort of US adults. *American Journal of Epidemiology*, 1997. 146(3): p. 214–222.

31. Huang, Z., W.C. Willett, J.E. Manson, B. Rosner, M.J. Stampfer, F.E. Speizer, and G.A. Colditz, Body weight, weight change, and risk for hypertension in women. *Annals of Internal Medicine*, 1998. 128(2): p. 81–88.

32. Wing, R. and J.O. Hill, Successful weight loss maintenance. *Annual Review of Nutrition*, 2001. 21: p. 323–341.

33. McGuire, M.T., R.R. Wing, M.L. Klem, W. Lang, and J.O. Hill, What predicts weight regain in a group of successful weight losers? *Journal of Consulting and Clinical Psychology*, 1999. 67(2): p. 177–185.

34. McGuire, M.T., R.R. Wing, M.L. Klem, and J.O. Hill, Behavioral strategies of individuals who have maintained long-term weight losses. *Obesity Research*, 1999. 7(4): p. 334–341.

35. Klem, M.L., R.R. Wing, M.T. McGuire, H.M. Seagle, and J.O. Hill, A descriptive study of individuals successful at long-term maintenance of substantial weight loss. *American Journal of Clinical Nutrition*, 1997. 66: p. 239–246.

36. Wing, R.R., M.D. Marcus, L.H. Epstein, and R. Salata, Type II diabetic subjects lose less weight than their overweight nondiabetic spouses. *Diabetes Care*, 1987. 10: p. 563–566.

37. Guare, J.C., R.R. Wing, and A. Grant, Comparison of obese NIDDM and nondiabetic women; short- and long-term weight loss. *Obesity Research*, 1995. 3(4): p. 329–335.

38. Davidson, M.H., J. Hauptman, M. DiGirolamo, J.P. Foreyt, C.H. Halsted, D. Heber, D.C. Heimburger, C.P. Lucas, D.C. Robbins, J. Chung, and S.B. Heymsfield, Weight control and risk factor reduction in obese subjects treated for 2 years with orlistat: a radomized controlled trial. *Journal of the American Medical Association*, 1999. 281(3): p. 235–242.

39. Kahn, M., J.V. St. Peter, G.A. Breen, G.G. Hartley, and J.T. Vessey, Diabetes disease stage predicts weight loss outcomes with long-term appetite suppressants. *Diabetes*, 1999. 48(Suppl 1): p. A308.

40. Block, G., A.M. Hartman, C.M. Dresser, M.D. Carroll, J. Gannon, and L. Gardner, A data-based approach to diet questionnaire design and testing. *American Journal of Epidemiology*, 1986. 124: p. 453–469.

41. Wyatt, H.R., G.K. Grunwald, C.L. Mosca, M. Klem, R.R. Wing, and J.O. Hill, Long-term weight loss and breakfast in subjects in the National Weight Control Registry. *Obesity Research*, 2002. 10(2): p. 78–82.

42. Raynor, H.A., R.W. Jeffery, S. Phelan, J.O. Hill, and R.R. Wing, Amount of food group variety consumed in the diet and long-term weight loss maintenance. *Obesity Research*, 2005. 13(5): p. 883–890.

43. Wing, R.R., Behavioral approaches to the treatment of obesity, in *Handbook of Obesity: Clinical Applications*, G. Bray and C. Bouchard, Editors. 2004, Marcel Dekker Inc.: New York, p. 147–167.

44. U.S. Department of Health and Human Services and U.S. Department of Agriculture, *Dietary Guidelines for Americans*, 2005. 6th ed. U.S. Government Printing Office: Washington, DC.

45. American Heart Association, *Heart and Stroke Statistical Update*. 2000, American Heart Association: Dallas, TX.

46. American Diabetes Association, Clinical practice recommendations 1999. *Diabetes Care*, 1999. 22(Suppl 1): p. S1–S114.

47. Jeffery, R.W., A. Drewnowski, L.H. Epstein, A. Stunkard, T.G. Wilson, R.R. Wing, and D.R. Hill, Long-term maintenance of weight loss: current status. *Health Psychology*, 2000. 19(1): p. 5–16.

48. Pascale, R.W., B.A. Butler, M. Mullen, and P. Bononi, Effects of a behavioral weight loss program stressing calorie restriction versus calorie plus fat restriction in obese individuals with NIDDM or a family history of diabetes. *Diabetes Care*, 1995. 18(9): p. 1241–1248.

49. Diabetes Prevention Program Research Group, The Diabetes Prevention Program: description of the lifestyle intervention. *Diabetes Care*, 2002. 25: p. 2165–2171.

50. Atkins, R.C., *Dr. Atkins' New Diet Revolution*, rev. ed. 1992, Avon Books: New York.

51. Bravata, D.M., L. Sanders, J. Huang, H.M. Krumholz, I. Olkin, C.D. Gardner, and D.M. Bravata, Efficacy and safety of low-carbohydrate diets: a systematic review. *Journal of the American Medical Association*, 2003. 289(14): p. 1837–1850.

52. Brehm, B.J., R.J. Seeley, S.R. Daniels, and D.A. D'Alessio, A randomized trial comparing a very low carbohydrate diet and a calorie-restricted low fat diet on body weight and cardiovascular risk factors in healthy women. *Journal of Clinical Endocrinology & Metabolism*, 2003. 88(4): p. 1617–1623.

53. Foster, G., H.R. Wyatt, J.O. Hill, B.G. McGuckin, C. Brill, S. Mohammed, P.O. Szapary, D.J. Rader, J.S. Edman, and S. Klein, A randomized trial of a low-carbohydrate diet for obesity. *New England Journal of Medicine*, 2003. 348(21): p. 2082–2090.

54. Samaha, F.F., N. Iqbal, P. Seshadri, K.L. Chicano, D.A. Daily, J. McGorory, T. Williams, M. Williams, E.J. Gracely, and L. Stern, A low-carbohydrate as compared with a low-fat diet in severe obesity. *New England Journal of Medicine*, 2003. 348(21): p. 2074–2081.

55. Stern, L., N. Iqbal, P. Seshadri, K.L. Chicano, D.A. Daily, J. McGrory, M. Williams, E.J. Gracely, and F.F. Samaha, The effects of low-carbohydrate versus conventional weight loss diets in severely obese adults: One-year follow-up of a randomized trial. *Annals of Internal Medicine*, 2004. 140(10): p. 778–785.

56. Yancy, W.S., M.K. Olsen, J.R. Guyton, R.P. Bakst, and E.C. Westman, A low-carbohydrate, ketogenic diet versus a low-fat diet to treat obesity and hyperlipidemia. *Annals of Internal Medicine*, 2004. 140: p. 769–777.

57. Raynor, H.A. and L.H. Epstein, Dietary variety, energy regulation, and obesity. *Psychological Bulletin*, 2001. 127(3): p. 325–341.

58. Barkeling, B., S. Rossner, and H. Bjorvell, Effects of a high-protein meal (meat) and a high-carbohydrate meal (vegetarian) on satiety measured by automated computerized monitoring of subsequent food intake, motivation to eat and food preferences. *International Journal of Obesity*, 1990. 14(9): p. 743–751.

59. Jeffery, R.W., R.R. Wing, C. Thornson, L.R. Burton, C. Raether, J. Harvey, and M. Mullen, Strengthening behavioral interventions for weight loss: A randomized trial of food provision and monetary incentives. *Journal of Consulting and Clinical Psychology*, 1993. 61(6): p. 1038–1045.

60. Wing, R.R., R.W. Jeffery, L.R. Burton, C. Thorson, K. Sperber Nissinoff, and J.E. Baxter, Food provision vs. structured meal plans in the behavioral treatment of obesity. *International Journal of Obesity*, 1996. 20: p. 56–62.

61. Ashley, J.M., S.T. St Jeor, S. Perumean-Chaney, J. Schrage, and V. Bovee, Meal replacements in weight intervention. *Obesity Research*, 2001. 9(Suppl 4): p. 312S–320S.

62. Ditschuneit, H.H. and M. Flechtner-Mors, Value of structured meals for weight management: risk factors and long-term weight maintenance. *Obesity Research*, 2001. 9(Suppl 4): p. 284S–289S.

63. Hannum, S.M., L. Carson, E.M. Evans, K.A. Canene, E.L. Petr, L. Bui, and J.W. Erdman, Use of portion-controlled entrees enhances weight loss in women. *Obesity Research*, 2004. 12(3): p. 538–546.

64. Yip, I., V.L. Go, S. DeShields, P. Saltsman, M. Bellman, G. Thames, S. Murray, H.J. Wang, R. Elashoff, and D. Heber, Liquid meal replacements and glycemic control in obese type 2 diabetes patients. *Obesity Research*, 2001. 9(Suppl 4): p. 341S–347S.

65. Redmon, J.B., S.K. Raatz, K.P. Reck, J.E. Swanson, C.A. Kwong, Q. Fan, W. Thomas, and J.P. Bantle, One-year outcome of a combination of weight loss therapies for subjects with type 2 diabetes: a randomized trial. *Diabetes Care*, 2003. 26(9): p. 2505–2511.

66. Redmon, J.B., K.P. Reck, S.K. Raatz, J.E. Swanson, C.A. Kwong, H. Ji, W. Thomas, and J.P. Bantle, Two-year outcome of a combination of weight loss therapies for type 2 diabetes. *Diabetes Care*, 2005. 28(6): p. 1311–1315.

67. Foreyt, J.P. and W.S. Poston II, The challenge of diet, exercise and lifestyle modification in the management of the obese diabetic patient. *International Journal of Obesity and Related Metabolic Disorders*, 1999. 23(Suppl 7): p. S5–S11.

68. Sigal, R.J., G.P. Kenny, D.H. Wasserman, and C. Castaneda-Sceppa, Physical activity/exercise and type 2 diabetes. *Diabetes Care*, 2004. 27(10): p. 2518–2539.

69. Boule, N.G., E. Haddad, G.P. Kenny, G.A. Wells, and R.J. Sigal, Effects of exercise on glycemic control and body mass in type 2 diabetes mellitus: A meta-analysis of controlled clinical trials. *Journal of the American Medical Association*, 2001. 286(10): p. 1218–1227.

70. Castaneda, C., J.E. Layne, L. Munoz-Orians, P.L. Gordon, J. Walsmith, M. Foldvari, R. Roubenoff, K.L. Tucker, and M.E. Nelson, A randomized controlled trial of resistance exercise training to improve glycemic control in older adults with type 2 diabetes. *Diabetes Care*, 2002. 25(12): p. 2335–2341.

71. Church, T.S., Y.J. Cheng, C.P. Earnest, C.E. Barlow, L.W. Gibbons, E.L. Priest, and S.N. Blair, Exercise capacity and body composition as predictors of mortality among men with diabetes. *Diabetes Care*, 2004. 27(1): p. 83–88.

72. Mayer-Davis, E.J., R. D'Agostino, Jr., A.J. Karter, S.M. Haffner, M.J. Rewers, M. Saad, and R.N. Bergman, Intensity and amount of physical activity in relation to insulin sensitivity: The Insulin Resistance Atherosclerosis Study. *Journal of the American Medical Association*, 1998. 279(9): p. 669–674.

73. Pronk, N.P. and R.R. Wing, Physical activity and long-term maintenance of weight loss. *Obesity Research*, 1994. 2(6): p. 587–599.

74. National Institutes of Health National Heart Lung and Blood Institute, Clinical Guidelines on the Identification, Evaluation, and Treatment of Overweight and Obesity in Adults–The Evidence Report. *Obesity Research*, 1998. 6(Suppl 2): p. 51S–209S.

75. Ballor, D.L. and R.E. Keesey, A meta-analysis of the factors affecting exercise-induced changes in body mass, fat mass and fat-free mass in males and females. *International Journal of Obesity*, 1991. 15: p. 717–726.

76. Garrow, J.S. and C.D. Summerbell, Meta-analysis: effect of exercise, with or without dieting, on the body composition of overweight subjects. *European Journal of Clinical Nutrition*, 1995. 49: p. 1–10.

77. Wing, R.R., Physical activity in the treatment of the adulthood overweight and obesity: Current evidence and research issues. *Medicine Science Sports and Exercise*, 1999. 31(Suppl 11): p. S547–S552.

78. Wing, R.R., L.H. Epstein, M. Paternostro-Bayles, A. Kriska, M.P. Nowalk, and W. Gooding, Exercise in a behavioural weight control programme for obese patients with type 2 (non-insulin-dependent) diabetes. *Diabetologia*, 1988. 31: p. 902–909.

79. Wood, P.D., M.L. Stefanick, P.T. Williams, and W.L. Haskell, The effects on plasma lipoproteins of a prudent weight-reducing diet, with or without exercise, in overweight men and women. *New England Journal of Medicine*, 1991. 325: p. 461–466.

80. Miller, W.C., D.M. Koceja, and E.J. Hamilton, A meta-analysis of the past 25 years of weight loss research using diet, exercise or diet plus exercise intervention. *International Journal of Obesity*, 1997. 21: p. 941–947.

81. Giannopoulou, I., L.L. Ploutz-Snyder, R. Carhart, R.S. Weinstock, B. Fernhall, S. Goulopoulou, and J.A. Kanaley, Exercise is required for isceral fat loss in postmenopausal women with type 2 diabetes. *Journal of Clinical Endocrinology & Metabolism*, 2005. 90: p. 1511–1518.

82. Anderson, R.E., T.A. Wadden, S.J. Bartlett, R.S. Vogt, and R.S. Weinstock, Relations of weight loss to change in serum lipids and lipoproteins in obese women. *American Journal of Clinical Nutrition*, 1995. 62: p. 350–357.

83. Svendsen, O.L., C. Hassager, and C. Christiansen, Six months follow-up on exercise added to a short-term diet in over-weight postmenopausal women - effects on body composition, resting metabolic rate, cardiovascular risk factors and bone. *International Journal of Obesity and Related Metabolic Disorders*, 1994. 18: p. 692–698.

84. Pavlou, K.N., S. Krey, and W.P. Steffee, Exercise as an adjunct to weight loss and maintenance in moderately obese subjects. *American Journal of Clinical Nutrition*, 1989. 49: p. 1115–1123.

85. Perri, M.G., A.D. Martin, E.A. Leermakers, S.F. Sears, and M. Notelovitz, Effects of group versus home-based exercise in the treatment of obesity. *Journal of Consulting and Clinical Psychology*, 1997. 65: p. 278–285.

86. Wadden, T.A., R.A. Vogt, R.E. Andersen, S.J. Bartlett, G.D. Foster, R.H. Kuehnel, J. Wilk, R. Weinstock, P. Buckenmeyer, R.I. Berkowitz, and S.N. Steen, Exercise in the treatment of obesity: Effects of four interventions on body composition, resting energy expenditure, appetite, and mood. *Journal of Consulting and Clinical Psychology*, 1997. 65: p. 269–277.

87. Wadden, T.A., R.A. Vogt, G.D. Foster, and D.A. Anderson, Exercise and maintenance of weight loss: 1-year follow-up of a controlled clinic trial. *Journal of Consulting & Clinical Psychology*, 1998. 66(2): p. 429–433.

88. Kayman, S., W. Bruvold, and J.S. Stern, Maintenance and relapse after weight loss in women: Behavioral aspects. *American Journal of Clinical Nutrition*, 1990. 52: p. 800–807.

89. Brill, J.B., A.C. Perry, L. Parker, A. Robinson, and K. Burnett, Dose-response effect of walking exercise on weight loss. How much is enough? *International Journal of Obesity*, 2002. 26: p. 1484–1493.

90. Jakicic, J., R. Wing, and C. Winters, Effects of intermittent exercise and use of home exercise equipment on adherence, weight loss, and fitness in overweight women. *Journal of the American Medical Association*, 1999. 282(16): p. 1554–1560.

91. Jeffery, R.W., R.R. Wing, N.E. Sherwood, and D.F. Tate, Physical activity and weight loss: does prescribing higher physical activity goals improve outcome? *American Journal of Clinical Nutrition*, 2003. 78(4): p. 684–689.

92. Paffenbarger, R.S., A.L. Wing, and R.T. Hyde, Physical activity as an index of heart attack risk in college alumni. *American Journal of Epidemiology*, 1978. 108: p. 161–175.

93. Jakicic, J.M., R.R. Wing, B.A. Butler, and R.J. Robertson, Prescribing exercise in multiple short bouts versus one continuous bout: Effects on adherence, cardiorespiratory fitness, and weight loss in overweight women. *International Journal of Obesity*, 1995. 19: p. 893–901.

94. Perri, M.G., W.G. McAdoo, P.A. Spevak, and D.B. Newlin, Effect of a multicomponent maintenance program on long-term weight loss. *Journal of Consulting and Clinical Psychology*, 1984. 52(3): p. 480–481.

95. Perri, M.G., D.A. McAllister, J.J. Gange, R.C. Jordan, W.G. McAdoo, and A.M. Nezu, Effects of four maintenance programs on the long-term management of obesity. *Journal of Consulting and Clinical Psychology*, 1988. 56(4): p. 529–534.

96. Wing, R., E. Blair, and M.D. Marcus, Year-long weight loss treatment for obese patients with type II diabetes: Does inclusion of intermittent very low calorie diet improve outcome? *American Journal of Medicine*, 1994. 97: p. 354–362.

97. Wing, R.R., E.M. Venditti, J.M. Jakicic, B.A. Polley, and W. Lang, Lifestyle intervention in overweight individuals with a family history of diabetes. *Diabetes Care*, 1998. 21(3): p. 350–359.

98. Harvey-Berino, J., S. Pintauro, P. Bulzzell, M. DiGiulio, B. Casey Gold, C. Moldovan, and E. Ramirez, Does using the Internet facilitate the maintenance of weight loss? *International Journal of Obesity*, 2002. 26: p. 1254–1260.

99. Tate, D.F., E.H. Jackvony, and R.R. Wing, Efects of Internet behavioral counseling on weight loss in adults at risk for type 2 diabetes. *Journal of the American Medical Association*, 2003. 289: p. 1833–1836.

100. Wing, R.R., R.W. Jeffery, W.L. Hellerstedt, and L.R. Burton, Effect of frequent phone contacts and optional food provision on maintenance of weight loss. *Annals of Behavioral Medicine*, 1996. 18: p. 172–176.

101. Jeffery, R.W., N.E. Sherwood, K. Brelje, N.P. Pronk, R. Boyle, J.L. Boucher, and K. Hase, Mail and phone interventions for weight loss in a managed-care setting: Weigh-To-Be one-year outcomes. *International Journal of Obesity and Related Metabolic Disorders*, 2003. 27(12): p. 1584–1592.

102. Kirkman, M.S., M. Weinberger, P.B. Landsman, G.P. Samsa, E.A. Shortliffe, D.L. Simel, and J.R. Feussner, A telephone-delivered intervention for patients with NIDDM: Effect on coronary risk factors. *Diabetes Care*, 1994. 17: p. 840–846.

103. Dansinger, M.L., J.A. Gleason, J.L. Griffith, H.P. Selker, and E.J. Schaefer, Comparison of the Atkins, Ornish, Weight Watchers, and Zone diets for weight loss and heart disease risk reduction: A randomized trial. *Journal of the American Medical Association*, 2005. 293(1): p. 43–53.

104. Djuric, Z., N.M. DiLaura, I. Jenkins, L. Darga, C.K. Jen, D. Mood, E. Bradley, and W.M. Hryniuk, Combining weight-loss counseling with the Weight Watchers plan for obese breast cancer survivors. *Obesity Research*, 2002. 10(7): p. 657–665.

105. Heshka, S., J.W. Anderson, R.L. Atkinson, F.L. Greenway, J.O. Hill, S.D. Phinney, R.L. Kolotkin, K. Miller-Kovach, and F.X. Pi-Sunyer, Weight loss with self-help compared with a structured commercial program: A randomized trial. *Journal of the American Medical Association*, 2003. 289(14): p. 1792–1798.

106. Womble, L.G., T. Wadden, B.G. McGuckin, S.L. Sargent, R.A. Rothman, and E.S. Krauthamer-Ewing, A randomized controlled trial of commercial Internet weight loss programs. *Obesity Research*, 2004. 12: p. 1011–1018.
107. Harvey-Berino, J., S. Pintauro, P. Buzzell, and E.C. Gold, Effect of Internet support on the long-term maintenance of weight loss. *Obesity Research*, 2004. 12: p. 320–329.

12 Unifying Hypothesis of Diabetic Complications

Takeshi Matsumura, MD, and Michael Brownlee, MD

SUMMARY

Over the past four decades, several molecular mechanisms have been implicated in glucose-mediated vascular damage: increased flux through the polyol pathway, accumulation of advanced glycation endproduct precursors, activation of protein kinase C isoforms, and increased hexosamine pathway activity. Each of these mechanisms has been studied independently of the others, and there has been no apparent common element linking them. Recent discoveries have made clear that all of these seemingly unrelated mechanisms arise from a single, hyperglycemia-induced process: the overproduction of reactive oxygen species by the mitochondrial electron transport chain.

Key Words: Hyperglycemia, reactive oxygen species, diabetic complications

INTRODUCTION

Chronic hyperglycemia and development of diabetes-specific microvascular complications in retina, peripheral nerve, and renal glomerulus are characteristic of all forms of diabetes. As a consequence of its microvascular

From: *Contemporary Endocrinology: Controversies in Treating Diabetes: Clinical and Research Aspects*
Edited by: D. LeRoith and A. I. Vinik © Humana Press, Totowa, NJ

pathology, diabetes is the leading cause of blindness, various debilitating neuropathies, and end-stage renal disease. Diabetics are the fastest growing group of renal dialysis and transplant recipients, and in the USA, their 5-year survival rate is only 21%, worse overall than that for all forms of cancer combined. Over 60% of diabetic patients suffer from neuropathy, which includes mononeuropathies, distal symmetrical polyneuropathy, and various autonomic neuropathies causing erectile dysfunction, urinary incontinence, gastroparesis, and nocturnal diarrhea. Fifty percent of all nontraumatic amputations in the USA are due to diabetic peripheral neuropathy, often in conjunction with lower extremity arterial disease (National Diabetes Data Group, Diabetes in America, 2nd edition, National Institutes of Health, NIH Publication 95–1468, 1995). Atherosclerotic macrovascular disease affecting arteries that supply the heart, brain, and lower extremities is also a characteristic feature of chronic diabetes. This condition resembles the macrovascular disease in nondiabetic patients; however, the atherosclerotic process is more extensive, more rapidly progressive, and characterized by a greater incidence of multi-vessel disease and an increased number of diseased vessel segments compared with nondiabetic patients *(1)*. As a consequence, patients with diabetes have a much higher risk of myocardial infarction, stroke, and limb amputation. Although macrovascular complications are often thought to occur primarily in type II diabetics, a recent study of type 1 diabetics in their 40s showed that coronary artery atheromatosis was present in all subjects *(2)*.

The Diabetes Control and Complications Trial (DCCT) and the U.K. Prospective Diabetes Study (UKPDS) established that hyperglycemia is the initiating cause of the diabetic tissue damage that we see clinically *(3,4)*. This process is modified by both genetic determinants of individual susceptibility and independent accelerating factors such as hypertension or hyperlipidemia. The mechanisms by which hyperglycemia causes micro- and macrovascular damages are discussed.

Increased Flux Through the Polyol Pathway

Aldose reductase normally has the function of reducing toxic aldehydes in the cell to inactive alcohols, but when the glucose concentration in the cell becomes too high, aldose reductase also reduces that glucose to sorbitol, which is later oxidized to fructose. In the process of reducing high intracellular glucose to sorbitol, the aldose reductase consumes the cofactor NADPH *(5)*. However, NADPH is also the essential cofactor for regenerating a critical intracellular antioxidant, reduced glutathione. By reducing the amount of reduced glutathione, we found that the polyol pathway increases susceptibility to intracellular oxidative stress. It has been reported that nerve conduction velocity in the diabetic dogs decreased over time as it does in patients; however, in diabetic dogs treated with an aldose reductase inhibitor, the diabetes-induced defect in nerve conduction velocity was prevented *(6)*.

Intracellular Production of Advanced Glycation Endproduct Precursors

Advanced glycation endproducts (AGEs) are found in increased amounts in diabetic retinal vessels *(7)* and renal glomeruli *(8)*, where they can cause damage. These AGEs were originally thought to arise from nonenzymatic reactions between extracellular proteins and glucose. However, it seems likely that intracellular hyperglycemia is the primary initiating event in the formation of both intracellular and extracellular AGEs *(9)*. These AGE precursors can diffuse out of the cell and modify extracellular matrix molecules nearby *(10)*, which changes signaling between the matrix and the cell and causes cellular dysfunction *(11)*. These AGE precursors also modify circulating proteins, such as albumin, in the blood. These modified circulating proteins can then bind to AGE receptors and activate them, thereby causing the production of inflammatory cytokines and growth factors, which in turn cause vascular pathology *(12–21)*. The potential importance of AGEs in the pathogenesis of diabetic complications is suggested by the observation in animal models that two structurally unrelated AGE inhibitors partially prevented various functional and structural manifestations of diabetic microvascular disease in retina, kidney, and nerve *(22–24)*. In endothelial cells exposed to high glucose, intracellular AGE formation occurs within 1 week *(25)*. Proteins involved in macromolecular endocytosis are modified by AGEs, as the increase in endocytosis induced by hyperglycemia is prevented by overexpression of the methylglyoxal-detoxifying enzyme glyoxalase I *(26)*. Glyoxalase-I overexpression also completely prevents the hyperglycemia-induced increase in Muller cell expression of angiopoietin-2 *(27)*, a factor that has been implicated in both pericyte loss and capillary regression *(28)*, suggesting that hyperglycemia-induced production of methylglyoxal is one of the accelerators of diabetic complication. Moreover, in a large randomized, double-blind, placebo-controlled, multi-center trial of the AGE inhibitor aminoguanidine in type I diabetic patients with overt nephropathy, aminoguanidine lowered total urinary protein and slowed progression of nephropathy, over and above the effects of existing optimal care. In addition, aminoguanidine reduced the progression of diabetic retinopathy (K.K. Bolton, personal communication).

Activation of Protein Kinase C

Protein kinase C (PKC) comprises a family of at least eleven isoforms, nine of which are activated by the lipid second messenger diacylglycerol (DAG). Hyperglycemia inside the cell increases DAG content primarily by increasing its de novo synthesis from the glycolytic intermediate dihydroxyacetonephosphate by reduction to glycerol-3-phosphate and stepwise acylation *(29)*. Increased de novo synthesis of DAG activates PKC in cultured vascular cells *(30,31)* as well as in retina and glomeruli of diabetic animals *(29,30)*. When PKC is activated by intracellular hyperglycemia, it has various effects on gene expression, examples of which are shown in the row of open boxes in Fig. 1. In each case, the things that are good for normal function are decreased and the things that are bad are increased. For example, starting from the far left of Fig. 1, the vasodilator-producing endothelial nitric oxide (NO) synthase (eNOS) is decreased, whereas the vasoconstrictor endothelin-1 is increased. Transforming growth factor-β and plasminogen activator inhibitor-1 are also increased. At the bottom of Fig. 1, the row of black boxes lists the pathological effects that may result from the abnormalities in the open boxes *(32–36)*. It is well known that hyperglycemia-induced PKC activation is important from many animal studies such as several published by George King, showing that inhibition of PKC prevented early changes in the diabetic retina and kidney *(33,37,38)*.

Increased Hexosamine Pathway Activity

Excess intracellular glucose may also cause several manifestations of diabetic complications by increasing flux through the hexosamine pathway *(39,40)*. As shown schematically in Fig. 2, when glucose is high inside a cell,

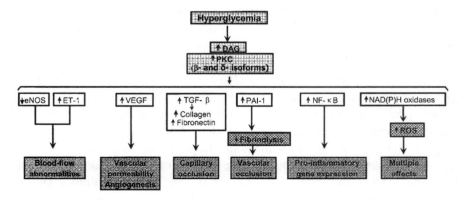

Fig. 1. Consequences of hyperglycemia-induced activation of protein kinase C (PKC).

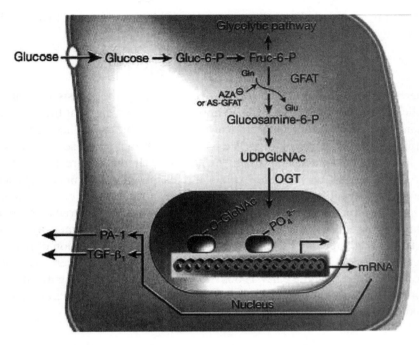

Fig. 2. Hyperglycemia increases flux through the hexosamine pathway. From ref. *45a.*

most of that glucose is metabolized through glycolysis, going first to glucose-6-phosphate, then fructose-6-phosphate, and then on through the rest of the glycolytic pathway. However, some of that fructose-6-phosphate gets diverted into a signaling pathway in which an enzyme called glutamine : fructose-6-phosphate amidotransferase (GFAT) converts the fructose-6-phosphate to glucosamine-6-phosphate and finally to uridine diphosphate (UDP) N-acetyl glucosamine. What happens after that is the N-acetyl glucosamine gets put onto serine and threonine residues of transcription factors, just like the more familiar process of phosphorylation, and overmodification by this glucosamine often results in pathologic changes in gene expression *(39–41)* For example, in Fig. 2, increased modification of the transcription factor Sp1 results in increased expression of transforming growth factor-β1 and plasminogen activator inhibitor-1, both of which are bad for diabetic blood vessels *(42).* Although this hexosamine pathway is the most recent to be recognized as a factor in the pathogenesis of diabetic complications, it has been shown to play a role both in hyperglycemia-induced abnormalities of glomerular cell gene expression *(39)* and in hyperglycemia-induced cardiomyocyte dysfunction in cell culture *(43).* In carotid artery plaques from type 2 diabetic subjects, modification of endothelial cell proteins by the hexosamine pathway is also significantly increased *(44)*.

A UNIFIED MECHANISM

There are many reports that are involved in the pathogenesis of diabetic complications. However, there was no apparent common element linking these mechanisms to each other, and clinical trials of inhibitors of these pathways in patients were all disappointing. We hypothesized that all these mechanisms were linked to a common upstream event and that the failure to block all the downstream pathways could explain the disappointing clinical trials with single-pathway inhibitors. We discovered this single unifying process, which is the overproduction of superoxide by the mitochondrial electron transport chain. We have reported that a consistent differentiating feature common to all cell types that are damaged by hyperglycemia is an increased production of reactive oxygen species (ROS) *(42,45)*. Although hyperglycemia had been associated with oxidative stress in the early 1960s *(46)*, neither the underlying mechanism that produced it nor its consequences for pathways of hyperglycemic damage were known.

How Does Hyperglycemia Increase Superoxide Production by the Mitochondria?

There are four protein complexes in the mitochondrial electron transport chain, called complexes I, II, III, and IV (Fig. 3). When glucose is metabolized through the tricarboxylic acid (TCA) cycle, it generates electron donors. The main electron donor is NADH, which gives electrons to complex I. The other electron donor generated by the TCA cycle is $FADH_2$, formed by succinate dehydrogenase, which donates electrons to complex II. Electrons from both these complexes are passed to coenzyme Q, and then from coenzyme Q they are transferred to complex III, cytochrome-C, complex IV, and finally to molecular oxygen, which they reduce to water. The electron transport system is organized in this way so that the level of ATP can be precisely regulated. As electrons are transported from left to right as shown in Fig. 3, some of the energy of those electrons is used to pump protons across the membrane at complexes I, III, and IV. This generates what is in effect a voltage across the mitochondrial membrane. The energy from this voltage gradient drives the synthesis of ATP by ATP synthase *(47,48)*. Alternatively, uncoupling proteins (UCPs; Fig. 3) can bleed down the voltage gradient to generate heat as a way of keeping the rate of ATP generation constant. On the contrary, in diabetic cells with high glucose inside, there is more glucose being oxidized in the TCA cycle, which in effect pushes more electron donors (NADH and $FADH_2$)

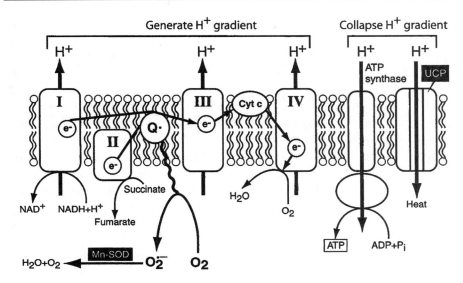

Fig. 3. Hyperglycemia-induced production of superoxide by the mitochondrial electron transport chain.

into the electron transport chain. As a result of this, the voltage gradient across the mitochondrial membrane increases until a critical threshold is reached. At this point, electron transfer inside complex III is blocked *(49)*, causing the electrons to back up to coenzyme Q, which donates the electrons one at a time to molecular oxygen, thereby generating superoxide (Fig. 3). The mitochondrial isoform of the enzyme superoxide dismutase (SOD) degrades this oxygen-free radical to hydrogen peroxide, which is then converted to H_2O and O_2 by other enzymes. Indeed, we looked at diabetic cells with a dye that changes color with increasing voltage of the mitochondrial membrane and found that intracellular hyperglycemia did indeed increase the voltage across the mitochondrial membrane above the critical threshold necessary to increase superoxide formation *(50)*. To prove that the electron transport chain indeed produces superoxide by the mechanism we proposed, we examined the effect of overexpressing either UCP-1 or manganese SOD (MnSOD) on hyperglycemia-induced ROS generation. Hyperglycemia caused a big increase in production of ROS. In contrast, an identical level of hyperglycemia does not increase ROS at all when we also collapse the mitochondrial voltage gradient by overexpressing UCP *(45)*. Similarly, hyperglycemia does not increase ROS at all when we degrade superoxide by overexpressing the enzyme MnSOD. These data demonstrate two things. First, the UCP effect shows that the mitochondrial electron transport chain is the source of the hyperglycemia-induced superoxide. Second, the MnSOD effect shows that the initial ROS formed is indeed superoxide. We further examined the effect of either UCP-1 overexpression or MnSOD overexpression on each of these four hyperglycemia-activated pathways. Hyperglycemia did not activate any of the pathways when either the voltage gradient across the mitochondrial membrane was collapsed by UCP-1 or the superoxide produced was degraded by MnSOD *(45)*. We have verified all these endothelial cell culture experiments in transgenic mice that overexpress MnSOD (M. Brownlee, personal communication). When wild-type animals are made diabetic, all four of the pathways are activated in tissues where diabetic complications occur. In contrast, when MnSOD transgenic mice are made diabetic, there is no activation of any of the four pathways. In endothelial cells, PKC also activates nuclear factor κB (NF κB), a transcription factor that itself activates many proinflammatory genes in the vasculature. As expected, hyperglycemia-induced PKC activation is prevented by either UCP-1 or MnSOD, both in cells and in animals. Importantly, inhibition of hyperglycemia-induced superoxide overproduction using a transgenic approach (SOD) also prevents long-term experimental diabetic nephropathy in the best animal model of this complication: the *db/db* diabetic mouse *(51)*.

Hyperglycemia-Induced Mitochondrial Superoxide Production Activates the Four Damaging Pathways by Inhibiting Glyceraldehyde-3-Phosphate Dehydrogenase

Figure 4 shows the scheme we proposed for how all these data link together. This model is based on a critical observation we made: diabetes in animals and patients, and hyperglycemia in cells, all decrease the activity of the key glycolytic enzyme glyceraldehyde-3-phosphate dehydrogenase (GAPDH). Inhibition of GAPDH activity by hyperglycemia does not occur when mitochondrial overproduction of superoxide is prevented by either UCP-1 or MnSOD *(42)*. As shown in Fig. 4, the level of all the glycolytic intermediates that are upstream of GAPDH increases. Increased levels of the upstream glycolytic metabolite glyceraldehyde-3-phosphate activates two of the four pathways. It activates the AGE pathway because the major intracellular AGE precursor methylglyoxal is formed from glyceraldehyde-3-phosphate. It also activates the classic PKC pathway, as the activator of PKC, DAG, is also formed from glyceraldehyde-3-phosphate. Further upstream, levels of the glycolytic metabolite fructose-6-phosphate increase, which increases flux through the hexosamine pathway, where fructose-6-phosphate is converted by the enzyme GFAT to UDP–N-acetylglucosamine (UDP–GlcNAc). Finally, inhibition of GAPDH increases intracellular levels of the first glycolytic metabolite, glucose. This increases flux through the polyol pathway, where

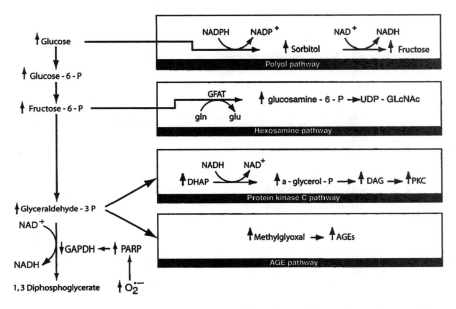

Fig. 4. Mitochondrial overproduction of superoxide activates four major pathways of hyperglycemic damage by inhibiting GAPDH. From ref. *45a.*

the enzyme aldose reductase reduces it, consuming NADPH in the process. To rule out the possibility that any other hyperglycemia-induced metabolic change accounted for these observations, we inhibited GAPDH activity using antisense DNA, so that the level of GAPDH activity in cells cultured in 5 mmol/L (90 mg/dL) glucose was reduced to that normally found in cells exposed to hyperglycemia. With reduced GAPDH activity, the only perturbation in these cells, the activity of each of the four pathways in 5 mmol/L glucose was elevated to the same extent as that induced by hyperglycemia *(52)*.

Hyperglycemia-Induced Mitochondrial Superoxide Production Inhibits GAPDH by Activating Poly(ADP-Ribose) Polymerase

To clarify the mechanism of inactivation of GAPDH, we next investigated the chemical modifications of GAPDH that correlated with the hyperglycemia-induced decrease in GAPDH activity. Hyperglycemia-induced superoxide inhibits GAPDH activity in vivo by modifying the enzyme with polymers of ADP-ribose (Fig. 5) *(52)*. By inhibiting mitochondrial superoxide production with either UCP-1 or MnSOD, we prevented both modification of GAPDH by ADP-ribose and reduction of its activity by hyperglycemia. Most importantly, both modification of GAPDH by ADP-ribose and reduction of its

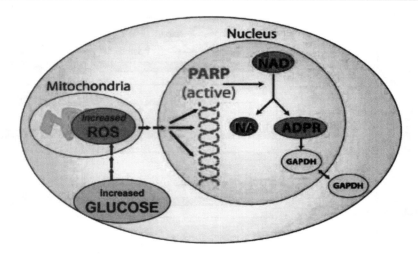

Fig. 5. Reactive oxygen species (ROS)-induced DNA damage activates poly(ADP-ribose) polymerase (PARP) and modifies GAPDH.

activity by hyperglycemia were also prevented by a specific inhibitor of poly(ADP-ribose) polymerase (PARP), the enzyme that makes these polymers of ADP-ribose. This established a cause-and-effect relationship between PARP activation and the changes in GAPDH. Normally, PARP resides in the nucleus in an inactive form, waiting for DNA damage to activate it (Fig. 5). When increased intracellular glucose generates increased ROS in the mitochondria, these free radicals induce DNA strand breaks, thereby activating PARP. Both hyperglycemia-induced processes are prevented by either UCP-1 or MnSOD *(52)*. Once activated, PARP splits the NAD$^+$ molecule into its two component parts: nicotinic acid and ADP-ribose. PARP then proceeds to make polymers of ADP-ribose, which accumulate on GAPDH and other nuclear proteins. Although GAPDH is commonly thought to reside exclusively in the cytosol, in fact it normally shuttles in and out of the nucleus, where it plays a critical role in DNA repair *(53,54)*. A schematic summary showing the elements of the unified mechanism of hyperglycemia-induced cellular damage is shown in Fig. 6. When intracellular hyperglycemia develops in target cells of diabetic complications, it causes increased mitochondrial production of ROS. The ROS cause strand breaks in nuclear DNA, which activate PARP. PARP then modifies GAPDH, thereby reducing its activity. Finally, decreased GAPDH activity activates the polyol pathway, increases intracellular AGE formation, activates PKC and subsequently NFκB, and activates hexosamine pathway flux.

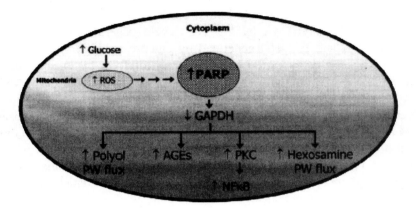

Fig. 6. The unifying mechanism of hyperglycemia-induced cellular damage.

How Does the Unifying Mechanism Explain Diabetic Macrovascular Disease?

Although the pathogenesis of diabetic microvascular complications can be explained by the unifying mechanism described in the preceding section (A UNIFYING MECHANISM), the relationship between a unifying mechanism and diabetic macrovascular disease is not fully understood. Using both cell culture and animal models, we found that the unappreciated consequence of insulin resistance is increased free fatty acid (FFA) flux from adipocytes into arterial endothelial cells (Fig. 7). In macrovascular, but not in microvascular, endothelial cells, we found that this increased flux results in increased FFA

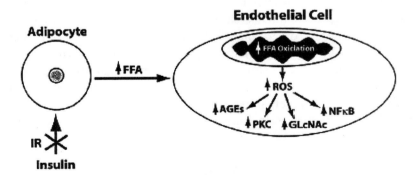

Fig. 7. Insulin resistance causes mitochondrial overproduction of reactive oxygen species (ROS) in macrovascular endothelial cells by increasing free fatty acid (FFA) flux and oxidation. From ref. *55a*.

oxidation by the mitochondria. As both β-oxidation of fatty acids and oxidation of FFA-derived acetyl CoA by the TCA cycle generate the same electron donors (NADH and FADH^2) generated by glucose oxidation, increased FFA oxidation causes mitochondrial overproduction of ROS by exactly the same mechanism described in the preceding section (A UNIFYING MECHANISM) for hyperglycemia. And, as with hyperglycemia, this FFA-induced increase in ROS activates the same damaging pathways: AGEs, PKC, the hexosamine pathway (GlcNAc), and NF κB. In insulin-resistant nondiabetic animal models, inhibition of either FFA release from adipocytes or FFA oxidation in arterial endothelium prevents the increased production of ROS and its damaging effects *(55)*. Although more work certainly needs to be done, these data support a major role for the unifying mechanism in the pathogenesis of diabetic macrovascular, as well as microvascular, complications.

NOVEL THERAPEUTIC APPROACHES

Transketolase Activators

When increased superoxide inhibits GAPDH activity, the glycolytic intermediates above the enzyme accumulate and are then shunted into the four pathways of hyperglycemic damage. Two of these glycolytic intermediates, fructose-6-phosphate and glyceraldehyde-3-phosphate, are also the final products of the transketolase reaction, which is the rate-limiting enzyme in another metabolic pathway, the pentose phosphate pathway *(56)*. Although this pathway is traditionally taught as flowing from pentose phosphates to glycolytic intermediates, in fact it can also flow from glycolytic intermediates to pentose phosphates, depending on the concentrations of substrate presented to the transketolase enzyme. As we know that in diabetes, the concentration of the glycolytic intermediates is high, we reasoned that if we could activate transketolase, then we could decrease the concentration of these two glycolytic metabolites and thus divert their flux away from three of the damaging pathways normally activated by hyperglycemia. As this enzyme requires the vitamin thiamine as a cofactor, we tried different thiamine derivatives and measured their effects. After 9 months of diabetic rats treated with benfotiamine, there was a complete prevention of hexosamine pathway activation and diabetes-induced increases in intracellular AGE formation, PKC activation, and NF κB activation *(56)*.

PARP Inhibitors

Although we had shown that increased superoxide produced by the mitochondria in response to both hyperglycemia and increased FFA activates PARP, and that this PARP activation then modifies and inhibits GAPDH

(Fig. 5), we predicted that that PARP inhibition would block the four major pathways of hyperglycemic damage that are activated by GAPDH inhibition. In cultured endothelial cells, a specific PARP inhibitor prevents hyperglycemia-induced activation of PKC, NF κB, intracellular AGE formation, and the hexosamine pathway *(48)*. In long-term experimental diabetes, treatment with a PARP inhibitor also completely prevented the major structural lesion of both human nonproliferative retinopathy and experimental diabetic retinopathy: acellular capillaries (H.P. Hammes, M. Brownlee, personal communications).

Catalytic Antioxidants

The enzymes that are particularly important for vascular biology are eNOS and prostacyclin synthase. eNOS is a very important antiatherogenic enzyme with great relevance to diabetic macrovascular disease. Prostacyclin synthase is also critical endothelial antiatherosclerotic enzyme. To prevent direct oxidative inactivation of these key enzymes, we must directly reduce the amount of superoxide. However, conventional antioxidants are unlikely to do this effectively. Conventional antioxidants neutralize reactive oxygen molecules on a one-for-one basis, whereas hyperglycemia-induced over production of superoxide is a continuous process. What is needed, then, is a new type of antioxidant, a catalytic antioxidant, such as an SOD/catalase mimetic *(57)*, that works continuously like the enzymes for which these compounds are named. Hyperglycemia-induced reactive oxygen overproduction directly reduces eNOS activity in diabetic aortas by 65%. However, when these diabetic animals are treated with an SOD/catalase mimetic, there is no reduction in activity of this antiatherogenic enzyme. Similarly, but more dramatically, hyperglycemia-induced reactive oxygen overproduction directly reduces prostacyclin synthase activity in diabetic aortas by 95%. Treatment of these diabetic animals with an SOD/catalase mimetic completely prevents diabetes-induced oxidative inactivation of aortic prostacyclin synthase. These data strongly suggest that therapeutic correction of diabetes-induced superoxide production may be a powerful new approach for preventing diabetic complications.

REFERENCES

1. Granger CB, Califf RM, Young S, Candela R, Samaha J, Worley S, Kereiakes DJ, Topol EJ. Outcome of patients with diabetes mellitus and acute myocardial infarction treated with thrombolytic agents. The Thrombolysis and Angioplasty in Myocardial Infarction (TAMI) Study Group. *J Am Coll Cardiol* 21: 920–925, 1993.
2. Larsen J, Brekke M, Sandvik L, Arnesen H, Hanssen KF, Dahl-Jorgensen K. Silent coronary atheromatosis in type 1 diabetic patients and its relation to long-term glycemic control. *Diabetes* 51: 2637–2641, 2002.

3. The Diabetes Control and Complications Trial Research Group. The effect of intensive treatment of diabetes on the development and progression of long-term complications in insulin-dependent diabetes mellitus. *N Engl J Med* 329: 977–86, 1993.

4. UK Prospective Diabetes Study (UKPDS) Group. Intensive blood-glucose control with sulphonylureas or insulin compared with conventional treatment and risk of complications in patients with type 2 diabetes (UKPDS 33). *Lancet* 352: 837–53, 1998.

5. Lee AY, Chung SS. Contributions of polyol pathway to oxidative stress in diabetic cataract. *FASEB J* 13: 23–30, 1999.

6. Engerman RL, Kern TS, Larson ME. Nerve conduction and aldose reductase inhibition during 5 years of diabetes or galactosaemia in dogs. *Diabetologia* 37: 141–144, 1994.

7. Stitt AW, Li YM, Gardiner TA, Bucala R, Archer DB, Vlassara H. Advanced glycation end products (AGEs) co-localize with AGE receptors in the retinal vasculature of diabetic and of AGE-infused rats. *Am J Pathol* 150: 523–531, 1997.

8. Horie K, Miyata T, Maeda K, Miyata S, Sugiyama S, Sakai H, van Ypersole de Strihou C, Monnier VM, Witztum JL, Kurokawa K. Immunohistochemical colocalization of glycoxidation products and lipid peroxidation products in diabetic renal glomerular lesions. Implication for glycoxidative stress in the pathogenesis of diabetic nephropathy. *J Clin Invest* 100: 2995–3004, 1997.

9. Degenhardt TP, Thorpe SR, Baynes JW. Chemical modification of proteins by methylglyoxal. *Cell Mol Biol (Noisy.-Le-Grand)* 44: 1139–1145, 1998.

10. McLellan AC, Thornalley PJ, Benn J, Sonksen PH. Glyoxalase system in clinical diabetes mellitus and correlation with diabetic complications. *Clin Sci (Lond)* 87: 21–29, 1994.

11. Charonis AS, Reger LA, Dege JE, Kouzi-Koliakos K, Furcht LT, Wohlhueter RM, Tsilibary EC. Laminin alterations after in vitro nonenzymatic glycosylation. *Diabetes* 39: 807–814, 1990.

12. Li YM, Mitsuhashi T, Wojciechowicz D, Shimizu N, Li J, Stitt A, He C, Banerjee D, Vlassara H. Molecular identity and cellular distribution of advanced glycation endproduct receptors: relationship of p60 to OST-48 and p90 to 80K-H membrane proteins. *Proc Natl Acad Sci USA* 93: 11047–11052, 1996.

13. Neeper M, Schmidt AM, Brett J, Yan SD, Wang F, Pan YC, Elliston K, Stern D, Shaw A. Cloning and expression of a cell surface receptor for advanced glycosylation end products of proteins. *J Biol Chem* 267: 14998–15004, 1992.

14. Smedsrod B, Melkko J, Araki N, Sano H, Horiuchi S. Advanced glycation end products are eliminated by scavenger-receptor-mediated endocytosis in hepatic sinusoidal Kupffer and endothelial cells. *Biochem J* 322: 567–573, 1997.

15. Vlassara H, Li YM, Imani F, Wojciechowicz D, Yang Z, Liu FT, Cerami A. Identification of galectin-3 as a high-affinity binding protein for advanced glycation end products (AGE): a new member of the AGE-receptor complex. *Mol Med* 1: 634–646, 1995.

16. Abordo EA, Thornalley PJ. Synthesis and secretion of tumour necrosis factor-alpha by human monocytic THP-1 cells and chemotaxis induced by human serum albumin derivatives modified with methylglyoxal and glucose-derived advanced glycation endproducts. *Immunol Lett* 58: 139–147, 1997.

17. Doi T, Vlassara H, Kirstein M, Yamada Y, Striker GE, Striker LJ. Receptorspecific increase in extracellular matrix production in mouse mesangial cells by advanced glycosylation end products is mediated via platelet derived growth factor. *Proc Natl Acad Sci USA* 89: 2873–2877, 1992.

18. Kirstein M, Aston C, Hintz R, Vlassara H. Receptor-specific induction of insulin-like growth factor I in human monocytes by advanced glycosylation end product-modified proteins. *J Clin Invest* 90: 439–446, 1992.

19. Schmidt AM, Hori O, Chen JX, Li JF, Crandall J, Zhang J, Cao R, Yan SD, Brett J, Stern D. Advanced glycation endproducts interacting with their endothelial receptor induce expression of vascular cell adhesion molecule-1 (VCAM-1) in cultured human endothelial cells and in mice: a potential mechanism for the accelerated vasculopathy of diabetes. *J Clin Invest* 96: 1395–1403, 1995.

20. Skolnik EY, Yang Z, Makita Z, Radoff S, Kirstein M, Vlassara H. Human and rat mesangial cell receptors for glucose-modified proteins: potential role in kidney tissue remodelling and diabetic nephropathy. *J Exp Med* 174: 931–939, 1991.

21. Vlassara H, Brownlee M, Manogue KR, Dinarello CA, Pasagian A. Cachectin/TNF and IL-1 induced by glucose-modified proteins: role in normal tissue remodeling. *Science* 240: 1546–1548, 1988.

22. Hammes HP, Martin S, Federlin K, Geisen K, Brownlee M. Aminoguanidine treatment inhibits the development of experimental diabetic retinopathy. *Proc Natl Acad Sci USA* 88: 11555–11558, 1991.

23. Nakamura S, Makita Z, Ishikawa S, Yasumura K, Fujii W, Yanagisawa K, Kawata T, Koike T. Progression of nephropathy in spontaneous diabetic rats is prevented by OPB-9195, a novel inhibitor of advanced glycation. *Diabetes* 46: 895–899, 1997.

24. Soulis-Liparota T, Cooper M, Papazoglou D, Clarke B, Jerums G. Retardation by aminoguanidine of development of albuminuria, mesangial expansion, and tissue fluorescence in streptozocin-induced diabetic rat. *Diabetes* 40: 1328–1334, 1991.

25. Giardino I, Edelstein D, Brownlee M. Nonenzymatic glycosylation in vitro and in bovine endothelial cells alters basic fibroblast growth factor activity. A model for intracellular glycosylation in diabetes. *J Clin Invest* 94: 110–117, 1994.

26. Shinohara M, Thornalley PJ, Giardino I, Beisswenger P, Thorpe SR, Onorato J, Brownlee M. Overexpression of glyoxalase-I in bovine endothelial cells inhibits intracellular advanced glycation endproduct formation and prevents hyperglycemia-induced increases in macromolecular endocytosis. *J Clin Invest* 101: 1142–1147, 1998.

27. Yao D, Taguchi T, Matsumura T, et al. (2007). Hyperglycemia Increases Angiopoietin-2 transcription in microvascular endothelial cell through methylglyoxal modification of mSin3A. *J Biol Chem* 2007, (*in press*).

28. Maisonpierre PC, Suri C, Jones PF, Bartunkova S, Wiegand SJ, Radziejewski C, Compton D, McClain J, Aldrich TH, Papadopoulos N, Daly TJ, Davis S, Sato TN, Yancopoulos GD. Angiopoietin-2, a natural antagonist for Tie2 that disrupts in vivo angiogenesis. *Science* 277: 55–60, 1997.

29. Koya D, King GL. Protein kinase C activation and the development of diabetic complications. *Diabetes* 47: 859–866, 1998.

30. Derubertis FR, Craven PA. Activation of protein kinase C in glomerular cells in diabetes. Mechanisms and potential links to the pathogenesis of diabetic glomerulopathy. *Diabetes* 43: 1–8, 1994.

31. Xia P, Inoguchi T, Kern TS, Engerman RL, Oates PJ, King GL. Characterization of the mechanism for the chronic activation of diacylglycerol-protein kinase C pathway in diabetes and hypergalactosemia. *Diabetes* 43: 1122–1129, 1994.

32. Koya D, Jirousek MR, Lin YW, Ishii H, Kuboki K, King GL. Characterization of protein kinase C beta isoform activation on the gene expression of transforming growth factor-beta, extracellular matrix components, and prostanoids in the glomeruli of diabetic rats. *J Clin Invest* 100: 115–126, 1997.

33. Ishii H, Jirousek MR, Koya D, Takagi C, Xia P, Clermont A, Bursell SE, Kern TS, Ballas LM, Heath WF, Stramm LE, Feener EP, King GL. Amelioration of vascular dysfunctions in diabetic rats by an oral PKC beta inhibitor. *Science* 272: 728–731, 1996.

34. Kuboki K, Jiang ZY, Takahara N, Ha SW, Igarashi M, Yamauchi T, Feener EP, Herbert TP, Rhodes CJ, King GL. Regulation of endothelial constitutive nitric oxide synthase gene expression in endothelial cells and in vivo: a specific vascular action of insulin. *Circulation* 101: 676–681, 2000.

35. Studer RK, Craven PA, Derubertis FR. Role for protein kinase C in the mediation of increased fibronectin accumulation by mesangial cells grown in high-glucose medium. *Diabetes* 42: 118–126, 1993.

36. Feener EP, Xia P, Inoguchi T, Shiba T, Kunisaki M, King GL. Role of protein kinase C in glucose- and angiotensin II-induced plasminogen activator inhibitor expression. *Contrib Nephrol* 118: 180–187, 1996.

37. Bishara NB, Dunlop ME, Murphy TV, Darby IA, Sharmini Rajanayagam MA, Hill MA. Matrix protein glycation impairs agonist-induced intracellular Ca^{2+} signaling in endothelial cells. *J Cell Physiol* 193: 80–92, 2002.

38. Koya D, Haneda M, Nakagawa H, Isshiki K, Sato H, Maeda S, Sugimoto T, Yasuda H, Kashiwagi A, Ways DK, King GL, Kikkawa R. Amelioration of accelerated diabetic mesangial expansion by treatment with a PKC beta inhibitor in diabetic db/db mice, a rodent model for type 2 diabetes. *FASEB J* 14: 439–447, 2000.

39. Kolm-Litty V, Sauer U, Nerlich A, Lehmann R, Schleicher ED. High glucose-induced transforming growth factor beta1 production is mediated by the hexosamine pathway in porcine glomerular mesangial cells. *J Clin Invest* 101: 160–169, 1998.

40. Sayeski PP, Kudlow JE. Glucose metabolism to glucosamine is necessary for glucose stimulation of transforming growth factor-alpha gene transcription. *J Biol Chem* 271: 15237–15243, 1996.

41. Wells L, Hart G. O-GlcNAc turns twenty: functional implications for posttranslational modification of nuclear and cytosolic protein with a sugar. *FEBS Lett* 546: 154–158, 2003.

42. Du XL, Edelstein D, Rossetti L, Fantus IG, Goldberg H, Ziyadeh F, Wu J, Brownlee M. Hyperglycemia-induced mitochondrial superoxide overproduction activates the hexosamine pathway and induces plasminogen activator inhibitor-1 expression by increasing Sp1 glycosylation. *Proc Natl Acad Sci USA* 97: 12222–12226, 2000.

43. Clark RJ, McDonough PM, Swanson E, Trost SU, Suzuki M, Fukuda M, Dillmann WH. Diabetes and the accompanying hyperglycemia impairs cardiomyocyte calcium cycling through increased nuclear O-GlcNAcylation. *J Biol Chem* 278: 44230–44237, 2003.

44. Federici M, Menghini R, Mauriello A, Hribal ML, Ferrelli F, Lauro D, Sbraccia P, Spagnoli LG, Sesti G, Lauro R. Insulin-dependent activation of endothelial nitric oxide synthase is impaired by O-linked glycosylation modification of signaling proteins in human coronary endothelial cells. *Circulation* 106: 466–472, 2002.

45. Nishikawa T, Edelstein D, Du, XL, Yamagishi S, Matsumura T, Kaneda Y, Yorek MA, Beebe D, Oates PJ, Hammes HP, Giardino I, Brownlee M. Normalizing mitochondrial superoxide production blocks three pathways of hyperglycaemic damage. *Nature* 404: 787–790, 2000.

45a. Brownlee M. Biochemistry and molecular cell biology of diabetic complications. *Nature* 414: 813–820, 2001.

46. Giugliano D, Ceriello A, Paolisso G. Oxidative stress and diabetic vascular complications. *Diabetes Care* 19: 257–267, 1996.

47. Wallace DC. Diseases of the mitochondrial DNA (Review). *Annu Rev Biochem* 61: 1175–1212, 1992.

48. Trumpower BL. The protonmotive Q cycle: energy transduction by coupling of proton translocation to electron transfer by the cytochrome bc1 complex. *J Biol Chem* 265: 11409–11412, 1990.

49. Korshunov SS, Skulachev VP, Starkov AA. High protonic potential actuates a mechanism of production of reactive oxygen species in mitochondria. *FEBS Lett* 416: 15–18, 1997.

50. Du, XL, Edelstein D, Dimmeler S, Ju Q, Sui C, Brownlee M. Hyperglycemia inhibits endothelial nitric oxide synthase activity by posttranslational modification at the Akt site. *J Clin Invest* 108: 1341–1348, 2001.

51. DeRubertis FR, Craven PA, Melhem MF, Salah EM. Attenuation of renal injury in db/db mice overexpressing superoxide dismutase: evidence for reduced superoxide–nitric oxide interaction. *Diabetes* 53: 762–768, 2004.

52. Du X, Matsumura T, Edelstein D, Rossetti L, Zsengeller Z, Szabo C, Brownlee M. Inhibition of GAPDH activity by poly(ADP-ribose) polymerase activates three major pathways of hyperglycemic damage in endothelial cells. *J Clin Invest* 112: 1049–1057, 2003.

53. Sawa A, Khan AA, Hester LD, Snyder SH. Glyceraldehyde-3-phosphate dehydrogenase: nuclear translocation participates in neuronal and nonneuronal cell death. *Proc Natl Acad Sci USA* 94: 11669 –11674, 1997.

54. Schmidtz HD. Reversible nuclear translocation of glyceraldehyde-3-phosphate dehydrogenase upon serum depletion. *Eur J Cell Biol* 80: 419–427, 2001.

55. Du X, Edelstein D, Obici S, Higham N, Zou MH, Brownlee M. Insulin resistance reduces arterial prostacyclin synthase and eNOS activities by increasing endothelial fatty acid oxidation. *J Clin Invest* 116: 1071–1080, 2006.

55a. Hofmann S, Brownlee M. Biochemistry and molecular cell biology of diabetic complications: a unifying mechanism. In Diabetes Mellitus: A Fundamental and Clinical Text. 3rd ed. LeRoith D, Taylor SI, Olefsky JM, Eds. Philadelphia, Lippincott Williams & Wilkins, pp. 1441–1457, 2004.

56. Hammes HP, Du, X, Edelstein D, Taguchi T, Matsumura T, Ju Q, Lin J, Bierhaus A, Nawroth P, Hannak D, Neumaier M, Bergfeld R, Giardino I, Brownlee M. Benfotiamine blocks three major pathways of hyperglycemic damage and prevents experimental diabetic retinopathy. *Nat Med* 9: 294–299, 2003.

57. Salvemini D, Wang ZQ, Zweier JL, Samouilov A, Macarthur H, Misko TP, Currie MG, Cuzzocrea S, Sikorski JA, Riley DP. A nonpeptidyl mimic of superoxide dismutase with therapeutic activity in rats. *Science* 286: 304–306, 1999.

13 The Diabetic Foot

Andrew J. M. Boulton, MD, DSC (HONS), FRPC

CONTENTS

SUMMARY

Diabetic foot problems remain all too common and are likely to increase in prevalence over the next few decades. It has been estimated that an individual with diabetes now has a 25% risk of developing a foot ulcer at some time during their lifespan. A number of controversies are discussed in this chapter starting with the key question of the best screening methods for the "at risk foot" for ulceration. The key message is that simple clinical techniques of examination of the feet and lower limbs are probably the most accurate way to assess for further risk of foot lesions. A foot ulcer will normally heal if the circulation is intact, infection is treated and pressure is taken off the lesion. Physicians find it hard to believe that patients with large plantar foot lesions would actually walk on this lesion, but they forget that sensory loss in the diabetic foot permits walking without discomfort. Thus offloading is frequently neglected and if applied properly, will lead to satisfactory healing

From: *Contemporary Endocrinology: Controversies in Treating Diabetes:
Clinical and Research Aspects*
Edited by: D. LeRoith and A. I. Vinik © Humana Press, Totowa, NJ

in most plantar neuropathic ulcers. In the area of infection, the key question is whether an ulcer is infected or colonized and this is discussed in some detail as is the differential diagnosis between osteomyelitis and Charcot neuroarthropathy. The use and abuse of expensive topical treatments is then discussed and finally the role of footwear in the prevention of recurrent ulcers is described.

Key Words: Diabetic neuropathy, diabetic foot ulceration, charcot neuroarthropathy, offloading, foot infection.

INTRODUCTION

2005 was an important year for the diabetic foot as the International Diabetes Federation chose the diabetic foot and reducing amputations as their focus topic for that year. It was estimated that in 2005, for every 30 s a lower limb is lost somewhere in the world as a consequence of diabetes *(1)*. This is a particularly depressing statistic because of all the late complications of diabetes, foot problems are probably the most preventable. Thus, over 70 years ago, Joslin wrote that "Diabetic gangrene is not heaven sent, but earth born." Thus, the development of foot ulceration results from the way we care for our patients or the way in which patients care for themselves. These observations suggest that early identification of those patients with risk factors for the development of foot problems, followed by their education in prevention, should ultimately lead to a reduction in foot ulcers and consequently amputations. This was the focus of the Year of the Diabetic Foot during which there were news conferences and publicity in every continent and the publication of a book "Time to Act" which focused on many aspects of the identification and management of those at risk of foot problems *(2)*.

As the lifetime incidence of foot ulceration in diabetic patients was recently estimated to be as high as 25% *(3)*, understanding the pathways that result in the development of an ulcer is increasingly important. A number of controversies regarding the diagnosis and management of diabetic foot problems will be included in this chapter. Surprisingly, controversy remains as how best to identify those at risk of foot problems: a clear understanding of the etiopathogenesis of ulceration is essential if we are to succeed in reducing the incidence of foot ulceration and ultimately amputations. As the vast majority of amputations are preceded by foot ulcers, a thorough understanding of the causative pathways to ulceration is important if we are to reduce the depressingly high incidences of ulceration and amputation *(4)*. Moreover, as lower limb complications are the commonest precipitants of hospitalization in diabetic patients in most Western countries, there are potential economic benefits to be gained from preventative strategies *(1)*.

Other controversies relating to the management of foot problems to be discussed in this chapter include the question of offloading the foot wound and how best to achieve this, the role of footwear in preventing foot ulcers, the question of infection and its management, the difference between Charcot neuroarthropathy (CN) and osteomyelitis, and finally, the place of some of the expensive adjunctive therapies in the management of diabetic foot wounds.

HOW TO SCREEN FOR THE "AT-RISK" FOOT

Pathway to Ulceration

Despite the increased attention that has been focused on the diabetic foot in recent years (5), particularly in 2005, routine screening for diabetic patients to assess their risk of foot lesions remains woefully inadequate. Tapp et al. (6), for example, reported that in a population-based study from Australia that foot screening remained poor with less than one half of the population reporting a regular examination for foot complications. A number of groups have programs in communities to improve screening of the diabetic foot: when such a system was established in Idaho, the proportion of patients receiving the recommended annual foot exam increased by 14% (7). However, much remains to be done: failure to screen and identify risk factors for foot ulceration may have disastrous consequences as illustrated in Fig. 1 (8). When discussing the optimal screening method for use in day-to-day clinical practice, it is important to have an understanding of the pathways that result in diabetic foot ulceration.

Foot ulceration invariably results from an interaction of a number of component causes, none of which is sufficient alone to cause ulceration but, when combined, complete the causal pathway to skin breakdown. Knowledge of these component causes and their potential to interact facilitates the design of preventive foot programs. These include all three components of diabetic neuropathy (sensory, motor, and autonomic), peripheral vascular disease, callus deformity, and high foot pressures and trauma. Chronic sensorimotor neuropathy is common as noted in Chapter 7, and it has been estimated that up to 50% of older type 2 diabetic patients have risk factors for foot ulceration (9). As many of these patients may have no neuropathic symptoms and be completely aware of their risk, the diagnosis can only be made by careful clinical examination. Sympathetic autonomic dysfunction affecting the lower limbs results in reduced sweating, dry skin, and the development of cracks and fissures. In the absence of large vessel arterial disease, there may be increased blood flow to the foot leading to the warm but "at-risk" foot. The importance of neuropathy is a major contributory cause to foot ulceration has been

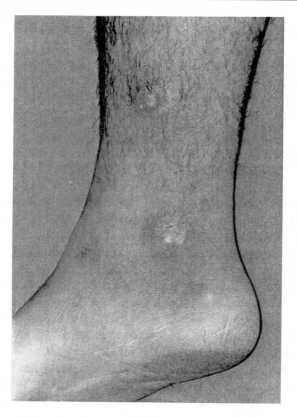

Fig. 1. This demonstrates the dangers of failing to screen the feet of diabetic patients regularly for foot ulcer risks. This patient had never had a foot screen, and when he developed neuropathic symptoms, he sought treatment from alternative medicine. These burns are caused by the inappropriate application of "moxibustion"—the application of a burning incense stick to meridians for people with vascular disease. This patient could feel no pain, and the burning sticks remained for too long and too close giving rise to symmetrical burns on the limb.

confirmed: the risk in those with neuropathy is seven-fold higher than in those without *(10)*.

Peripheral vascular disease is also more common in diabetic patients, and in combination with minor trauma, this may lead to ulceration. Early identification of those at risk for peripheral vascular disease is essential, and appropriate investigation involving non-invasive studies together with arteriography may lead to bypass surgery or angioplasty to improve blood flow to the extremities.

Motor dysfunction, with imbalance of the flex or extensor muscles in the foot, frequently results in foot deformity, with prominent metatarsal heads and clawing of the toes. In turn, the combination of proprioceptive loss due to neuropathy and prominence of the metatarsal heads may lead to increased foot pressures and loads under the diabetic foot, whereas plantar callus has been shown in cross-sectional and prospective studies to be a significant marker of foot ulcer risk, removal of plantar callus is associated with the reduction in foot pressures and thus a reduction in foot ulcer risk *(11)*.

It is the combination of two or more of the earlier described risk factors that usually results in diabetic foot ulceration. In 1999, a North American/UK collaborative study assessed risk factors that resulted in ulceration in more than 150 consecutive foot ulcer cases. From this study, a number of causal pathways were identified but the most common triad of component causes that was present in nearly two-thirds of ulcers comprised neuropathy, deformity, and trauma *(12)*. This summarizes the risk factors and pathways that result in ulceration, but it must also be remembered that the most "at-risk" patient is the individual with a past history of foot ulceration or amputation (Fig. 2).

Suggestions for Screening

It is essential that all patients with diabetes should have at least annually an assessment of their risk for the development of foot problems. Those found to have risk factors require more frequent review, education in self foot care, and podiatric assessment. There is, however, no universal consensus as to how this screening should be carried out. The following are recommended:

HISTORY

1. Neuropathic symptoms.
2. Past history of ulcer.
3. Other diabetic problems, especially retinopathy/impaired vision.
4. History of claudication/rest pain/vascular surgery.
5. Home circumstances—for example, living alone.

EXAMINATION

Inspection. Shoes and socks must be removed.

1. Skin status: thickness, dryness, and cracking.
2. Infection: check between the toes as well.
3. Ulceration.
4. Deformity: for example, Charcot changes or clawing of the toes.
5. Foot shape.
6. Skin temperature: compare the feet. A unilateral, warm swollen foot with intact skin would suggest the possibility of acute CN. Moreover, prior to neuropathic ulceration, there is a local increase in temperature *(13)*.

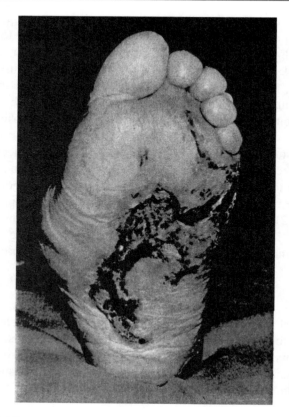

Fig. 2. The "at-risk" neuropathic foot. This demonstrates wasting of muscles in the lower tibial region and in the intrinsic muscles of the foot. There are signs of diabetic dermopathy on the lower shins, dystrophic nails, and prominent metatarsal heads. There is some clawing of the lateral toes.

7. The patient's footwear and gait should also be assessed. Walking without a limp with a plantar ulcer is diagnostic of neuropathy.

Neurological Assessment

1. Neuropathy can easily be documented by a simple clinical examination of large fiber function (e.g., 128-Hz tuning fork for vibration), small fiber function (e.g., pin prick and hot/cold rods), and ankle reflexes. A simple composite score comprising these measures has been shown to be useful in the prediction of those at risk of future ulceration (10).
2. Ten-gram monofilament—this tests pressure perception and is frequently used to assess foot ulcer risk status (14). Although simple to perform, general agreement is lacking as to which site should be tested, and not all filaments accurately assess pressure at 10 g (15). Moreover, the number of sites that

should be tested is unknown: for example, the 128-Hz tuning fork vibration assessment tested at two sites was recently shown to be as sensitive as the monofilament tested at eight sites *(16)*.

Vascular Assessment

1. Posterior tibial and dorsalis pedis pulses should be palpated.
2. Bedsides, assessment of the circulation using a doppler ultrasound probe can be useful. However, the presence of diabetes and neuropathy make the usual tests such as the ankle brachial index (AB1) less efficacious: wave form analysis and toe pressures are more effective *(17)*. Although it was suggested in a recent American Diabetes Association Consensus Statement *(18)* that all patients over 50 years of age with diabetes should have an annual measurement of the ABI, this has not been universally accepted. As noted above, neuropathy and vascular calcification might lead to false elevation in the ABI inaccurate. Thus, a patient with neuropathy and "stiffened arteries" might have an apparently normal ABI in the presence of peripheral vascular disease. In summary, for the vascular assessment, a careful clinical examination of the foot assessing the peripheral pulses and skin temperature may be sufficient for the annual review.

OTHER ASSESSMENTS

Other more detailed assessments such as quantitative sensory testing (QST) and foot pressure studies may be added in specialist centers but are not necessary in routine clinical practice *(9)*. The use of simple semi-quantitative mat systems for assessment of foot pressure may be useful. PressureStat, for example, is an inexpensive and semi-quantitative foot print mat that takes only a minute or two to measure, and higher pressures are associated with darker areas. This can provide a powerful educational tool to help patients understand which areas under their foot are at particular risk *(19)*. In summary, although some controversy remains regarding which particular simple clinical test should be used in the annual foot screening, the most important step that could be taken to reduce amputations in diabetes as emphasized during the Year of the Diabetic Foot *(1)*would be that every time a patient with diabetes was seen by a physician or any other health care professional, the shoes and socks should be removed and a careful clinical inspection of the foot should be made.

QST

1. Vibration assessment: The biothesiometer, neurothesiometer, and vibration perception threshold (VPT) meters are simple, hand-held tests of vibration perception that can easily be used in the outpatient setting: loss of vibration as assessed with these instruments is strongly predictive of subsequent ulceration *(19)*.

2. Temperature perception: A new hand-held instrument, the NeuroQuick *(20)*, that tests cold sensation is now available. This may in future be useful in screening for early neuropathy.
3. Other QST instruments: Other more elaborate equipments to assess distal sensory function are available *(16)*. However, most of these are expensive and time consuming and restricted to clinical research usage.
4. Electrophysiology: Although nerve conduction studies strongly predict future ulcers *(20)*, their use is generally restricted to clinical research studies.

OFFLOADING: ITS IMPORTANCE AND APPLICATION

It is generally accepted that a diabetic foot wound will heal if three factors are attended to:

1. There is adequate arterial inflow to the foot.
2. The wound is debrided and any infection treated with appropriate antibiotics.
3. Pressure over the wound and surrounding area is minimized.

It is the last of these three points that is frequently neglected. A normal individual with a foot wound will limp to avoid putting pressure on the wound as this is painful, hence the early observation in leprosy that a patient who walks on a plantar wound without limping must have neuropathy. Peripheral sensory loss in patients with diabetes therefore permits weight bearing on an active plantar ulcer, which in turn impairs healing. Thus, the use of a total contact cast (TCC) was proposed first in leprosy and second in diabetes to manage the patient with a plantar neuropathic ulcer. The principal of this treatment is that pressure is mitigated, but in addition, as the device is irremovable, adherence with the treatment is enforced and mobility is reduced. Following a number of published case series, the first randomized trial of casting was published by Mueller et al. in 1989. In this study, significantly faster healing was reported in the TCC compared with accommodative footwear with an absolute risk reduction of 59%. Subsequent to this and previous studies, the TCC was accepted as the gold standard for managing the plantar neuropathic ulcer by the American Diabetes Association *(22)*, although a systematic review concluded that further confirmatory studies were required. A second, larger randomized trial was performed in which the TCC was compared with a removable cast walker (RCW) and half shoe *(23)*. Again, the TCC proved superior to the other two modalities. Surprisingly, previous gait laboratory studies had confirmed that the RCW reduces pressure to approximately the same degree as the TCC *(24)*, leaving the question as to why the TCC was consistently superior in terms of wound healing compared to the RCW.

The most likely answer is related to patient adherence to wearing the RCW. A subsequent study tested this hypothesis and confirmed that although patients with plantar diabetic foot ulcers were asked to wear the RCW whenever they were walking, in practice they only wore the device for 28% of all footsteps *(25)*. Thus, the main reason for the poorer performance of the RCW in clinical trials was indeed due to the fact that these were frequently not worn while walking. Accordingly, an alternative to the TCC was proposed by Armstrong et al. *(26)* and named the "instant total contact cast" (iTCC). This technique involves taking an RCW and rendering it irremovable by wrapping it with one or two bands of plaster of paris, therefore addressing most of the disadvantages of the TCC but preserving irremovability. Two recent randomized controlled trials using the iTCC have confirmed that (i) the iTCC has equal efficacy to the TCC in healing plantar foot wounds *(27)* and (ii) that the iTCC is superior in terms of healing rates when compared with the RCW *(28)*.

Evidence from Italy suggests that maintained pressure on a wound maintains the chronicity of a lesion: after a period of offloading, a chronic neuropathic foot ulcer has many of the histopathological features of an acute wound, with angiogenesis and granulation *(29)*. These important observations strongly suggest that repetitive pressure on a neuropathic foot wound contributes to the chronicity of the wound, and offloading therefore can help to promote wound healing. It was therefore proposed in an editorial that future trials of new treatments for diabetic foot ulcers should have standardized offloading, preferably irremovable using a TCC or iTCC, thereby removing one of the most important confounding variables that has probably contributed to many negative clinical trials of proposed new therapies for neuropathic foot ulcers *(30)*.

Two recent publications provide further help in the use of total contact casting. First, it was shown that the TCC can be used not only in neuropathic ulcers but also effectively in neuroischemic ulcers, provided that there is no evidence of infection *(31)*. The same group later confirmed that it is safe to use TCC recurrently in patients who have repetitive episodes of foot ulcer *(32)*.

INFECTION OR COLONIZATION

Controversy has existed for many years regarding the management of infection in diabetic foot wounds, regarding whether or not the wound is infected, and regarding which antibiotics to use and for how long to continue treatment.

Some help in this difficult area has come from the International Consensus Working Group on diagnosing and treating the infected diabetic foot, which published guidelines in 2004 *(33)*. With respect to the diagnosis of infection, it must be remembered that all skin wounds harbor microorganisms, and therefore, the diagnosis of infection is a clinical one and not a microbiological one. Help in the diagnosis can be made by looking for clinical systemic signs of infection such as purulent secretions or at least two local findings of inflammation (including redness, warmth, induration, pain, and tenderness). Other signs that might suggest infection include the presence of necrosis, a foul odor, or failure of a properly treated wound to heal.

Any wound showing clinical signs suggestive of infection should be cultured, and this is best achieved using a curette, a wound biopsy, wound aspiration that should be obtained aseptically from the base of a wound after debridement.

With respect to treatment, those with a severe infection should usually be hospitalized for possible surgical intervention, control of metabolic derangement, and other forms of resuscitation.

For less severe infection, outpatient treatment is possible remembering that management of infection is only one of the aspects of wound management. The initial choice of antibiotic regimen is usually empirical, and commonly used agents would include Clindamycin, Augmentin (Amoxycillin and Clavulanic acid), or a cephalosporin.

Detailed management of diabetic foot infections is beyond the scope of this chapter, and readers are directed to some excellent recent reviews (33,34). Another rhetorical question relates to the duration of antibiotic treatment: again, this should be judged clinically, but there is little evidence to suggest that antibiotics should be continued until complete wound healing is achieved.

One of the dangers of overuse of antibiotics is the development of resistant organisms such as Methicillin-resistant staphylococcus Aureus (MRSA). Reports suggest that MRSA is increasing in diabetic foot clinics (35,36). However, the presence of MRSA is usually suggestive of opportunistic colonization rather than true pathogenetic infections. There is generally no indication to use specific agents active against MRSA unless this organism is clinically suspected as the primary pathogen.

OSTEOMYELITIS OR CHARCOT NEUROARTHROPATHY?

CN is a progressive condition affecting the bones and joints of the foot and is characterized by joint dislocation, subluxation, and pathological fractures of the foot in neuropathic patients resulting often in debilitating deformities. Permissive features for the development of CN include both peripheral and autonomic neuropathy, an intact peripheral circulation, and some form of trauma although this may go unnoticed in neuropathic patients. CN typically presents with a unilateral warm, swollen, and sometimes painful foot. Diagnosis at this stage and early intervention may prevent the progression to the typical deformities seen in chronic CN (Fig. 3). Unfortunately, as many such cases are painless, acute CN is often misdiagnosed as a variety of other conditions

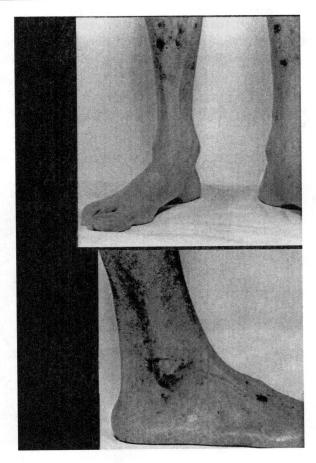

Fig. 3. Healing burn to Charcot foot. This shows chronic deformity due to Charcot neuroarthropathy at the cuneiform-metatarsal joints. This patient felt that his feet were cold, so he sat in front of the fire but unfortunately fell asleep. An example of a preventable deformity and a preventable injury.

including cellulitus, osteomyelitis, or even an inflammatory arthropathy. The differential diagnosis from osteomyelitis can be difficult as both can be associated with local warmth, erythema, and swelling. However, in a patient with a history of minor trauma and the absence of any skin breaks in the foot, the clinical diagnosis should be that of CN until proven otherwise. A further problem can be that the x-ray might be normal in the early stages of both osteomyelitis and CN.

    In contrast, the diagnosis of osteomyelitis is more likely if there is active ulceration, particularly if bone is visible or palpable at the base of the ulcer. If the involved area is one of the toes, the so-called sausage toe, a red swollen digit *(37)*, frequently indicates underlying osteomyelitis. The "probe-to-bone" test using a sterile blunt metal probe that is positive when the distinctive gritty or stony feeling of bone is encountered is highly suggestive of osteomyelitis *(38)*. Although osteomyelitis has typical radiological changes, these tend to occur late (Fig. 4) and therefore are not particularly helpful in the early differential diagnosis between CN and osteomyelitis.

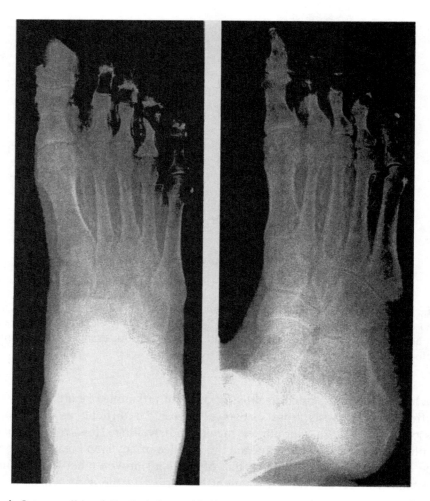

Fig. 4. Osteomyelitis of distal phalanx of hallux. Note, first, the extensive vascular calcification and even periarticular calcification. A soft tissue defect is seen at the apex of the hallux with bony destruction typical of osteomyelitis.

Perhaps, the most useful tests in differentiating between these two conditions in the acute or early stages are the three-phase ^{111}In-labelled leukocyte (white blood cell) scan and magnetic resonance imaging (MRI) *(34)*.

ARE EXPENSIVE ADJUNCTIVE THERAPIES JUSTIFIED TO HEAL THE DIABETIC FOOT WOUND?

A number of new and mostly expensive adjunctive therapies have been proposed to enhance wound healing in the diabetic foot *(20,21)*. These include platelet-derived growth factors, skin substitutes, negative pressure wound therapy (NPWT) and hyperbaric oxygen (HBO): this review considers the last two of these.

Over the last few years, NPWT has emerged as a commonly employed option in the treatment of complex wounds including diabetic foot lesions. This involves the delivery of intermittent or continuous sub-atmospheric pressure through a specialized pump connected to a resilient open-celled foam surface dressing covered with an adhesive drape to maintain a closed environment. NPWT appears to optimize blood flow, decrease local tissue oedema, remove excessive discharge, and exudate and promote the development of healthy granulation tissue. Until recently, the only support for the use of this therapy in complex diabetic foot wounds has come from published case series. A recent study *(39)*, however, provides evidence from a randomized controlled clinical trial to support the use of NPWT in complex wounds usually after surgery in the diabetic foot. Patients were randomized either to NPWT or standard therapy that comprised moist wound care according to consensus guidelines. NPWT was delivered through the vacuum-assisted closure (VAC) therapy system. This study confirmed more rapid healing in the NPWT group and a trend toward fewer amputations in the NPWT group compared with standard treatment.

A recent consensus conference focusing entirely on targeting diabetic foot wounds considered the use of NPWT and agreed that this should be reserved for larger, deeper, and often post-surgical debridement/partial foot amputation wounds. It was also agreed that NPWT should be used until there is healthy granulation tissue: NPWT may even be used in conjunction with removable offloading by bridging the tubing from the plantar surface to the dorsum of the foot *(40)*. In conclusion, it appears that NPWT is a useful adjunct to healing complex diabetic foot wounds often in the post-operative situation.

Even more controversy surrounds the use of HBO in diabetic foot wounds. The evidence for HBO in the diabetic foot was reviewed by Bakker in 2000, and it was concluded that multiple anecdotal reports and retrospective studies of HBO therapy in diabetic foot wounds suggested some efficacy, but because most of these published studies suffered from methodological problems, HBO could not be recommended at this time as standard therapy in patients with foot ulcers *(41)*. If HBO was to be used, Bakker suggested that those most likely to benefit would have ischemic lesions treated unsuccessfully by standard methods when amputation seems a possibility. This review has been followed by several further randomized controlled trials. The first of these *(42)* was in patients without vascular disease and suggested that HBO might improve the healing rate. However, as many of these ulcers were plantar lesions, they may well have been better treated with appropriate offloading rather than expensive HBO. Another randomized trial looked at patients with ischemic non-healing lower extremity ulcers and provided evidence that HBO might enhance healing of such lesions and could be a valuable adjunct to conventional treatment.

A subsequent Cochrane analysis suggested that there might be some benefit for HBO in patients with ischemic lesions, the modest number of patients, methodological shortcomings, and poor reporting in trials suggested that such results need to be interpreted with caution. Thus in this area, there is still a need for an appropriately powered trial with high methodological rigor to confirm the potential benefits of HBO in ischemic diabetic foot wounds.

THE ROLE OF FOOTWEAR

It may seem surprising that the role of footwear appears as a controversial issue in overall diabetic foot care. However, although it is well recognized that inappropriate footwear is a major cause of injury to the insensate foot *(3,4,12)*, the role of special shoes in the protection of the neuropathic feet from recurrent ulceration is far less clear *(43)* although there is almost universal clinical opinion and experience that appropriate therapeutic footwear can reduce the incidence of primary and recurrent ulceration. Several small studies have suggested that patients randomized to therapeutic footwear after ulcer healing had a lower incidence of recurrent ulcers *(43,44)*. The most recent trial *(45)* by Reiber et al. *(43)* surprisingly found no benefit of specialist footwear in reducing recurrent ulcer rates although this study was somewhat controversial because of the unusual patient population recruited and the type of shoe gear chosen. Moreover, guidelines for the prescription of footwear are not well established, and few practitioners measure plantar pressures at previous ulcer sites to ensure that high pressures are reduced by the footwear *(20,43)*. Research is ongoing into the use of computer-aided design and manufacture of specialist therapeutic shoes. The future might herald the use of "intelligent footwear design" with "on-board systems" available to monitor features of the foot-ground interface *(43)*.

WHAT DOES THE FUTURE HOLD?

Recent technological developments have led to promising breakthroughs in the treatment of chronic wounds *(21)*. There is great potential in the delivery of stem or progenitor cells, either applied topically or recruited from the circulation *(46)*. Preliminary work suggests that topically applied autologous bone marrow-cultured cells and the subsequent grafting of epidermal sheets might accelerate wound healing in intractable diabetic foot ulcers *(21,47)*.

Thus, there is good reason to believe that in the near future, further therapy to advances will further aid in the healing of chronic diabetic foot ulcers. However, this will never be achieved without a dedicated clinical team of individuals working together to try and reduce the morbidity and even mortality associated with diabetic foot problems.

REFERENCES

1. Boulton AJM, Vileikyte L, Ragrnarson-Tennvall G, Apelqvist J. (2005) The global burden of diabetic foot disease. *Lancet* **366**, 1719–1724.
2. International Diabetes Federation. *Diabetes and Foot Care: Time to Act.* Brussels, Belgium: International Diabetes Federation 2005.
3. Singh N. Armstrong DG, Lipsky BA. (2005) Preventing foot ulcers in patients with diabetes. *JAMA* **293**, 217–228.
4. Boulton AJM, Kirsner RS, Vileikyte L. (2004) Neuropathic diabetic foot ulcers. *N Engl J Med* **351**, 48–55.
5. Boulton AJM. (2004) The diabetic foot: from art to science. *Diabetologia* **47**, 1343–1353.
6. Tapp RJ, Zimmet PZ, Harper CA, Taylor HR, Welborn TA, Shaw JE. (2004) Diabetes care in an Australian population: frequency of screening examinations for eye and foot complications of diabetes. *Diabetes Care* **27**, 688–693.
7. Beem SE, Machala M, Holman C, Wraalstad R, Bybee A. (2004). Aiming at "de feet" and diabetes: a rural model to increase annual foot examinations. *Am J Public Health* **94**, 1664–1666.
8. Ewins DL, Bakker K, Young MJ, Boulton AJM. (1993) Alternative medicine: potential dangers for the diabetic foot. *Diabet Med* **10**, 980–982.
9. Boulton AJM. (2006) The pathway to foot ulceration. In: Boulton AJM, Cavanagh PR, Rayman G (eds). *The Foot in Diabetes*, 4th edn. Chichester: Wiley.
10. Abbott CA, Carrington AL, Ashe H, Van Ross ER, Boulton AJM. (2002) The North-West diabetes foot care study: incidence of, and risk factors for, new diabetic foot ulceration in a community-based cohort. *Diabet Med* **20**, 377–384.
11. Murray HJ, Young MJ, Boulton AJM. (1996) The relationship between callus formation, high foot pressures and neuropathic in diabetic foot ulceration. *Diabet Med* **16**, 979–982.
12. Reiber GE, Vileikyte, Boyko EJ, Lavery LA, Boulton AJM. (1999) Causal pathways for incident lower extremity ulcers in patients with diabetes from two settings. *Diabetes Care* **22**, 157–162.
13. Lavery LA, Higgins KR, Lanctot DR. (2004) Home monitoring of foot skin temperatures to prevent ulceration. *Diabetes Care* **27**, 2642–2647.

14. Mayfield JE, Sugarman JR. (2000) The use of Semmes-Weinstein monofilament and other threshold tests for preventing foot ulceration and amputation in people with diabetes. *J Fam Pract* **49 (suppl)**, S17–S29.

15. Booth J, Young MJ. (2000) Differences in the performance of commercially available monofilaments. *Diabetes Care* **23**, 984–988.

16. Miranda-Palma B, Sosenko JM, Bowker JH, Mizel M, Boulton AJM. (2005) A comparison of the monofilament with other testing modalities for foot ulcer susceptibility. *Diabetes Clin Pract* **70**, 8–12.

17. Williams DT, Harding KG, Price P. (2005) An evaluation of methods used in screening for lower limb arterial disease in diabetes. *Diabetes Care* **28**, 1169–1174.

18. American Diabetes Association. (2003) Peripheral arterial disease in people with diabetes. *Diabetes Care* **26**, 3333–3341.

19. Van Schie CH, Abbott CA, Vileikyte L, Boulton AJM. (1999) A comparative study of the Podotrack and the optical pedobarograph in the assessment of pressures under the diabetic foot. *Diabet Med* **16**, 154–159.

20. Boulton AJM, Malik RA, Arezzo JC, Sosenko JM. Diabetic Somatic Neuropathy. *Diabetes care* 2004; 27: 1458–1486.

21. Ziegler D, Siekerka-Klaiser E, Meyer B, Schweers M. Validation of a novel screening device, Neuroquick for quantitative assessment of small nerve fibre dysfunction as an early feature of diabetic poly neuropathy. *Diabetes care* 2005; 28:1169–1174.

22. Mueller MJ, Diamond JE, Sinacore DR (1989). Total contact casting in the treatment of diabetic plantar ulcers; controlled clinical trial. *Diabetes Care* **12**, 384–388.

23. American Diabetes Association. (1999) Consensus development conference on diabetic wound care. *Diabetes Care* **22**, 1354–1360.

24. Armstrong DG, Nguyen HC, Lavery LA, Van Schie CHM, Boulton AJM, Harkless LB. (2001). Offloading the diabetic foot wound: a randomized clinical trial. *Diabetes Care* **24**, 1019–1022.

25. Braumhauer JF, Wervery R, McWilliams J, Harris GF, Shereff MJ. (1997) A comparative study of plantar foot pressure in a standardized shoe, total contact cast prefabricated pneumatic walking brace. *Foot Ankle Int* **18**, 26–33.

26. Armstrong DG, Lavery LA, Kimbriel HR, Boulton AJM (2003). Activity patterns of patients with diabetic foot ulceration: patients with active ulceration may not adhere to a standard pressure offloading regimen. *Diabetes Care* **26**, 2595–2597.

27. Armstrong DG, Short B, Espensen EH, Abu-Ramman PL, Nixon BP, Boulton AJM. (2002). Technique for fabrication of an 'instant total contact cast' for treatment of neuropathic diabetic foot ulcers. *J Am Podiatr Assoc* 92, 405–408.

28. Katz IA, Harlan A, Miranda-Palma B, Prieto-Sanchez L, Armstrong DG, Bowker JH, Mizel MS, Boulton AJM. (2005) A randomized trial of two irremovable off-loading devices in the management of plantar neuropathic diabetic foot ulcers. *Diabetes Care* **28**, 555–559.

29. Armstrong DG, Lavery LA, Wu S, Boulton AJM (2005). Evaluation of removable and irremovable cast walkers in the healing of the diabetic foot wounds: a randomized controlled trial. *Diabetes Care* **28**, 551–554.

30. Piaggesi A, Viacava P, Rizzo L, del Prato S. (2003) Semi-quantitative analysis of the histopathological features of the neuropathic foot ulcer – effects of pressure relief. *Diabetes Care* **26**, 3123–3128.

31. Boulton AJM, Armstrong DG. (2003) Trials in neuropathic diabetic foot ulceration: time for a paradigm shift? *Diabetes Care* **26**, 2689–2690.

32. Nabuurs-Franssen MH, Sleegers R, Huijberts MS, Sanders AP, Schaper NC. (2005) Total contact casting of the diabetic foot in daily practice: a prospective follow-up study. *Diabetes Care* **28**, 243–247.

33. Nabuurs-Franssen MH, Sleegers R, Huijberts MS, Schaper NC. (2005) Casting of recurrent diabetic foot ulcers: effective and safe? *Diabetes Care* **28**, 1493–1494.

34. Lipsky BA. (2004) A report from the international consensus on diagnosing and treating the infected diabetic foot. *Diabet Metab Res Rev* **20(suppl 1)**, S68–S77.

35. Lipsky BA, Berendt AR, Embil J, De Lalla F. (2004) Diagnosing and treating diabetic foot infections. *Diabet Metab Res Rev* **20(suppl 1)**, S56–S64.

36. Tentolouris N, Jude EB, Smirnoff I, Knowles EA, Boulton AJM. (1999) Methicillin-resistant Staphylococcus aureus: an increasing problem in a diabetic foot clinic. *Diabet Med* **16**, 767–771.

37. Dang CN, Prasad YD, Boulton AJM, Jude EB. (2003) Methicillin-resistant Staphylococcus aureus in the diabetic foot clinic: a worsening problem. *Diabet Med* **20**, 159–161.

38. Rajbhandari SM, Sutton M, Davies C, Tesfaye S, Ward JD. (2000) 'Sausage toe': a reliable sign of underlying osteomyelitis. *Diabet Med* **17**, 74–77.

39. Grayson ML, Gibbons GW, Balogh K, Levin E, Karchmer AW. (1995) Probing to bone in infected pedal ulcers. A clinical sign of underlying osteomyelitis in diabetic patients. *JAMA* **9**, 721–723.

40. Armstrong DG, Lavery LA. (2005) Negative pressure wound therapy after partial diabetic foot amputation: a multicentre, randomized controlled trial. *Lancet* **366**, 1704–1710.

41. Armstrong DG, Attinger CF, Boulton AJM, Frykberg RG, Kirsner RS, Lavery LA. (2004) Guidelines regarding negative wound therapy (NPWT) in the diabetic foot. *Ostomy Wound Manage* **50(4B suppl)**, 3S–27S.

42. Bakker DJ. (2000) Hyperbaric oxygen therapy and the diabetic foot. *Diabet Metal Res Rev* **16(suppl 1)**, S55–S58.

43. Kessler I, Bilbault P, Ortega F, Crasso C, Passemard R, Stephan D, Pinget M, Schneider F. (2003) Hyperbaric oxygenation accelerates the healing rate of non-ischemic chronic diabetic foot ulcers: a prospective randomized study. *Diabetes Care* **26**, 2378–2382.

44. Cavanagh PR. (2004) Therapeutic footwear for people with diabetes. *Diabet Metab Res Rev* **20(suppl 1)**, S51–S55.

45. Uccioli L, Faglia E, Monticone G, Menzinger G. (1995) Manufactured shoes in the prevention of diabetic foot ulcers. *Diabetes Care* **18**, 1376–1378.

46. Reiber GE, Smith DG, Wallace C, Sullivan K, Hayes S, LeMaster J. (2002) Effect of therapeutic footwear on foot reulceration in patients with diabetes: a randomized controlled trial. *JAMA* **28**, 2552–2558.

47. Conrad C, Huss R. (2005) Adult stem cell lines in regenerative medicine and reconstructive surgery. *J Surg Res* **124**, 201–208.

48. Yamaguchi Y, Yoshida S, Sumikawa Y, Hosokawa K, Hearing VJ, Itami S. (2004) Rapid healing of intractable diabetic foot ulcers with exposed bones following a novel therapy of exposing bone marrow cells and then grafting epidermal sheets. *Br J Dermatol* **151**, 1019–1028.

49. Mason J, O'Keeffe C, Hutchinson A, McIntosh A, Young R, Booth A (1999). A systematic review of foot ulcers in patients with type 2 diabetes mellitus II treatment. *Diabet Med* **16**, 889–909.

50. Abidia A, Laden G, Kuhan G, Johnson BF, Wilkinson AR, Renwick PM, Masson EA, McCollum PT. (2003) The role of hyperbaric oxygen therapy in ischaemic diabetic lower extremity ulcers: a double-blind randomized-controlled trial. *Eur J Vasc Endovasc Surg* **25**, 513–518.

51. Kranke P, Bennett M, Rocckl-Wiedmann I, Debus S. (2004) Hyperbaric oxygen therapy for chronic wounds. *Cochrane Database Syst Rev* **2**, CD004123.

14 Coming of Age for the Incretins

Jens Juul Holst, MD, and Carolyn F. Deacon, DR. MED SCI

CONTENTS

SUMMARY

The incretin hormones, glucose-dependent insulinotropic polypeptide (GIP) and glucagon-like peptide-1 (GLP-1), may be responsible for up to 70% of postprandial insulin secretion. In type 2 diabetes (2DM), the incretin effect is severely reduced. Secretion of GIP is normal, but its effect on insulin is lost. GLP-1 secretion may be impaired, but its actions may restore insulin secretion to near normal levels. Substitution therapy with GLP-1 might therefore be possible. GLP-1 actions include potentiation of glucose-induced insulin secretion, up-regulation of insulin and other ß-cell genes, stimulation of ß-cell proliferation and neogenesis and inhibition of ß-cell apoptosis, inhibition of glucagon secretion, inhibition of gastric emptying, and inhibition of appetite and food intake. It may also have cardioprotective and neuroprotective actions. These actions make GLP-1 particularly attractive as a therapeutic agent for 2DM, but GLP-1 is rapidly destroyed in the body by the enzyme, dipeptidyl peptidase IV (DPP-IV). Clinical strategies therefore include (i) the development of metabolically stable activators of the GLP-1 receptor and (ii) inhibition of DPP-IV. Orally active DPP-IV inhibitors are currently undergoing clinical trials, and recent clinical studies have provided

From: *Contemporary Endocrinology: Controversies in Treating Diabetes:
Clinical and Research Aspects*
Edited by: D. LeRoith and A. I. Vinik © Humana Press, Totowa, NJ

long-term proof of concept. Metabolically stable analogs/activators include the structurally related lizard peptide, exendin-4, or analogs thereof, as well as GLP-1-derived molecules that bind to albumin and thereby assume the pharmacokinetics of albumin. These molecules are effective in animal experimental models of 2DM and have been employed successfully in clinical studies of up to 82 weeks' duration, and exendin-4 has just been approved for add-on therapy of 2DM.

Key Words: GLP-1 (glucagon-like peptide-1), GIP (glucose-dependent insulinotropic polypeptide), DPP-IV (dipeptidyl peptidase IV), glucagon, insulin, type 2 diabetes mellitus.

INTRODUCTION: THE INCRETIN EFFECT

"The incretin effect" designates the amplification of insulin secretion elicited by hormones secreted from the gastrointestinal tract. In the most strict sense, it is quantified by comparing insulin responses to oral and intravenous glucose administration, where the intravenous infusion is adjusted so as to result in the same (isoglycemic) peripheral (preferably arterialized) plasma glucose concentrations *(1,2)*. In healthy subjects, oral administration causes a two-fold to three-fold larger insulin response compared with the intravenous route. The increase is mainly due to the actions of insulinotropic gut hormones, although changing hepatic uptake of insulin may play a minor role. The same gut hormones are also released by mixed meals, and given that their postprandial concentrations in plasma are similar and that the elevations in glucose concentrations are also similar, it is generally assumed that the incretin hormones are playing a similarly important role for the meal-induced insulin secretion. If the analysis is based on measurements of C-peptide instead of insulin, it is possible to avoid errors introduced by hepatic extraction of insulin (since C-peptide is not taken up by the liver), and such measurements applied to isoglycemic glucose challenges indicate a similar amplification of beta cell secretion. By applying C-peptide kinetics and deconvolution it is possible to calculate the actual prehepatic insulin secretion rate, which shows a similar increase after oral compared with intravenous glucose *(3)*.

Many hormones have been suspected to be responsible for the incretin effect *(4)*, but today, there is ample evidence to suggest that the two most important incretins are glucose-dependent insulinotropic polypeptide (GIP), previously designated gastric inhibitory polypeptide, and glucagon-like peptide-1 (GLP-1). Both have been established as important incretin hormones in mimicry experiments in humans, where the hormones were infused together with intravenous glucose to concentrations approximately corresponding to those observed during oral glucose tolerance tests. Both hormones powerfully enhanced insulin secretion, actually to an extent that could fully explain the insulin response *(5,6)*. Likewise, administration of GLP-1 and GIP receptor antagonists to rodents or immunoneutralization has clearly indicated that both hormones play an important role for the incretin effect *(7,8)*. Recent human experiments, involving clamping of blood glucose at fasting and postprandial levels, exact copying of the meal-induced concentrations of both GLP-1 and GIP indicated that both are active with respect to enhancing insulin secretion from the beginning of a meal (even at fasting glucose levels) and that they contribute almost equally, but with the effect of GLP-1 predominating at higher glucose levels *(9)*. The effects of the two hormones with respect to insulin secretion have been shown to be additive in humans *(10)*. From studies in mice with targeted lesions of the both GLP-1 and GIP receptors, it was concluded that both hormones are essential for a normal glucose tolerance and that the effect of deletion of one receptor was "additive" to the effect of deleting the other *(11)*. Thus, there is little doubt that the incretin effect plays an important role in postprandial insulin secretion and, therefore, glucose tolerance in humans and animals.

It is now well established that type 2 diabetes (2DM) is characterized not only by insulin resistance but also by a beta cell defect , which renders the beta cells incapable of responding adequately to the insulin resistance *(12)*. Therefore, it is relevant to ask how the incretin effect functions in these patients. Careful studies by Nauck et al. *(13)* indicated that the incretin effect is severely reduced or lost in type 2 diabetic patients. In a similar study carried out in our own laboratory in obese subjects with 2DM (those studied by Nauck et al. were relatively lean), we could confirm the loss of the incretin effects and also observed that the amount of intravenous glucose required for copying of the oral glucose response was similar to the oral dose, another indication that in these patients, the route of administration did not result in different handling of the glucose (unpublished studies). Thus, there is little doubt that the loss of the incretin effect contributes to the glucose intolerance of these patients.

Given that GLP-1 and GIP are the most important incretin hormones, it is possible also to dissect their contribution to the defective incretin action in diabetic patients. Such contributions could consist in defects with respect to secretion, action, or metabolism. Detailed studies of the secretion of GIP and GLP-1 in response to mixed meals in patients with 2DM revealed a slightly impaired secretion of GIP but a more pronounced impairment with respect to the secretion of GLP-1. In fact, the GLP-1 response, expressed as the incremental area under the curve, was reduced to approximately 50% in the patients compared with healthy glucose tolerant controls. The decreased response was related to both BMI (lower the higher the BMI) and to the actual diabetic state but was independent of the presence of neuropathy. Thus, an impaired secretion of GLP-1 may contribute to the failing incretin effect.

The metabolism of GIP and GLP-1 was compared by Vilsboll et al. *(14)* in diabetic patients and controls, but both hormones were metabolized at similar rates (and unpublished studies). With respect to the effects of the incretin hormones, it was discovered in 1993 *(15)* that infusion of GLP-1 resulted in near normal insulin responses in patients with 2DM, whereas GIP had no significant effect. Similar observations were made by Elahi and coworkers *(16)*. In subsequent studies involving infusion of various doses of GLP-1 during stepwise increases in plasma glucose, it was possible to analyse the influence of GLP-1 on the beta cell sensitivity to glucose *(17)*. It was found that although GLP-1 at a low infusion rate (0.5 pmol/kg x min) was capable of restoring beta cell sensitivity to glucose to completely normal values, the sensitivity of the diabetic islets to GLP-1 was nevertheless severely decreased. Combined with the finding that the secretion of GLP-1 is reduced, one may infer that the insulinotropic effects of endogenous GLP-1 may be severely compromised in 2DM. Therefore, it can be concluded that decreased efficacy characterizes the incretin action of both GLP-1 and GIP in 2DM. On the other hand, whereas GIP is ineffective regardless of dose *(18)*, GLP-1 retains the capability to enhance glucose-induced secretion, raising the possibility that GLP-1, in pharmacological doses, could be used clinically to enhance insulin secretion in 2DM. The following sections describe the extent to which this is possible in clinical practice. Finally, one may ask whether the incretin defect is a primary event, perhaps a major etiological contributor to the beta cell failure that characterizes 2DM. Several observations, however, suggest that this is not the case. Thus, the impaired secretion of GLP-1 seems to be a consequence of diabetes *(19)*. In identical twins, that were discordant for type 2DM, meal-induced GLP-1 secretion was reduced only in the diabetic twin *(20)*, and in first-degree relatives of patients with 2DM, 24-h incretin hormone profiles were normal (actually there was a significant increase in the secretion of GIP but no difference for GLP-1) *(21)*. A reduced insulinotropic action of GIP to almost diabetic levels was observed in about 50% of first-degree relatives of patients with 2DM, suggesting that this might represent a primary, genetic defect *(22)*. However, subsequent observations have questioned this interpretation. Vilsboll et al. *(23)* studied insulin responses to GIP in patients with diabetes of different etiologies, including diabetes secondary to pancreatitis. In these patients, there was a similar loss of insulinotropic effects of GIP as observed in the classical type 2 diabetic subjects. These findings suggest that the lost effect of GIP is also secondary to the diabetic condition. Similarly, in women with previous gestational diabetes, which constitute a high risk group for diabetes development, GIP secretion and action was completely normal, precluding an early GIP defect to play a role for subsequent diabetes development (24).

Thus, although a therapeutic strategy based on incretin hormones may restore beta cell responsiveness to glucose in 2DM, the incretin defect is not a primary cause of diabetes.

It should be emphasized that it is currently unknown whether the lost effects of GIP are permanent in 2DM. This is relevant because reports have recently appeared showing that stabilized analogs of GIP may have antidiabetic potential in animal models of 2DM, notably ob/ob mice (25).

EFFECTS OF NATIVE GLP-1 IN 2DM

The acute insulinotropic effects of GLP-1 raised interest for the use of this peptide in diabetes treatment. Moreover, the peptide possesses a number of additional effects which in the context of diabetes treatment must be considered favorable.

Effects on the Islets

Not only does GLP-1 stimulate insulin secretion in a glucose-dependent manner (thereby minimizing the risk of causing hypoglycemia), it also enhances all steps of insulin biosynthesis as well as insulin gene transcription (26), thereby providing continued and augmented supplies of insulin for secretion. Important steps in the GLP-1 receptor signaling include activation of adenylate cyclase with subsequent accumulation of cAMP as well as increases in intracellular calcium levels. However, many of the subsequent changes that occur in the beta cells are protein kinase A independent. Thus, cAMP-regulated guanine nucleotide exchange factors (in particular Epac 2) appear to act as downstream mediators (27). Also the actions of GLP-1 on the insulin gene promoter appear to be mediated by both PKA-dependent and PKA-independent mechanisms, the latter possibly involving the MAP kinase pathway (28). The transcription factor pancreatic duodenal homeobox-1 (PDX-1), a key regulator of islet growth and insulin gene transcription, appears to be essential for most of the glucoregulatory, proliferative, and cytoprotective actions of GLP-1 (29). In addition, GLP-1 up-regulates the genes for the cellular machinery involved in insulin secretion, such as the glucokinase and glucose transporter-4 (GLUT-2) genes (30). Much attention was aroused by the finding that GLP-1 appeared to be essential for conveying "glucose competence" to the beta cells, that is, without GLP-1 signaling, beta cells would not be responsive to glucose (31,32). However, the beta cells of mice with disruption of the GLP-1 receptor gene show preserved glucose competence (33).

Finally, GLP-1 also has trophic effects on ß-cells *(34)*. Not only does it stimulate ß-cell proliferation *(35,36)*, it also enhances the differentiation of new ß-cells from progenitor cells in the pancreatic duct epithelium *(37)*. Most recently, GLP-1 has been shown to be capable of inhibiting apoptosis of beta cells including human beta cells*(38)*. As the normal number of beta cells is maintained in a balance between apoptosis and proliferation, this observation is of considerable interest and also raises the possibility that GLP-1 could be useful in conditions with increased beta cell apoptosis. The complicated mechanisms whereby GLP-1 may exert these effects on the beta cells were reviewed recently *(39,40)*.

GLP-1 also strongly inhibits glucagon secretion *(41)*. As in patients with 2DM, there is fasting hyperglucagonemia as well as exaggerated glucagon responses to meal ingestion *(19)*, and as it is likely that the hyperglucagonemia contributes to the hyperglycemia of the patients *(42)*, this effect may be as important as the insulinotropic effects. Indeed, in patients with type 1 diabetes and complete lack of beta cell activity (C-peptide negative), GLP-1 is still capable of lowering fasting plasma glucose concentrations, presumably as a consequence of a powerful lowering of the plasma glucagon concentration *(43)*.

Effects on the Gastrointestinal Tract

Further important effects of GLP-1 include inhibition of gastrointestinal secretion and motility, notably gastric emptying *(44,45)*. By this mechanism, GLP-1 may curtail postprandial glucose excursions *(46)* and thereby reduce the number of episodes with high postprandial glucose levels. There has been concern that the powerful inhibitory effect could represent a problem in patients with gastroparesis, but so far, there has not been a single reported case. It has also been speculated that the capability of high doses of GLP-1 to cause nausea and eventually vomiting might be a consequence of its actions of the stomach. However, GLP-1 may also cause nausea in the fasting state, so this is unlikely. Furthermore, in studies where GLP-1 infusions caused complete arrest of gastric emptying of a meal for several hours, the subjects were not nauseated and incapable of sensing the inhibition *(46)*. Recent studies by Schirra et al. *(47)*, involving administration of the GLP-1 receptor antagonist to humans, have clearly shown that the inhibitory actions of GLP-1 on gastric motility are among the physiological actions of the hormone.

Effects on Appetite and Food Intake

GLP-1 inhibits appetite and food intake in normal subjects *(48)* as well as in obese subjects with 2DM *(49,50)*, and it is thought that GLP-1 is one of the gastrointestinal hormones that normally regulates food intake *(50)*.

Other Effects

It has been known for some time that there are GLP-1 receptors in the heart *(51)*. A physiological function for these receptors was indicated in recent studies in mice lacking the GLP-1 receptor, which exhibits impaired left ventricular contractility and diastolic functions as well as impaired responses to exogenous epinephrine *(52)*. Recent studies in rats showed that GLP-1 protects the ischemic and reperfused myocardium in rats by mechanisms independent of insulin *(53)*. These findings may have important clinical implications. Thus, Nikolaidis et al. *(54)* studied patients treated with angioplasty after acute myocardial infarction but with postoperative left ventricular ejection fractions as low as 29%. In these patients, GLP-1 administration significantly improved the ejection fraction to 39% and improved both global and regional wall motion indices. Recently, GLP-1 was reported to dramatically improve left ventricular and systemic hemodynamics in dogs with induced dilated cardiomyopathy, and it was suggested that GLP-1 may be a useful metabolic adjuvant in decompensated heart failure *(55)*. Finally, GLP-1 was recently found to improve endothelial dysfunction in type 2 diabetic patients with coronary heart disease, again a finding with interesting therapeutic perspectives *(56)*. GLP-1 may also possess *neurotropic* effects. Thus, intracerebroventricular GLP-1 administration was associated with improved learning in rats and also displayed neuroprotective effects *(57,58)*, and GLP-1 has been proposed as a new therapeutic agent for neurodegenerative diseases, including Alzheimer's disease *(59)*.

In agreement with the findings of preserved insulinotropic actions of GLP-1 in 2DM *(15)*, intravenous infusion of GLP-1 at 1 pmol/kg × min was demonstrated to be able to completely normalize plasma glucose in patients with longstanding severe disease, admitted to hospital for insulin treatment *(60)*. Subsequent studies in patients with moderate disease showed that plasma glucose concentrations could be near normalized by an intravenous GLP-1 infusion covering the night time and the next day including two meals *(61)*. In another study, a continuous intravenous administration of GLP-1 for 7 consecutive days was demonstrated to dramatically lower both fasting and postprandial glucose concentrations with no sign of tachyphylaxis over 7 days *(62)*. In this study, which included four different infusion rates, glucose concentrations were not completely normalized at the two lowest infusion rates (4 and 8 ng/kg × min approximately corresponding to 1 and 2 pmol/kg × min), whereas the higher rates (16 and 24 ng/kg × min) had to be discontinued because of side effects (nausea and vomiting). So in these studies, it was not possible within the therapeutic window to completely normalize plasma glucose concentrations.

Clearly, continuous intravenous infusion is clinically irrelevant, but the effect of subcutaneous injections of GLP-1 given to both patients and healthy subjects *(63)* on plasma glucose and insulin concentrations turned out to be very short lasting, even after maximally tolerated doses (1.5 nmol/kg—higher doses resulted in nausea and vomiting) *(64)*. The short duration of action was demonstrated to be due to an extremely rapid and extensive metabolism of GLP-1 in the body *(65,66)* leaving the intact peptide with an apparent half-life of 1–2 min in the body and a plasma clearance amounting to two to three times cardiac plasma output *(14)*. The degradation is due to the actions of the ubiquitous enzyme, DPP-IV, which catalyses the removal of the two N-terminal amino acids of the molecule rendering it inactive *(65)*. It has been demonstrated that the metabolite, GLP-1 (9–36) amide, may act as a GLP-1 receptor antagonist *(67)* and that prevention of its generation might enhance the antidiabetic actions of GLP-1. Recent studies, however, clearly showed that glucose-lowering effects of GLP-1 in humans were the same whether the metabolite was present or not *(68)*.

The metabolic instability of GLP-1 clearly restricts its clinical usefulness, but Zander et al. *(69)* carried out a clinical study in which GLP-1 or saline was administered as a continuous subcutaneous infusion (using insulin pumps) for 6 weeks to a group of 2DM patients. The patients were evaluated before, after 1 week, and after 6 weeks of treatment. No changes were observed in the saline-treated control group, whereas in the GLP-1 group, fasting and average plasma glucose concentrations were lowered by approximately 5 mmol/l, hemoglobin A1c [glycated hemoglobin, a long-term (months) measure of mean plasma glucose concentrations] decreased by 1.2%, free fatty acids were significantly lowered, and the patients had a gradual weight loss of approximately 2 kg. In addition, insulin sensitivity, determined by a hyperinsulinamic euglycemic clamp, almost doubled, and insulin secretion capacity (measured using a 30 mmol/l glucose clamp + arginine) greatly improved. There was no significant difference between results obtained after 1 and 6 weeks of treatment, but there was a tendency toward further improvement of plasma glucose as well as insulin secretion. There were very few side effects and no differences between saline-treated and GLP-1-treated patients in this respect. Despite the marked metabolic improvement, plasma glucose levels were not completely normalized, but the dose given (4.8 pmol/kg × min) may not have been optimal. Thus, in a different study, higher infusion rates were actually more efficacious and still did not elicit prohibitive side effects *(70)*.

This study, therefore, provided "proof-of-concept" for the principle of GLP-based therapy of 2DM, and further attempts to utilize the therapeutic potential of GLP-1 have included on one hand the development of stable, DPP-IV-resistant analogs *(71)*, and on the other hand, inhibitors of DPP-IV demonstrated to be capable of protecting the peptide from degradation and thereby augmenting its insulinotropic activity *(72)*.

GLP-1 ANALOGS (INCRETIN MIMETICS)

Stable peptide agonists of the GLP-1 receptor have given great hope with respect to future diabetes therapy. The compound most advanced with respect to clinical development is exenatide, produced by the Amylin Corporation, Amylin, San Diego, Ca, US in collaboration with Eli Lilly, Indiana polis, Indiana, US a synthetic replica of exendin 4, a peptide derived from the salivary glands of a lizard, the Gila Monster. It has 53% sequence homology with GLP-1 but is not the GLP-1 of the Gila monster and is therefore designated a GLP-1 receptor activator or incretin mimetic. It activates the GLP-1 receptor with about the same potency as native GLP-1 but survives much longer in the circulation, both because of its resistance to DPP-IV and because of reduced renal elimination *(73,74)*. Upon single subcutaneous injection of 10 µg, the recommended dose, there is an exposure for about 6–7 h in humans *(75)*. Exenatide is therefore given twice daily. Otherwise, exenatide seems to share all of the effects of native GLP-1 *(73)*. The compound has been tested in several clinical trials, most recently in three controlled pivotal trials comprising 1494 patients. Exenatide was given for 30 weeks as an add-on therapy to type 2 diabetic patients inadequately treated with sulfonylureas *(76)*, metformin *(77)* or a combination of metformin and sulfonylureas *(78)*. After 30 of weeks treatment, fasting blood glucose concentrations were significantly reduced, HbA1c levels were reduced by approximately 0.8% in all groups, and to or below 7% (a recommended value) in 41, 46, and 34% of the patients in the three groups. Adverse effects were mild and generally gastrointestinal. Mild hypoglycemia was noted in 28–36% of patients also receiving sulfonylurea. An important result was a significant, dose-dependent and progressive weight loss of 1.6 kg (SU and SU + metformin) and 2.8 kg (metformin) from baseline. In open-label extensions of these studies, exenatide has been given for a total of 82 weeks with continued effects on HbA1c and body weight (http://www.amylin.com). However, some patients (about 38% of patients after 30 weeks) appear to develop low titre antibodies against exenatide, and 6% developed antibodies with higher titres. In about half of these, the glucose-lowering effect of exenatide appeared attenuated. The three pivotal studies provided the basis for an application for approval of exenatide as a new drug for the treatment of diabetes, and this was approved by the FDA in April 2005. Information about the new drug, which is named "Byetta," is available on the web site of the company (http://www.BYETTA.com). It appears from the label that an increased rate of benign C-cell adenomas were observed with a dose-dependent frequency in female rats, whereas a study in mice was negative. As there are GLP-1 receptors on the C-cells in several species *(79)*, including humans, this could represent a class effect and will require careful observation, although apparently such adenomas have not been observed in humans. Calcitonin levels were not affected during the 6 weeks of continuous GLP-1 administration to diabetic patients mentioned above (unpublished studies). Most recently, the Amylin Corporation has developed a slow release formulation of exenatide *(80)*. Exenatide long-acting release (LAR) is a poly-lactide-glycolide microsphere suspension containing 3% exenatide that exhibits sustained dose-dependent glycemic control in diabetic fatty Zucker rats for up to 28 days following a single subcutaneous injection. In 30 patients with 2DM previously treated with diet/exercise and/or metformin, weekly injections of exenatide LAR for 15 weeks was reported to reduce fasting plasma glucose by ~3 mmol/l, to reduce HbA1c by 1.7%, and to cause a weight loss of 3.8 kg in the group with the highest dose. Notably, the enhanced efficacy was associated with a markedly reduced incidence of side effects (nausea). This supports the concept that it is essential to maintain a constant level of high GLP-1 activity for optimal treatment results. In conclusion, exenatide represents an efficacious supplement to failing conventional oral antidiabetic agents, and the sustained effect observed in the extension studies and its continued weight-lowering effects must be considered very promising.

Other analogs currently in clinical development include slightly modified versions of the GLP-1 molecule that, by various means, attach to albumin and thereby acquire the pharmacokinetic profile of albumin. One such analog is Liraglutide produced by NovoNordisk, Bagsværd, Denmark. It consists of a slightly modified GLP-1 sequence to which is attached a palmitoyl chain. Thereby, the molecule obtains affinity for and binds to albumin and, as a result, escapes both DPP-IV and renal elimination. The plasma half-life of this compound is approximately12 h, and it therefore provides exposure for more than 24 h after a single injection *(81)*. The compound seems to possess all of the activities of native GLP-1*(82)*. A recent report describes administration of increasing doses of Liraglutide to patients with 2DM for 3 months *(83)*. Liraglutide lowered fasting blood glucose and HbA1c dose-dependent manner (by up to 0.75% points from a base line level of 7.6%) and also significantly lowered body weight in some doses. There were very few side effects and no antibody formation. The strength of this compound seems to be its attractive pharmacokinetic profile, providing a rather stable plateau of active compound in plasma upon single daily injections. In this way, side effects (nausea and vomiting) associated with large excursions in the plasma concentration of more rapidly metabolized compounds after s.c. injection may be avoided. In a recent study *(84)*, Liraglutide was given in doses up to 2 mg OD in a 5-week period with weekly up titrations to patients with high HbA1c levels (8–10%). In particular when added on to metformin, Liraglutide powerfully reduced fasting glucose levels (from 13 to 9 mmol/l) and caused a weight loss (of 2.4%). Gastrointestinal side effects were transient and led to withdrawal in only 4%. Most recently, results from a 14-week trial of Liraglutide given once daily as monotherapy to 165 patients were reported on the company's web site (http://www.novonordisk.com). HbA1c was reported to decrease by 1.5–2%, fasting blood glucose by >3 mmol/l and body weight to decrease by 3 kg from 90 kg. Notably, there were very few side effects, primarily a low rate of very mild nausea initially and decreasing with time.

Other compounds include the Conjuchem compound, C-1131, composed of a D-alanine-8-substituted GLP-1 molecule with a linker and a reactive moiety (maleimidoproprionic acid) attached to the C-terminus, but the development of this compound has recently been terminated.

The Albugon compound from Human Genome Sciences, Rockville, MD, US which is a fusion protein between human albumin and a resistant GLP-1 analog, has recently attracted interest, because it was demonstrated (85) that this large molecule not only had antidiabetic activity in animal models of diabetes but also was capable of activating the neural mechanisms whereby the much smaller molecules, GLP-1 or exenatide, influence gastrointestinal motility, appetite, and food intake. In glucose-intolerant mice and in diabetic rats, a single injection near normalized glucose levels for 24 h. The half-life was said to be 3 days in monkeys (86).

INHIBITORS OF DPP-IV

The therapeutic use of inhibitors of the enzyme responsible for the inactivation of GLP-1 as antidiabetic agents was first proposed in 1995 (66) based on the finding that GLP-1 seems uniquely sensitive to cleavage by DPP-IV, and compounds of this class have now reached phase III clinical trials. DPP-IV inhibition results in the N-terminal degradation of GLP-1, which normally occurs in vivo being completely prevented, leading to significant enhancement of its insulinotropic activity (72) . Studies in Vancouver diabetic fatty rats have shown that chronic oral administration of the Probiodrug DPP-IV inhibitor, isoleucine thiazolidide (P32/98), for 12 weeks improves glucose tolerance, insulin sensitivity, and β-cell responsiveness (87). The longer acting Ferring inhibitor, FE 999-011, continuously inhibited plasma DPP-IV activity and not only normalized the glucose excursion after oral glucose administration in insulin-resistant Zucker obese rats but also delayed the onset of hyperglycemia in Zucker diabetic fatty rats (88). These effects were, at least partly, due to increased intact GLP-1 concentrations that were also implicated in the improved islet function seen after chronic treatment of high fat-fed (glucose intolerant and insulin resistant) mice with valine-pyrrolidide (89). Further support for the involvement of DPP-IV in mediating glucose tolerance comes from studies in animal models, which lack DPP-IV activity (Fischer rats, which have a mutation in the catalytic site, and CD26 knockout mice, in which the gene encoding DPP-IV has been disrupted). Such animals have improved glucose tolerance compared with their wild-type counterparts (90–92). The impairment in glucose tolerance that normally accompanies aging is prevented in DPP-IV-negative Fischer rats and DPP-IV inhibitor-treated control animals(92,93), whereas both Fischer rats and CD26 knockout mice are protected against diet (high fat)-induced insulin resistance and glucose intolerance (93–95) . Again, the mechanism of action is thought to involve preservation of endogenous GLP-1 levels, because the concentrations of intact GLP-1 are elevated.

After these promising preclinical studies, the first clinical proof-of-concept was obtained using the short-acting Novartis inhibitor, NVP-DPP728 (96). When given twice or thrice daily for 4 weeks in patients with relatively mild 2DM (mean HbA1c of 7.4%), both fasting and prandial glucose levels were lowered significantly, resulting in a reduction in HbA1c of 0.5%, and despite the fall in glycemia, fasting and post-prandial insulin levels were sustained. NVP-DPP728 appeared to be well tolerated, with only minor adverse events being reported. However, some of these symptoms (pruritis and nasopharyn-gitis) may be a property of the compound itself rather than being class specific, because they were not reported for another inhibitor, LAF237, subsequently developed by Novartis. NVP-DPP728 has now been dropped in favor of LAF237, which is longer acting and suitable for once-daily administration. A clinical study with this compound was recently reported, showing it to have a pharmacodynamic profile upon once daily administration which was similar to that of its predecessor given two or three times daily (97). The mechanism of action was suggested to be incretin mediated, because LAF237 treatment increased both baseline and prandial active GLP-1 levels. As with NVP-DPP78, insulin levels were not actually increased, but interestingly, glucagon levels were significantly suppressed. Most recently, clinical data from long-term studies, namely a 12-week controlled study in patients already on metformin treatment, followed up by an extension period of 40 weeks, were published (98). LAF 237 significantly lowered HbA1c levels from 7.7 to approximately 7% after 3 of months treatment, and this level was maintained for the remaining period, whereas in the control group a significant increase was noted, resulting in a difference between placebo-treated and LAF 237-treated patients of 1.1%. In addition, meal-induced insulin secretion was impaired in the placebo group and remained unaltered in the treatment group despite significantly lower glucose levels. A post hoc analysis of these data indicated that the treatment lead to significant and progressive improvements in beta cell function and insulin sensitivity (99). This could indicate that LAF 237 exerted a beta cell protective effect not noted in the placebo groups. Side effects were mild, and importantly, hypoglycemia was not reported. However, in contrast to the GLP-1 analogs, there was no change in body weight. Details regarding the binding kinetics, type of inhibition, and selectivity with respect to other peptidases for the inhibitor, which is now called Vildagliptin or Galvus®, were recently published (100). In a recent clinical study, details regarding its action on beta cell function and hormone levels were studied. The inhibitor significantly increased insulin secretion rate at 7 mmol/l glucose (the so-called insulin secretory tone) and inhibited glucagon secretion while increasing levels of active GLP-1 and GIP (101). A New Drug Application was filed with the FDA in the spring of 2006 but approval has so far been delayed. In a recent news release from the company, some of the phase III results were described. Vildagliptin given once or twice daily was as effective as rosiglitazone in a direct comparison study, and nearly as effective as metformin, and gave further improvements when added to either metformin or rosiglitazone. Interestingly, when added to existing but insufficient insulin therapy, vildagliptin improved HbA1c levels, was associated with decreased insulin use, and completely prevented hypoglycemia.

The Merck company (Merck & Co., Inc., Whitehouse Station, NJ, US) has an inhibitor (MK-0431, now known as sitagliptin or Januvia®) and recently filed a new drug application with the FDA (http://www.msd.com), but so far, less is known about this compound (102). Results of placebo-controlled, single-dose studies were recently published (103). MK-0431 was well-tolerated and caused significant reductions in the glycemic excursion following an oral glucose tolerance test (OGTT), associated with increases in intact GLP-1 and insulin, and reductions in glucagon secretion. According to websites, several other companies are developing DPP-IV inhibitors, including Bristol-Meyer-Squibb (www.bms.com) (Phase III) and Prosidion (www.prosidion.com) (P93/01; phase II). Single doses of P93/01 were reported to have good tolerability and result in dose-related reductions in prandial glucose in type 2 diabetic subjects when HbA1c was above 6% (104).

The clinical studies with DPP-IV inhibitors which have been reported so far have not been associated with any serious adverse side effects, but there has been understandable concern that undesirable side effects could arise from inhibiting an enzyme with multiple substrates or because of non-mechanism-based actions (i.e., not related to the selective inhibition of DPP-IV). With regard to the former, although a number of regulatory and neuropeptides, chemokines, and cytokines have been identified as potential substrates from in vitro kinetic studies [reviewed by (105)], it is uncertain how many of them are actually endogenous substrates, and if so, whether DPP-IV-mediated degradation is their primary route of elimination. In addition to GLP-1, the other incretin hormone, GIP, is an endogenous DPP-IV substrate, as is the neuropeptide pituitary adenylate cyclase activating peptide (PACAP) *(106)*, but inhibition of their degradation would be expected to contribute to the antidiabetic effects of DPP-IV inhibitors *(107)*. The evidence for a physiological role for DPP-IV in the degradation of many of the other potential substrates remains to be demonstrated. DPP-IV also has some other roles that potentially could be compromised by DPP-IV inhibition. It is present on the surface of T-cells (where it is usually known as the T-cell marker CD26) and contributes to T-cell activation and proliferation through its interaction with other membrane-expressed molecules such as CD45, although it is uncertain whether the enzymatic activity is involved or even whether its presence is mandatory *(108)*. In this context, a family of DPP-IV-related enzymes is now known to exist, which have similar catalytic activities. Selective inhibition of two of these enzymes (DPP 8 and DPP 9) was recently reported to affect T-cell activation in vitro and be associated with severe, even lethal, side effects in preclinical species *(109)*, whereas selective DPP-IV inhibition was not, suggesting that DPP 8 and 9 could be responsible for some of the functions previously ascribed to DPP-IV. In turn, this raises the possibility that some of the potential or reported side effects of DPP-IV inhibition could be due to inhibition of DPP 8 and 9 rather than DPP-IV itself. It is, therefore, highly relevant that the rodents that lack DPP-IV enzymatic activity (the Fischer rat and the CD26 knockout mouse) are completely viable and seem to suffer no ill effects because of the lack of DPP-IV. Selectivity data for the inhibitors in development has so far only been released for the Merck compound, which is reported to have >2500-fold selectivity for DPP-IV relative to DPP 8 and 9 *(110)* and for vildagliptin, which has 75-fold selectivity for DPP-IV relative to DPP 8 *(100)* and between 32-fold and 250-fold relative to DPP 9 (Novartis website).

CONCLUSION

As detailed in the sections on GLP-1 analogs and DPP-IV inhibitors, there is ample evidence to suggest that treatment of 2DM will be feasible using either DPP-IV inhibitors or GLP-1 analogs/receptor activators. One GLP-1 receptor activator (Byetta) and one of the DPP-IV inhibitors are already on the market and other compounds are in late phases of development or awaiting approval. The question arises which principle to choose. If the DPP-IV inhibitors continue to show minimal side effects, it would be tempting to suggest their use for the treatment of very early 2DM, perhaps even prevention in groups with a high risk for 2DM (familial disposition, obesity, glucose intolerance, and previous gestational diabetes). On the other hand, as their ability to elevate the levels of active endogenous GLP-1 is limited, it may be preferable to chose an injectable GLP-1 analog in patients with long-standing disease and limited beta cell capacity. The DPP-IV inhibitors are weight neutral in patients with 2DM, which in itself is an attractive feature, but the analogs appear to provide a reliable weight loss. The most important parameter, however, is undoubtedly the potential of the compounds to protect beta cells and, thereby, possibly break the otherwise inevitable progression of disease. Although hard data regarding this in humans are still lacking, the stable HbA1c levels observed in patients treated long-term with both inhibitors and analogs as opposed to increasing levels in placebo-treated controls may indeed indicate that progression has been halted. Future studies directly addressing the beta cell protective effects of either group of compounds will be of the greatest interest, also regarding the choice of therapeutic principle.

REFERENCES

1. McIntyre, N., Holdsworth, C. D., Turner, D. S. New interpretation of oral glucose tolerance. *Lancet* 1964, **2**, 20–21.
2. Perley, M., Kipnis, D. M. Plasma insulin responses to oral and intravenous glucose: studies in normal and diabetic subjects. *J Clin Invest* 1967, **46**, 1954–1962.
3. Mari, A., Schmitz, O., Gastaldelli, A., Oestergaard, T., Nyholm, B., Ferrannini, E. Meal and oral glucose tests for assessment of beta-cell function: modeling analysis in normal subjects. *Am J Physiol Endocrinol Metab* 2002, **283**(6), E1159–E1166.
4. Holst, J. J., Orskov, C. Incretin hormones–an update. *Scand J Clin Lab Invest Suppl* 2001, **234**, 75–85.
5. Nauck, M., Schmidt, W. E., Ebert, R., Strietzel, J., Cantor, P., Hoffmann, G., Creutzfeldt, W. Insulinotropic properties of synthetic human gastric inhibitory polypeptide in man: interactions with glucose, phenylalanine, and cholecystokinin-8. *J Clin Endocrinol Metab* 1989, **69**(3), 654–662.
6. Kreymann, B., Williams, G., Ghatei, M. A., Bloom, S. R. Glucagon-like peptide-1 7–36: a physiological incretin in man. *Lancet* 1987, **2**(8571), 1300–1304.
7. Kolligs, F., Fehmann, H. C., Goke, R., Goke, B. Reduction of the incretin effect in rats by the glucagon-like peptide 1 receptor antagonist exendin (9-39) amide. *Diabetes* 1995, **44**(1), 16–19.
8. Gault, V. A., O'Harte, F. P., Harriott, P., Mooney, M. H., Green, B. D., Flatt, P. R. Effects of the novel (Pro3)GIP antagonist and exendin(9-39)amide on GIP- and GLP-1-induced cyclic AMP generation, insulin secretion and postprandial insulin release in obese diabetic (ob/ob) mice: evidence that GIP is the major physiological incretin. *Diabetologia* 2003, **46**(2), 222–230.
9. Vilsboll, T., Krarup, T., Madsbad, S., Holst, J. J. Both GLP-1 and GIP are insulinotropic at basal and postprandial glucose levels and contribute nearly equally to the incretin effect of a meal in healthy subjects. *Regul Pept* 2003, **114**(2–3), 115–121.
10. Nauck, M. A., Bartels, E., Orskov, C., Ebert, R., Creutzfeldt, W. Additive insulinotropic effects of exogenous synthetic human gastric inhibitory polypeptide and glucagon-like peptide-1-(7-36) amide infused at near-physiological insulinotropic hormone and glucose concentrations. *J Clin Endocrinol Metab* 1993, **76**(4), 912–917.

11. Hansotia, T., Baggio, L., Delmeire, D., Hinke, S. A., Preitner, F., Yamada, Y., Tsukiyama, K., Thorens, B., Seino, Y., Holst, J. J., Schuit, F., Drucker, D. J. Double incretin receptor knockout (DIRKO) mice reveal an essential role for the enteroinsular axis in transducing the glucoregulatory action of DPP-IV inhibitors. *Diabetes*, 2004, **53:** 1326–1335.

12. Pratley, R. E., Weyer, C. The role of impaired early insulin secretion in the pathogenesis of type II diabetes mellitus. *Diabetologia* 2001, **44**(8), 929–945.

13. Nauck, M., Stockmann, F., Ebert, R., Creutzfeldt, W. Reduced incretin effect in type 2 (non-insulin-dependent) diabetes. *Diabetologia* 1986, **29**(1), 46–52.

14. Vilsboll, T., Agerso, H., Krarup, T., Holst, J. J. Similar elimination rates of glucagon-like peptide-1 in obese type 2 diabetic patients and healthy subjects. *J Clin Endocrinol Metab* 2003, **88**(1), 220–224.

15. Nauck, M. A., Heimesaat, M. M., Orskov, C., Holst, J. J., Ebert, R., Creutzfeldt, W. Preserved incretin activity of glucagon-like peptide 1 [7–36 amide] but not of synthetic human gastric inhibitory polypeptide in patients with type-2 diabetes mellitus. *J Clin Invest* 1993, **91**(1), 301–307.

16. Elahi, D., McAloon Dyke, M., Fukagawa, N. K., Meneilly, G. S., Sclater, A. L., Minaker, K. L., Habener, J. F., Andersen, D. K. The insulinotropic actions of glucose-dependent insulinotropic polypeptide (GIP) and glucagon-like peptide-1 (7–37) in normal and diabetic subjects. *Regul Pept* 1994, **51**(1), 63–74.

17. Kjems, L. L., Holst, J. J., Volund, A., Madsbad, S. The influence of GLP-1 on glucose-stimulated insulin secretion: effects on beta-cell sensitivity in type 2 and nondiabetic subjects. *Diabetes* 2003, **52**(2), 380–386.

18. Vilsboll, T., Krarup, T., Madsbad, S., Holst, J. J. Defective amplification of the late phase insulin response to glucose by GIP in obese type II diabetic patients. *Diabetologia* 2002, **45**(8), 1111–1119.

19. Toft-Nielsen, M. B., Damholt, M. B., Madsbad, S., Hilsted, L. M., Hughes, T. E., Michelsen, B. K., Holst, J. J. Determinants of the impaired secretion of glucagon-like peptide-1 in type 2 diabetic patients. *J Clin Endocrinol Metab* 2001, **86**(8), 3717–3723.

20. Vaag, A. A., Holst, J. J., Volund, A., Beck-Nielsen, H. B. Gut incretin hormones in identical twins discordant for non-insulin-dependent diabetes mellitus (NIDDM)–evidence for decreased glucagon- like peptide 1 secretion during oral glucose ingestion in NIDDM twins. *Eur J Endocrinol* 1996, **135**(4), 425–432.

21. Nyholm, B., Walker, M., Gravholt, C. H., Shearing, P. A., Sturis, J., Alberti, K. G., Holst, J. J., Schmitz, O. Twenty-four-hour insulin secretion rates, circulating concentrations of fuel substrates and gut incretin hormones in healthy offspring of Type II (non-insulin-dependent) diabetic parents: evidence of several aberrations. *Diabetologia* 1999, **42**(11), 1314–1323.

22. Meier, J. J., Hucking, K., Holst, J. J., Deacon, C. F., Schmiegel, W. H., Nauck, M. A. Reduced insulinotropic effect of gastric inhibitory polypeptide in first-degree relatives of patients with type 2 diabetes. *Diabetes* 2001, **50**(11), 2497–2504.

23. Vilsboll, T., Knop, F. K., Krarup, T., Johansen, A., Madsbad, S., Larsen, S., Hansen, T., Pedersen, O., Holst, J. J. The pathophysiology of diabetes involves a defective amplification of the late-phase insulin response to glucose by glucose-dependent insulinotropic polypeptide-regardless of etiology and phenotype. *J Clin Endocrinol Metab* 2003, **88**(10), 4897–4903.

24. Meier, J. J., Gallwitz, B., Askenas, M., Vollmer, K., Deacon, C. F., Holst, J. J., Schmidt, W. E., Nauck, M. A. Secretion of incretin hormones and the insulinotropic

effect of gastric inhibitory polypeptide in women with a history of gestational diabetes. *Diabetologia* 2005, **48**(9), 1872–1881.

25. Irwin, N., Green, B. D., Mooney, M. H., Greer, B., Harriott, P., Bailey, C. J., Gault, V. A., O'Harte, F. P., Flatt, P. R. A novel, long-acting agonist of glucose dependent insulinotropic polypeptide (GIP) suitable for once daily administration in type 2 diabetes. *J Pharmacol Exp Ther* 2005, **314**(3): 1181–1194.

26. Fehmann, H. C., Habener, J. F. Insulinotropic hormone glucagon-like peptide-I(7-37) stimulation of proinsulin gene expression and proinsulin biosynthesis in insulinoma beta TC-1 cells. *Endocrinology* 1992, **130**(1), 159–166.

27. Holz, G. G. Epac: a new cAMP-binding protein in support of glucagon-like peptide-1 receptor-mediated signal transduction in the pancreatic beta-cell. *Diabetes* 2004, **53**(1), 5–13.

28. Kemp, D. M., Habener, J. F. Insulinotropic hormone glucagon-like peptide 1 (GLP-1) activation of insulin gene promoter inhibited by p38 mitogen-activated protein kinase. *Endocrinology* 2001, **142**(3), 1179–1187.

29. Li, Y., Cao, X., Li, L. X., Brubaker, P. L., Edlund, H., Drucker, D. J. Beta-cell Pdx1 expression is essential for the glucoregulatory, proliferative, and cytoprotective actions of glucagon-like peptide-1. *Diabetes* 2005, **54**(2), 482–491.

30. Buteau, J., Roduit, R., Susini, S., Prentki, M. Glucagon-like peptide-1 promotes DNA synthesis, activates phosphatidylinositol 3-kinase and increases transcription factor pancreatic and duodenal homeobox gene 1 (PDX-1) DNA binding activity in beta (INS-1)-cells. *Diabetologia* 1999, **42**(7), 856–864.

31. Holz, G. H., Kuhtreiber, W. M., Habener, J. F. Induction of glucose competence in pancreatic beta cells by glucagon-like peptide-1(7–37). *Trans Assoc Am Physicians* 1992, **105**, 260–267.

32. Gromada, J., Holst, J. J., Rorsman, P. Cellular regulation of islet hormone secretion by the incretin hormone glucagon-like peptide 1. *Pflugers Arch* 1998, **435**(5), 583–594.

33. Flamez, D., Van Breusegem, A., Scrocchi, L. A., Quartier, E., Pipeleers, D., Drucker, D. J., Schuit, F. Mouse pancreatic beta-cells exhibit preserved glucose competence after disruption of the glucagon-like peptide-1 receptor gene. *Diabetes* 1998, **47**(4), 646–652.

34. Egan, J. M., Bulotta, A., Hui, H., Perfetti, R. GLP-1 receptor agonists are growth and differentiation factors for pancreatic islet beta cells. *Diabetes Metab Res Rev* 2003, **19**(2), 115–123.

35. Xu, G., Stoffers, D. A., Habener, J. F., Bonner-Weir, S. Exendin-4 stimulates both beta-cell replication and neogenesis, resulting in increased beta-cell mass and improved glucose tolerance in diabetic rats. *Diabetes* 1999, **48**(12), 2270–2276.

36. Stoffers, D. A., Kieffer, T. J., Hussain, M. A., Drucker, D. J., Bonner-Weir, S., Habener, J. F., Egan, J. M. Insulinotropic glucagon-like peptide 1 agonists stimulate expression of homeodomain protein IDX-1 and increase islet size in mouse pancreas. *Diabetes* 2000, **49**(5), 741–748.

37. Zhou, J., Wang, X., Pineyro, M. A., Egan, J. M. Glucagon-like peptide 1 and exendin-4 convert pancreatic AR42J cells into glucagon- and insulin-producing cells. *Diabetes* 1999, **48**(12), 2358–2366.

38. Buteau, J., El-Assaad, W., Rhodes, C. J., Rosenberg, L., Joly, E., Prentki, M. Glucagon-like peptide-1 prevents beta cell glucolipotoxicity. *Diabetologia* 2004, **47**(5), 806–815.

39. Brubaker, P. L., Drucker, D. J. Minireview: glucagon-like peptides regulate cell proliferation and apoptosis in the pancreas, gut, and central nervous system. *Endocrinology* 2004, **145**(6), 2653–2659.

40. Sinclair, E. M., Drucker, D. J. Proglucagon-derived peptides: mechanisms of action and therapeutic potential. *Physiology (Bethesda)* 2005, **20**, 357–365.

41. Orskov, C., Holst, J. J., Nielsen, O. V. Effect of truncated glucagon-like peptide-1 [proglucagon-(78–107) amide] on endocrine secretion from pig pancreas, antrum, and nonantral stomach. *Endocrinology* 1988, **123**(4), 2009–2013.

42. Shah, P., Vella, A., Basu, A., Basu, R., Schwenk, W. F., Rizza, R. A. Lack of suppression of glucagon contributes to postprandial hyperglycemia in subjects with type 2 diabetes mellitus. *J Clin Endocrinol Metab* 2000, **85**(11), 4053–4059.

43. Creutzfeldt, W. O., Kleine, N., Willms, B., Orskov, C., Holst, J. J., Nauck, M. A. Glucagonostatic actions and reduction of fasting hyperglycemia by exogenous glucagon-like peptide I(7–36) amide in type I diabetic patients. *Diabetes Care* 1996, **19**(6), 580–586.

44. Wettergren, A., Schjoldager, B., Mortensen, P. E., Myhre, J., Christiansen, J., Holst, J. J. Truncated GLP-1 (proglucagon 78-107-amide) inhibits gastric and pancreatic functions in man. *Dig Dis Sci* 1993, **38**(4), 665–673.

45. Nauck, M. A., Niedereichholz, U., Ettler, R., Holst, J. J., Orskov, C., Ritzel, R., Schmiegel, W. H. Glucagon-like peptide 1 inhibition of gastric emptying outweighs its insulinotropic effects in healthy humans. *Am J Physiol* 1997, **273**(5 Pt 1), E981–E988.

46. Willms, B., Werner, J., Holst, J. J., Orskov, C., Creutzfeldt, W., Nauck, M. A. Gastric emptying, glucose responses, and insulin secretion after a liquid test meal: effects of exogenous glucagon-like peptide-1 (GLP-1)-(7–36) amide in type 2 (noninsulin-dependent) diabetic patients. *J Clin Endocrinol Metab* 1996, **81**(1), 327–332.

47. Schirra, J., Nicolaus, M., Roggel, R., Katschinski, M., Storr, M., Woerle, H. J., Goke, B. Endogenous glucagon-like peptide 1 controls endocrine pancreatic secretion and antro-pyloro-duodenal motility in humans. *Gut* 2006, **55**(2), 243–251.

48. Naslund, E., Barkeling, B., King, N., Gutniak, M., Blundell, J. E., Holst, J. J., Rossner, S., Hellstrom, P. M. Energy intake and appetite are suppressed by glucagon-like peptide-1 (GLP-1) in obese men. *Int J Obes Relat Metab Disord* 1999, **23**(3), 304–311.

49. Gutzwiller, J. P., Drewe, J., Goke, B., Schmidt, H., Rohrer, B., Lareida, J., Beglinger, C. Glucagon-like peptide-1 promotes satiety and reduces food intake in patients with diabetes mellitus type 2. *Am J Physiol* 1999, **276**(5 Pt 2), R1541–R1544.

50. Verdich, C., Flint, A., Gutzwiller, J. P., Naslund, E., Beglinger, C., Hellstrom, P. M., Long, S. J., Morgan, L. M., Holst, J. J., Astrup, A. A meta-analysis of the effect of glucagon-like peptide-1 (7–36) amide on ad libitum energy intake in humans. *J Clin Endocrinol Metab* 2001, **86**(9), 4382–4389.

51. Bullock, B. P., Heller, R. S., Habener, J. F. Tissue distribution of messenger ribonucleic acid encoding the rat glucagon-like peptide-1 receptor. *Endocrinology* 1996, **137**(7), 2968–2978.

52. Gros, R., You, X., Baggio, L. L., Kabir, M. G., Sadi, A. M., Mungrue, I. N., Parker, T. G., Huang, Q., Drucker, D. J., Husain, M. Cardiac function in mice lacking the glucagon-like peptide-1 receptor. *Endocrinology* 2003, **144**(6), 2242–2252.

53. Bose, A. K., Mocanu, M. M., Mensah, K. N., Brand, C. L., Carr, R. D., Yellon, D. M. GLP-1 protects schemic and reperfused myocardium via PI3Kinase and p42/p44 MAPK signalling pathways. *Diabetes* 2004, **53**(suppl. 2), A1.

54. Nikolaidis, L. A., Mankad, S., Sokos, G. G., Miske, G., Shah, A., Elahi, D., Shannon, R. P. Effects of glucagon-like peptide-1 in patients with acute myocardial infarction and left ventricular dysfunction after successful reperfusion. *Circulation* 2004, **109**(8), 962–965.

55. Nikolaidis, L. A., Elahi, D., Hentosz, T., Doverspike, A., Huerbin, R., Zourelias, L., Stolarski, C., Shen, Y. T., Shannon, R. P. Recombinant glucagon-like peptide-1 increases myocardial glucose uptake and improves left ventricular performance in conscious dogs with pacing-induced dilated cardiomyopathy. *Circulation* 2004, **110**(8), 955–961.

56. Nystrom, T., Gutniak, M. K., Zhang, Q., Zhang, F., Holst, J. J., Ahren, B., Sjoholm, A. Effects of glucagon-like peptide-1 on endothelial function in type 2 diabetes patients with stable coronary artery disease. *Am J Physiol Endocrinol Metab* 2004, **287**(6): 1209–1215.

57. Perry, T., Haughey, N. J., Mattson, M. P., Egan, J. M., Greig, N. H. Protection and reversal of excitotoxic neuronal damage by glucagon-like peptide-1 and exendin-4. *J Pharmacol Exp Ther* 2002, **302**(3), 881–888.

58. During, M. J., Cao, L., Zuzga, D. S., Francis, J. S., Fitzsimons, H. L., Jiao, X., Bland, R. J., Klugmann, M., Banks, W. A., Drucker, D. J., Haile, C. N. Glucagon-like peptide-1 receptor is involved in learning and neuroprotection. *Nat Med* 2003, **9**(9), 1173–1179.

59. Perry, T. A., Greig, N. H. A new Alzheimer's disease interventive strategy: GLP-1. *Curr Drug Targets* 2004, **5**(6), 565–571.

60. Nauck, M. A., Kleine, N., Orskov, C., Holst, J. J., Willms, B., Creutzfeldt, W. Normalization of fasting hyperglycaemia by exogenous glucagon-like peptide 1 (7–36 amide) in type 2 (non-insulin-dependent) diabetic patients. *Diabetologia* 1993, **36**(8), 741–744.

61. Rachman, J., Barrow, B. A., Levy, J. C., Turner, R. C. Near-normalisation of diurnal glucose concentrations by continuous administration of glucagon-like peptide-1 (GLP-1) in subjects with NIDDM. *Diabetologia* 1997, **40**(2), 205–211.

62. Larsen, J., Hylleberg, B., Ng, K., Damsbo, P. Glucagon-like peptide-1 infusion must be maintained for 24 h/day to obtain acceptable glycemia in type 2 diabetic patients who are poorly controlled on sulphonylurea treatment. *Diabetes Care* 2001, **24**(8), 1416–1421.

63. Nauck, M. A., Wollschlager, D., Werner, J., Holst, J. J., Orskov, C., Creutzfeldt, W., Willms, B. Effects of subcutaneous glucagon-like peptide 1 (GLP-1 [7–36 amide]) in patients with NIDDM. *Diabetologia* 1996, **39**(12), 1546–1553.

64. Ritzel, R., Orskov, C., Holst, J. J., Nauck, M. A. Pharmacokinetic, insulinotropic, and glucagonostatic properties of GLP-1 [7–36 amide] after subcutaneous injection in healthy volunteers. Dose-response-relationships. *Diabetologia* 1995, **38**(6), 720–725.

65. Deacon, C. F., Johnsen, A. H., Holst, J. J. Degradation of glucagon-like peptide-1 by human plasma in vitro yields an N-terminally truncated peptide that is a major endogenous metabolite in vivo. *J Clin Endocrinol Metab* 1995, **80**(3), 952–957.

66. Deacon, C. F., Nauck, M. A., Toft-Nielsen, M., Pridal, L., Willms, B., Holst, J. J. Both subcutaneously and intravenously administered glucagon-like peptide I are rapidly degraded from the NH2-terminus in type II diabetic patients and in healthy subjects. *Diabetes* 1995, **44**(9), 1126–1131.

67. Knudsen, L. B., Pridal, L. Glucagon-like peptide-1-(9–36) amide is a major metabolite of glucagon-like peptide-1-(7–36) amide after in vivo administration to dogs, and it acts as an antagonist on the pancreatic receptor. *Eur J Pharmacol* 1996, **318**(2–3), 429–435.

68. Zander, M., Madsbad, S., Deacon, C. F., Holst, J. J. The metabolite generated by dipeptidyl-peptidase 4 metabolism of glucagon-like peptide-1 has no influence on plasma glucose levels in patients with type 2 diabetes. *Diabetologia* 2006, **49**(2), 369–374.

69. Zander, M., Madsbad, S., Madsen, J. L., Holst, J. J. Effect of 6-week course of glucagon-like peptide 1 on glycaemic control, insulin sensitivity, and beta-cell function in type 2 diabetes: a parallel-group study. *Lancet* 2002, **359**(9309), 824–830.

70. Ehlers, M. R. W., Roderick, E. H., Schneider, R. L., Kipnes, M. S. Continuous subcutaneous infusion of recombinant GLP-1 for 7 days dose-dependently improved glycemic controls in type 2 diabetes. *Diabetes* 2002, **51**(suppl 2), A579.

71. Deacon, C. F., Knudsen, L. B., Madsen, K., Wiberg, F. C., Jacobsen, O., Holst, J. J. Dipeptidyl peptidase IV resistant analogues of glucagon-like peptide-1 which have extended metabolic stability and improved biological activity. *Diabetologia* 1998, **41**(3), 271–278.

72. Deacon, C. F., Hughes, T. E., Holst, J. J. Dipeptidyl peptidase IV inhibition potentiates the insulinotropic effect of glucagon-like peptide 1 in the anesthetized pig. *Diabetes* 1998, **47**(5), 764–769.

73. Edwards, C. M., Stanley, S. A., Davis, R., Brynes, A. E., Frost, G. S., Seal, L. J., Ghatei, M. A., Bloom, S. R. Exendin-4 reduces fasting and postprandial glucose and decreases energy intake in healthy volunteers. *Am J Physiol Endocrinol Metab* 2001, **281**(1), E155–E161.

74. Simonsen, L., Holst, J. J., Deacon, C. F. Exendin-4, but not glucagon-like peptide-1, is cleared exclusively by glomerular filtration in anaesthetised pigs. *Diabetologia* 2006, **49**(4): 706–712.

75. Kolterman, O. G., Kim, D. D., Shen, L., Ruggles, J. A., Nielsen, L. L., Fineman, M. S., Baron, A. D. Pharmacokinetics, pharmacodynamics, and safety of exenatide in patients with type 2 diabetes mellitus. *Am J Health Syst Pharm* 2005, **62**(2), 173–181.

76. Buse, J. B., Henry, R. R., Han, J., Kim, D. D., Fineman, M. S., Baron, A. D. Effects of exenatide (exendin-4) on glycemic control over 30 weeks in sulfonylurea-treated patients with type 2 diabetes. *Diabetes Care* 2004, **27**(11), 2628–2635.

77. Defronzo, R. A., Ratner, R. E., Han, J., Kim, D. D., Fineman, M. S., Baron, A. D. Effects of exenatide (exendin-4) on glycemic control and weight over 30 weeks in metformin-treated patients with type 2 diabetes. *Diabetes Care* 2005, **28**(5), 1092–1100.

78. Kendall, D. M., Riddle, M. C., Rosenstock, J., Zhuang, D., Kim, D. D., Fineman, M. S., Baron, A. D. Effects of exenatide (exendin-4) on glycemic control over 30 weeks in patients with type 2 diabetes treated with metformin and a sulfonylurea. *Diabetes Care* 2005, **28**(5), 1083–1091.

79. Lamari, Y., Boissard, C., Moukhtar, M. S., Jullienne, A., Rosselin, G., Garel, J. M. Expression of glucagon-like peptide 1 receptor in a murine C cell line: regulation of calcitonin gene by glucagon-like peptide. *FEBS Lett* 1996, **393**(2–3), 248–252.

80. Gedulin, B. R., Smith, P., Prickett, K. S., Tryon, M., Barnhill, S., Reynolds, J., Nielsen, L. L., Parkes, D. G., Young, A. A. Dose-response for glycaemic and metabolic changes 28 days after single injection of long-acting release exenatide in diabetic fatty Zucker rats. *Diabetologia* 2005, **48**(7), 1380–1385.

81. Degn, K. B., Juhl, C. B., Sturis, J., Jakobsen, G., Brock, B., Chandramouli, V., Rungby, J., Landau, B. R., Schmitz, O. One week's treatment with the long-acting glucagon-like peptide 1 derivative liraglutide (NN2211) markedly improves 24-h glycemia and alpha- and beta-cell function and reduces endogenous glucose release in patients with type 2 diabetes. *Diabetes* 2004, **53**(5), 1187–1194.

82. Knudsen, L. B., Agersø, H., Bjenning, C., Bregenholt, S., Gotfredsen, C., Holst, J. J., Huusfeldt, P. O., Larsen, M. Ø., Larsen, P. J., Nielsen, P. F., Ribel, U., Rolin, B., Rømer, J., Wilken, M., Kristensen, P. GLP-1 derivatives as novel compounds for the treatment of type 2 diabetes. *Drugs Future* 2001, **26**, 677–685.

83. Madsbad, S., Schmitz, O., Ranstam, J., Jakobsen, G., Matthews, D. R. Improved glycemic control with no weight increase in patients with type 2 diabetes after once-daily treatment with the long-acting glucagon-like peptide 1 analog liraglutide (NN2211): a 12-week, double-blind, randomized, controlled trial. *Diabetes Care* 2004, **27**(6), 1335–1342.

84. Nauck, M., Hompesch, M., Filipczak, R., Le, T. T. D., Nielsen, L., Zdravkovic, M., Gumprecht, J. Liraglutide as add-on to metformin in type 2 diabetes: significant improvement in glycaemic control with a reduction in body weight compared with glimepiride. Diabetologia 2004, **47**(suppl 1) A281.

85. Baggio, L. L., Huang, Q., Brown, T. J., Drucker, D. J. A recombinant human glucagon-like peptide (GLP)-1-albumin protein (Albugon) mimics peptidergic activation of GLP-1 receptor-dependent pathways coupled with satiety, gastrointestinal motility, and glucose homeostasis. *Diabetes* 2004, **53**(9), 2492–2500.

86. Bloom, M., Bock, J., Duttaroy, A., Grzegorzewski, K., Moor, P., Ou, Y., Wojcik, S., Zhou, X., Bell, A. Albugon fusion protein: a long acting analogue of GLP-1 that provides lasting antidiabetic effect in animals. *Diabetes* 2003, **52**(suppl 1), A112.

87. Pospisilik, J. A., Stafford, S. G., Demuth, H. U., Brownsey, R., Parkhouse, W., Finegood, D. T., McIntosh, C. H., Pederson, R. A. Long-term treatment with the dipeptidyl peptidase IV inhibitor P32/98 causes sustained improvements in glucose tolerance, insulin sensitivity, hyperinsulinemia, and beta-cell glucose responsiveness in VDF (fa/fa) Zucker rats. *Diabetes* 2002, **51**(4), 943–950.

88. Sudre, B., Broqua, P., White, R. B., Ashworth, D., Evans, D. M., Haigh, R., Junien, J. L., Aubert, M. L. Chronic inhibition of circulating dipeptidyl peptidase IV by FE 999011 delays the occurrence of diabetes in male zucker diabetic fatty rats. *Diabetes* 2002, **51**(5), 1461–1469.

89. Reimer, M. K., Holst, J. J., Ahren, B. Long-term inhibition of dipeptidyl peptidase IV improves glucose tolerance and preserves islet function in mice. *Eur J Endocrinol* **2002**, **146**(5), 717–727.

90. Nagakura, T., Yasuda, N., Yamazaki, K., Ikuta, H., Yoshikawa, S., Asano, O., Tanaka, I. Improved glucose tolerance via enhanced glucose-dependent insulin secretion in dipeptidyl peptidase IV-deficient Fischer rats. *Biochem Biophys Res Commun* 2001, **284**(2), 501–506.

91. Marguet, D., Baggio, L., Kobayashi, T., Bernard, A. M., Pierres, M., Nielsen, P. F., Ribel, U., Watanabe, T., Drucker, D. J., Wagtmann, N. Enhanced insulin secretion and improved glucose tolerance in mice lacking CD26. *Proc Natl Acad Sci USA* 2000, **97**(12), 6874–6879.

92. Mitani, H., Takimoto, M., Kimura, M. Dipeptidyl peptidase IV inhibitor NVP-DPP728 ameliorates early insulin response and glucose tolerance in aged rats but not in aged Fischer 344 rats lacking its enzyme activity. *Jpn J Pharmacol* 2002, **88**(4), 451–458.

93. Mitani, H., Takimoto, M., Hughes, T. E., Kimura, M. Dipeptidyl peptidase IV inhibition improves impaired glucose tolerance in high-fat diet-fed rats: study using a Fischer 344 rat substrain deficient in its enzyme activity. *Jpn J Pharmacol* 2002, **88**(4), 442–450.

94. Yasuda, N., Nagakura, T., Yamazaki, K., Inoue, T., Tanaka, I. Improvement of high fat-diet-induced insulin resistance in dipeptidyl peptidase IV-deficient Fischer rats. *Life Sci* 2002, **71**(2), 227–238.

95. Conarello, S. L., Li, Z., Ronan, J., Roy, R. S., Zhu, L., Jiang, G., Liu, F., Woods, J., Zycband, E., Moller, D. E., Thornberry, N. A., Zhang, B. B. Mice lacking dipeptidyl peptidase IV are protected against obesity and insulin resistance. *Proc Natl Acad Sci USA* 2003, **100**(11), 6825–6830.

96. Ahren, B., Simonsson, E., Larsson, H., Landin-Olsson, M., Torgeirsson, H., Jansson, P. A., Sandqvist, M., Bavenholm, P., Efendic, S., Eriksson, J. W., Dickinson, S., Holmes, D. Inhibition of dipeptidyl peptidase IV improves metabolic control over a 4-week study period in type 2 diabetes. *Diabetes Care* 2002, **25**(5), 869–875.

97. Ahren, B., Landin-Olsson, M., Jansson, P. A., Svensson, M., Holmes, D., Schweizer, A. Inhibition of dipeptidyl peptidase-4 reduces glycemia, sustains insulin levels, and reduces glucagon levels in type 2 diabetes. *J Clin Endocrinol Metab* 2004, **89**(5), 2078–2084.

98. Ahren, B., Gomis, R., Standl, E., Mills, D., Schweizer, A. Twelve- and 52-week efficacy of the dipeptidyl peptidase IV inhibitor LAF237 in metformin-treated patients with type 2 diabetes. *Diabetes Care* 2004, 27(12), 2874–2880.

99. Ahren, B., Pacini, G., Foley, J. E., Schweizer, A. Improved meal-related beta-cell function and insulin sensitivity by the dipeptidyl peptidase-IV inhibitor vildagliptin in metformin-treated patients with type 2 diabetes over 1 year. *Diabetes Care* 2005, **28**(8), 1936–1940.

100. Brandt, I., Joossens, J., Chen, X., Maes, M. B., Scharpe, S., Meester, I. D., Lambeir, A. M. Inhibition of dipeptidyl-peptidase IV catalyzed peptide truncation by Vildagliptin ((2S)-{[(3-hydroxyadamantan-1-yl)amino]acetyl}-pyrrolidine-2-carbonitrile). *Biochem Pharmacol* 2005, **70**(1), 134–143.

101. Mari, A., Sallas, W. M., He, Y. L., Watson, C., Ligueros-Saylan, M., Dunning, B. E., Deacon, C. F., Holst, J. J., Foley, J. E. Vildagliptin. A dipeptidyl peptidase-iv inhibitor, improves model-assessed {beta}-cell function in patients with type 2 diabetes. *J Clin Endocrinol Metab* 2005, **90**(8): 4888-4894.

102. Deacon, C. F. MK-431 (Merck). *Curr Opin Investig Drugs* 2005, **6**(4), 419–426.

103. Herman, G. A., Stevens, C., Van, D. K., Bergman, A., Yi, B., De, S. M., Snyder, K., Hilliard, D., Tanen, M., Tanaka, W., Wang, A. Q., Zeng, W., Musson, D., Winchell, G., Davies, M. J., Ramael, S., Gottesdiener, K. M., Wagner, J. A. Pharmacokinetics and pharmacodynamics of sitagliptin, an inhibitor of dipeptidyl peptidase IV, in healthy subjects: results from two randomized, double-blind, placebo-controlled studies with single oral doses. *Clin Pharmacol Ther* 2005, **78**(6), 675–688.

104. Heins, J., Glund, K., Hoffmann, T., Metzner, J., Demuth, H.-U. The DP-IV inhibitor P93/01 improves glucose tolerance in humans with HbA1c gerater than 6.0. *Diabetes* 2004, **53**(suppl 2), A128.

105. Lambeir, A. M., Durinx, C., Scharpe, S., De, M., I Dipeptidyl-peptidase IV from bench to bedside: an update on structural properties, functions, and clinical aspects of the enzyme DPP-IV. *Crit Rev Clin Lab Sci* 2003, **40**(3), 209–294.

106. Zhu, L., Tamvakopoulos, C., Xie, D., Dragovic, J., Shen, X., Fenyk-Melody, J. E., Schmidt, K., Bagchi, A., Griffin, P. R., Thornberry, N. A., Sinha, R. R. The role of dipeptidyl peptidase IV in the cleavage of glucagon family peptides: in vivo metabolism of pituitary adenylate cyclase activating polypeptide-(1–38). *J Biol Chem* 2003, **278**(25), 22418–22423.

107. Ahren, B., Hughes, T. E. Inhibition of dipeptidyl peptidase-4 augments insulin secretion in response to exogenously administered glucagon-like peptide-1, glucose-dependent insulinotropic polypeptide, pituitary adenylate cyclase-activating polypeptide, and gastrin-releasing peptide in mice. *Endocrinology* 2005, **146**(4), 2055–2059.

108. von Bonin, A., Huhn, J., Fleischer, B. Dipeptidyl-peptidase IV/CD26 on T cells: analysis of an alternative T-cell activation pathway. *Immunol Rev* 1998, **161**, 43–53.

109. Lankas, G. R., Leiting, B., Roy, R. S., Eiermann, G. J., Beconi, M. G., Biftu, T., Chan, C. C., Edmondson, S., Feeney, W. P., He, H., Ippolito, D. E., Kim, D., Lyons, K. A., Ok, H. O., Patel, R. A., Petrov, A. N., Pryor, K. A., Qian, X., Reigle, L., Woods, A., Wu, J. K., Zaller, D., Zhang, X., Zhu, L., Weber, A. E., Thornberry, N. A. Dipeptidyl peptidase iv inhibition for the treatment of type 2 diabetes: potential importance of selectivity over dipeptidyl peptidases 8 and 9. *Diabetes* 2005, **54**(10), 2988–2994.

110. Weber, A. E., Kim, D., Beconi, M., et.al. MK-0431 is a potent, selective dipeptidyl peptidase IV inhibitor for the treatment of type 2 diabetes. *Diabetes* 2004, **53**(suppl 2), A151.

15

Controversies in Evaluation and Management of Lipid Disorders in Diabetes

Ronald B. Goldberg, MD

CONTENTS

From: *Contemporary Endocrinology: Controversies in Treating Diabetes: Clinical and Research Aspects*
Edited by: D. LeRoith and A. I. Vinik © Humana Press, Totowa, NJ

SUMMARY

Dyslipidemia is a key factors contributing to the high risk of cardiovascular disease (CVD) in diabetes and its management is of prime importance. However there are a number of controversies in this area which are dealt with in this chapter. One of these is the extent to which diabetes increases CVD risk, which turns out to vary considerably. A second question deals with the preferred dietary and other weight loss therapies and their benefits in dyslipidemic subjects. The third topic discussed deals with the question of "how low to go" with LDL-cholesterol lowering, and in a fourth issue the indications and approach to the use of second or third lipid-modifying agents in combination with statin therapy is discussed. Finally the controversial issue of whether apolipoprotein or lipoprotein subfraction measurements add to the value of the standard lipid profile is debated.

Key Words: Diabetic dyslipidemia, management, cardiovascular disease

INTRODUCTION

Cardiovascular disease (CVD) is the major cause of morbidity and mortality in diabetes *(1)*, and thus identification and effective management of its determinants are crucial in the effort to improve health status and extend survival in people with diabetes. Dyslipidemia is one of the major risk factors predisposing to CVD *(2)*, and over the past decade, controlled clinical trials with lipid-modifying agents have led to considerable advances in our understanding of the relationships between the predictive value of lipids and lipoproteins for CVD and the extent to which these interventions produce benefit *(3)*. Despite this, the evidence indicates that the majority of diabetic subjects are not at lipid and lipoprotein targets *(4)*, and given the fact that progress in reducing CVD events in diabetic subjects over the past decade or two has been minimal *(5)*, more attention is required to convey to health care providers the requisite urgency needed in targeting and achieving optimal lipoprotein levels. It is with these considerations in mind that this discussion of controversial issues in the evaluation and management of dyslipidemia in diabetes is presented.

IS DIABETES REALLY A CORONARY HEART DISEASE RISK EQUIVALENT?

The advent of the National Cholesterol Education Program's (NCEP) Adult Treatment Panel III (ATP III) guidelines for management of hypercholesterolemia did more than any other program to promote a risk-based approach to the problem of CVD and its prevention *(6)*. In particular, the concept of a coronary heart disease (CHD) risk equivalent state (≥20% 10-year risk of "hard CHD events") introduced the idea that individuals without heart disease, but with the same risk for an event as those with established CHD, should be as aggressively treated as the latter. Although this strategy has not formally been accepted for management of other risk factors, the results of clinical intervention trials in subjects with CHD statins has led to widespread support for this approach as far as low-density lipoprotein cholesterol (LDL-C) levels and therapeutic decision-making are concerned. Thus, the report from Finland in 1998 that type 2 diabetic subjects without CHD had essentially the same risk of myocardial infarction (MI) as did non-diabetic subjects who had already experienced an MI *(7)* prompted the NCEP ATP III panel to label essentially all type 2 diabetic subjects as having a CHD equivalent risk *(6)*. This finding garnered support quite soon from the Organization to Assess Strategies for Ischemic Syndromes (OASIS) study *(8)*, although an Australian study found that the risk for CHD in diabetic individuals without CHD was significantly lower than that in non-diabetic subjects with CHD *(9)*. Since then, there have been at least five reports indicating that men and women with diabetes but no evident CHD have approximately a third to a quarter less relative risk for CHD than do non-diabetic individuals with established CHD *(9–13)*. The reason for these discrepancies are unknown but likely have to do with differences in the diabetic populations being surveyed, including factors such as age, severity, and duration of diabetes *(10,11)*.

More people with type 2 diabetes are being diagnosed at a younger age, and age is a powerful CVD risk factor even in diabetes. In a prospective observational study *(14)* of the incidence of macrovascular disease in 7844 newly diagnosed diabetic subjects in a large health maintenance organization (mean follow-up 3.9 years), individuals diagnosed before the age of 45 years (mean age at diagnosis was 38 years) had an MI incidence of 4.6% as compared with 23.4% in those diagnosed after 45 years of age (mean age 60 years). The respective incidences of stroke were 1.6 and 11.1%. There is far less clear-cut evidence on how to grade the CVD risk of subjects with type 1 diabetes. The Joslin clinic experience indicates that juvenile onset type 1 diabetic subjects begin to develop a significant increase in CVD events by 40 years of age irrespective of whether the onset of their disease was in the first or second decade of life *(15)*. It seems likely that in most diabetic subjects under the age of 30 years, the 10-year risk of CHD events is considerably <20%, and health care providers may wish to treat such individuals as they would the population with intermediate risk.

Another issue of increasing importance, as the global explosion of diabetes takes hold and with the expansion in numbers of immigrants and minority groups, is the effect of ethnicity. In the Center for Disease Control and Prevention data set *(16)*, White men had a CVD prevalence of 38.7% (26% more frequent than White women), Black men 31.3% (7.6% more frequent than Black women), and Hispanic men 29.9% (26% more frequent than Hispanic women). In a 20-year cohort study reported in 1996 from London, compared with Europeans, Afro-Caribbean diabetic subjects had a risk ratio for CVD of 0.33 and for CHD of 0.37 *(17)*, and in two studies from the Netherlands, both Moroccan and Turkish immigrants with diabetes had significantly lower CVD mortality rates than did diabetic subjects in the indigenous population *(18,19)*. In the USA, earlier data had suggested that despite greater rates of obesity and diabetes, Mexican-Americans had lower CVD mortality rates than did non-Hispanic Whites, giving rise to the so-called Hispanic paradox. However, this was likely due to migration factors and selection, because a more recent study indicated that Mexican-American diabetic subjects born in the USA had higher CVD mortality rates than Mexican-born individuals and indigenous non-Hispanic Whites *(20)*. It is also well-recognized that in the USA, Black subjects have a higher risk of stroke than do Whites, but this does not appear to be the case for diabetic individuals *(21)*. Other factors influencing incidence of CVD include the presence of hypertension *(22,23)* and, perhaps most significantly, renal disease *(24,25)*. Ultimately, the implications of these differences may be important for individualized therapeutic decisions, but they do not significantly minimize concern for the heightened risk of CVD in diabetic subjects.

ARE LOW CARBOHYDRATE DIETS MORE EFFECTIVE THAN LOW FAT DIETS IN THE INITIAL MANAGEMENT OF DIABETIC DYSLIPIDEMIA, AND SHOULD GREATER USE BE MADE OF WEIGHT LOSS MEDICINES AND BARIATRIC SURGERY IN OBESE DIABETIC SUBJECTS WITH COMORBIDITIES?

To begin with, it is important to be clear what the goals of lifestyle intervention in the management of diabetic dyslipidemia are. Most subjects with type 2 diabetes are overweight or obese, and moderate weight loss may improve diabetic dyslipidemia and other CVD risk factors as well lower glucose levels. Therefore, weight loss is an important therapeutic strategy in targeting all overweight or obese dyslipidemic individuals with diabetes. The primary approach for achieving weight loss, in the vast majority of cases, is therapeutic lifestyle change, which includes a reduction in energy intake and an increase in physical activity, both of which are more likely to be facilitated in the setting of a behavior modification program. A moderate decrease in caloric balance (500–1000 kcal/day) will result in a slow but progressive weight loss (1–2 lb/week). For most patients, weight loss diets should supply at least 1000–1200 kcal/day for women and 1200–1600 kcal/day for men, and very low-calorie diets are not generally recommended. A low-fat diet is the conventional approach to initiating weight reduction as these have shown long-term success *(26)*. However, there is a recent interest in the use of low-carbohydrate hypocaloric diets, because in the short term, they may result in greater weight loss and better control of glycemia and dyslipidemia than conventional weight-reducing diets *(27)* as discussed further in this section. Physical activity is an important component of a comprehensive weight management program *(28)*. Regular, moderate intensity, physical activity enhances long-term weight maintenance. Regular activity also improves insulin sensitivity, glycemic control, and dyslipidemia, and increased aerobic fitness decreases the risk of CHD. Initial physical activity recommendations should be modest, based on the patient's willingness and ability, gradually increasing the duration and frequency to 30–45 min of moderate aerobic activity 3–5 days per week when possible *(29)*. Greater activity levels of at least 1 h/day of moderate (walking) or 30 min/day of vigorous (jogging) activity may be needed to achieve successful long-term weight loss; however, exercise testing should be performed at the discretion of the primary care physician before vigorous exercise, particularly in patients with diabetes.

With respect to the effects of diet composition on improvement of diabetic dyslipidemia, both NCEP and American Diabetes Association (ADA) guidelines give first priority to lowering of LDL-C in the management of diabetic dyslipidemia as discussed further in the next section. They further concur in recommending that the intake of saturated fatty acids and trans-saturated fatty acids be reduced to lower LDL-C levels *(6,30)*. ATP III recommends limiting the intake of saturated fat to less than 7% of the daily calories and the intake of cholesterol to less than 200mg/day. This diet, also known as the step 2 diet, has been shown in a meta-analysis to be associated with a 16% LDL-C reduction *(31)*. Additional dietary options to lower LDL-C include increasing the amount of soluble dietary fiber to 10–25 grams daily, adding 2 grams daily of plant stanols/sterols, and including soy protein in the diet. These interventions have been associated with a 5–15% reduction in LDL-C values *(32–35)*. However, as mentioned already in relation to dietary weight loss approaches, the distribution of macronutrients in the diet is a matter of debate particularly in individuals with diabetic dyslipidemia. Low-fat, high-carbohydrate (>60% of total caloric intake) diets have been associated with an increase in triglyceride and a fall in high-density lipoprotein cholesterol (HDL-C) levels *(36)*. When monounsaturated fat is substituted for saturated fat in the diet, the LDL-lowering effect is similar to that obtained with a low-fat, high-carbohydrate diet without the raise in triglyceride and the fall in HDL levels *(37)*. ATP III recommends limiting the intake of carbohydrates to less than 60% in individuals with the metabolic syndrome and type 2 diabetes. Furthermore, for individuals with elevated triglyceride and low HDL-C levels, lower carbohydrate intake (i.e., 50% of calories) could be considered, but very low carbohydrate intake is not recommended. The ADA also recommends replacing saturated fat with carbohydrates or monounsaturated fat (30) but does not formally recommend very low-carbohydrate diets.

Low-carbohydrate diets have been used for many years and have recently become even more popular. Though these diets may have short-term beneficial effects on serum lipids, fasting glucose, and weight reduction (27), these apparent benefits have not been shown to persist over a more lengthy period and do not appear to lower LDL-C compared with higher carbohydrate, lower fat diets (38). Furthermore, low-carbohydrate diets have not been adequately evaluated in individuals with diabetes and hyperlipidemia, and their long-term safety and efficacy remain unknown. Additional research is needed to clarify the long-term efficacy and safety of low-carbohydrate diets, particularly in patients with diabetes.

The role of weight loss medications and bariatric surgery in the management of obesity in diabetes has not been well defined. Although there is clinical trial evidence showing that the two currently available prescription medications with an indication for weight reduction, sibutramine and orlistat plus dietary recommendations do increase weight loss, reduce HbA1c, and improve lipids in subjects with type 2 diabetes compared with placebo and diet (39,40); the question as to whether or when patients should receive these medications long-term given their side effects, expense and unproven benefit except in short-term studies, is unknown. Similarly, although bariatric surgery is reported to lead to withdrawal of antihyperglycemic medications in approximately 60% of cases and to reductions of medicines in many others, most of these procedures are performed for reasons other than for management of diabetes and its complications (41), and most reports have been uncontrolled or inadequately controlled. What is needed are long-term controlled clinical trials with the primary objective of assessing whether bariatric surgery is more efficacious, safe, and cost effective in the management of diabetes compared with standard medical therapy.

THE FIRST PRIORITY IN THE PHARMACOTHERAPY OF DIABETIC DYSLIPIDEMIA IS TO LOWER LDL-C WITH A STATIN; THE TARGET SHOULD BE AN LDL-C OF <100 MG/DL, AND THE BENEFIT IS DUE TO LDL LOWERING

At first glance, this statement appears to be non-controversial, but each part of it has been and continues to be a subject of considerable debate, and the issues at stake are considered to be crucial to a full understanding of modern therapeutic strategies. Although the lipid profile in subjects with type 1 diabetes is usually unremarkable, it is well-recognized that the typical abnormality in the lipid profile in subjects with type 2 diabetes is that of elevated triglyceride and/or reduced HDL-C occurring together with average LDL-C levels *(42)*. It may be tempting therefore to view the high triglyceride/low HDL-C abnormality as the primary target for treatment. This would require the preferential use of fibrates and niacin in pharmacotherapy after lifestyle intervention rather than statins that have more modest effects on triglycerides and HDL-C. However, the MRFIT study demonstrated that the total cholesterol—a surrogate of LDL-C—is a powerful predictor of CVD mortality in diabetic individuals *(22)*, and the United Kingdom Prospective Diabetes Study (UKPDS) established that in newly diagnosed type 2 diabetic subjects, LDL-C was the most important predictor of CVD events, followed by HDL-C, and then the HbA1c *(43)*. The triglyceride level was not a significant predictor, as is the case in most epidemiologic studies of CVD risk factors. Whether lipoprotein subfractions are more powerful CVD risk factors than traditional lipid measures as discussed in the section dealing with newer lipoprotein measurements.

For many years, LDL-C lowering in diabetes was included together with the treatment of all subjects with elevated LDL-C levels, and diabetes (without evident heart disease) was just another risk factor that helped to set the boundary between what was an acceptable LDL-C level and what required medical treatment. In 2001, when the ATP III panel recommended that diabetes be considered a CHD-risk equivalent *(6)*, treatment strategies changed. Given the importance of LDL-C as a CVD predictor in diabetes even though LDL-C levels typically are not elevated in these subjects, the concept developed that highly active atherogenesis might progress in the presence of even below average LDL-C levels because of ramped up arterial wall inflammation and that this scenario operates in individuals with diabetes. Even though LDL-C levels might be low, highly atherogenic small LDL particle numbers are frequently elevated, and this has been advanced as a potentially important factor driving progression of vascular disease (as discussed in the last section). Whatever the mechanisms, the results of recent statin trials in high-risk and very high-risk subjects has borne out the correctness of this idea, demonstrating that benefit accrues from the use of statins in subjects with relatively and recently, absolutely low LDL-C levels irrespective of their triglyceride or HDL-C levels. The modern paradigm, best illustrated in the Heart Protection Study (HPS) appears to be that whatever the LDL-C level is in subjects with a CHD-risk equivalent, statin therapy will reduce CVD if it achieves at least a 30% LDL-C lowering *(44)*. In HPS, the relative risk reduction from 40 mg/day simvastatin treatment in subjects with CHD and/or diabetes and with a baseline LDL-C $\geq$ 130 mg/dl was the same as in those with an LDL-C $\leq$ 100 mg/dl, namely approximately 25%. Although there were only a small number of diabetic subjects who fitted criteria for type 1 diabetes in HPS, they appeared to benefit from simvastatin therapy in similar fashion to the rest of the diabetic cohort. The participants in HPS were a mixed group of mostly non-diabetic individuals with CVD, as well as of diabetic subjects with and without heart disease, and therefore, the study was not able to address the question as to whether this conclusion applied specifically to the majority of diabetic subjects (60–75%) who do not have overt CVD and whose absolute CHD risk may be somewhat lower than 20% over 10 years. However, the Collaborative Atorvastatin Diabetes Study (CARDS) only randomized diabetic subjects without evident CVD (and with one CVD risk factor) and with a baseline LDL-C < 160 mg/dl to atorvastatin 10 mg/day versus placebo treatment *(45)*. They were able to show that subjects above and below the mean LDL-C of 118 mg/dl had the same relative risk reduction ($\sim 35\%$) attributable to atorvastatin treatment. This gives support to the notion that primary prevention in subjects with diabetes should be considered even in subjects with below average LDL-C levels.

Based on the HPS results as well as those from PROVE-IT, a study demonstrating in a cohort with an acute coronary syndrome that subjects with atorvastatin 80 mg/day treated down to a median LDL-C of approximately 70 mg/dl benefited more than those treated with pravastatin 40 mg/day whose median LDL-C was approximately 100 mg/dl *(46)*, the NCEP ATP III panel proposed an optional lower LDL-C target of 70 mg/dl in very high-risk patients. The panel continues to recommend a standard target of <100 mg/dl for subjects with a CHD-risk equivalent, which includes those with diabetes but no CVD *(47)*. Although the PROVE-IT trial included subjects with diabetes plus CHD, the results of this study in individuals presenting with an acute coronary syndrome that is associated with a very high event rate cannot be extrapolated to the majority of high-risk subjects with stable CHD. However, definitive evidence that additional benefit accrues to subjects with stable CHD (as opposed to the very high-risk group with an acute coronary syndrome) and average LDL-C (~ 130 mg/dl) levels treated down to a mean LDL-C of 77 mg/dl compared with those treated to a mean of 101 mg/dl has now been demonstrated in the Treatment to New Targets (TNT) Study *(48)*. Although similar results were demonstrated in the TNT subgroup with diabetes to that of the entire cohort *(49)*, there were no diabetic subjects without evident CHD in that study. Thus, although the evidence may point to added benefit resulting from statin treatment down to an LDL-C of 77 mg/dl in diabetic subjects with a clear CHD equivalent, this is not established for younger, less complicated diabetic subjects without CHD. It is also appears from TNT that the 22% relative risk reduction achieved in lowering LDL-C from approximately 100 to 70 mg/dl is somewhat smaller than what has been reported in previous statin intervention trials with baseline LDL-C levels of ≥115 mg/dl, where it is typically 25–35%. In addition, despite the efficacy of modern LDL-C lowering treatment, achievement of these very low LDL-C levels may not always be attained. For example, at LDL-C levels ≥145 mg/dl, no more than 50% of subjects will attain an LDL-C of 70 mg/dl despite maximum doses of potent statins in combination with ezetemibe *(50)*. Finally, there is a greater risk of adverse events at maximum statin doses. Like the NCEP ATP III, the primary treatment strategy recommended by the ADA is directed at LDL-C. The recommended LDL-C target is <100 mg/dl in individuals without established CHD and in those >40 years of age or in those with overt CVD, the ADA recommends achieving an LDL-C reduction of approximately 30–40% regardless of baseline LDL-C levels; in addition, an optional target of 70 mg/dl is indicated for those with CVD *(51)*.

There has been considerable evidence that statins have pleiotropic anti-inflammatory and antithrombotic effects *(52)*, and the recognition that atherosclerosis is characterized by inflammatory change in the vascular wall has raised the possibility that statins might reduce CVD events through their pleiotropic actions, in addition to effects on lowering of LDL-C. Although it seems clear from statin intervention trials that there is a close relationship between CVD event reduction and the degree of LDL-C lowering that is either linear or more likely curvilinear *(6)*, several clinical trials have provided some suggestive evidence that there may be therapeutically important statin effects independent of LDL-C lowering. Use of high-dose statin therapy in the 4-month myocardial ischemia reduction with aggressive cholesterol lowering (MIRACL) study trial that demonstrated beneficial effects of statins in subjects with an acute coronary syndrome *(53)* suggested the possible induction of acute and subacute beneficial vascular changes not easily explained by the traditional concepts of how statins reduce events, namely by slowing of plaque progression through LDL-C reduction. Furthermore, subanalyses of the coronary atherosclerosis and recurrent events (CARE) *(54)* and PROVE-IT *(55)* trials showed that statin-induced decreases in levels of high-sensitivity C reactive protein (CRP), a marker of subclinical inflammation and a powerful predictor of CVD events, appear to predict benefit independently of LDL-C lowering. In the PROVE-IT trial, the investigators showed that the benefit achieved in lowering LDL-C levels below 70 mg/dl with statin treatment as compared to those with values >70 mg/dl, approximated the benefit accruing to those whose CRP levels were reduced to <2 mg/l by statin therapy relative to those with CRP levels >2 mg/l and that the LDL-C-lowering and CRP-lowering effects were additive. More support for this concept may be obtained if similar results are obtained in the JUPITER trial in which subjects without CVD and with levels of LDL-C < 130 mg/dl and CRP > 2 mg/l have been randomized to either 20 mg rosuvastatin or placebo treatment for a 3- to 4-year period *(56)*. This issue may have special importance for the prevention of CVD in diabetic subjects in whom circulating markers and vascular levels of inflammation are known to be elevated compared with non-diabetic comparators *(57,58)*.

SHOULD ANTIDYLIPIDEMIC AGENTS SUCH AS FIBRATES, NIACIN OR FISH OIL BE ADDED TO STATIN TREATMENT FOR MOST PATIENTS GIVEN THE FREQUENCY OF HYPERTRIGLYCERIDEMIA AND/OR LOW HDL-C IN TYPE 2 DIABETES?

The prevalence of dyslipidemia in individuals with diabetes depends on the criteria used to define it. Overall, 30–40% of patients with type 2 diabetes have triglyceride levels >200 mg/dl and 10% >400 mg/dl *(59)*. Sixty two percent of participants with diabetes in NHANES III aged 50 years and older had triglyceride levels >150 mg/dl and 60% had low HDL cholesterol levels (<40mg/dl in men and <50 mg/dl in women) *(60)*. In the UKPDS, baseline HDL-C levels were 9% lower in newly diagnosed men with type 2 diabetes and 23% lower in diabetic women compared with non-diabetic controls *(61)*. Triglyceride levels were 50% higher in diabetic subjects than in controls, whereas LDL-C values were similar in diabetic men and higher in diabetic women compared with their non-diabetic controls. The frequency of LDL phenotype B (preponderance of small-dense LDL particles) in diabetic subjects is two-fold higher than in the rest of the population *(62)*. As a comparison, in subjects with impaired glucose tolerance 46% have triglyceride levels >150 mg/dl, 57% have HDL-C < 40 mg/dl in men and <50 mg/dl in women, and 41% of men and 25% of women have the small dense LDL phenotype *(63)*.

After achieving LDL-C targets, NCEP ATP-III and ADA guidelines for dyslipidemia management differ somewhat. That there is a need for further antidyslipidemic therapy arises from the recognition that while benefits from statin intervention trials are significant and robust, despite statin therapy, CHD continues to develop in treated diabetic subjects at rates greater than that in the general population. In addition, statins do not typically restore all components of the lipid profile to an acceptable range. It has also been demonstrated that achievement of all three lipid goals is more likely with combination therapy *(64–66)* in short-term studies. However, the added complexity and risks of combination therapy in the absence of robust clinical trial evidence for additional CVD benefit should place some limitations on the use of these combinations. The presence of CVD would appear to be such an indication because of the very large risk for recurrent events in these diabetic subjects; in those without evident CVD, it would seem appropriate for subjects above the age of 40 years and/or with other major CVD risk factors, such as hypertension or albuminuria. The presence of renal disease is a relative contraindication to statin–fibrate combinations.

According to ATP-III, for individuals with triglyceride levels >200mg/dl, the secondary lipid target is the non-HDL-C (total cholesterol—HDL-C). Non-HDL-C correlates well with apoB levels and includes the cholesterol content of all atherogenic lipoproteins that contain apo B, namely, LDL, lipoprotein (a), intermediate-density lipoprotein, and very low-density lipoprotein (VLDL) *(6)*. The goal for non-HDL-C is set 30 mg/dL higher than the LDL target (<130 mg/dl for diabetic subjects). When triglyceride values are ≥500 mg/dl, triglyceride lowering becomes the first priority because of concerns about the risk of pancreatitis. Low HDL-C is the third priority for management and HDL-C-raising strategies may be considered in "high-risk" individuals with HDL-C levels <40 mg/dl. However, in the NCEP guidelines, HDL-C target levels were not established. By contrast, after achievement of LDL-C targets, the ADA guidelines recommend raising reduced HDL-C and lowering elevated triglyceride levels as the second and third priorities, respectively, with low-risk levels for HDL-C of >40 mg/dl in men and >50 mg/dl in women and for triglyceride <150 mg/dl *(51)*. The ADA guidelines also emphasize the importance of glycemic control and lifestyle interventions such as weight loss, exercise, and smoking cessation in the management of hypertriglyceridemia and low HDL-C levels. Improved glycemic control regardless of type of treatment is associated with improved lipid values in individuals with moderate to severe hyperglycemia. In the Veterans Affairs Cooperative Study in type II diabetes, intensive glycemic control with insulin therapy, in which HbA1c was reduced from 9.3 to 7.2%, was associated with a 31% reduction in triglyceride levels after 1 year and 23% reduction at 2 years *(67)*. LDL-C and HDL-C did not change significantly from baseline in the intensive treatment group. Metformin has been shown to lower triglyceride concentrations between 10 and 29%, with beneficial changes of lesser magnitude in LDL-C and HDL in some but not all studies *(68)*. Both rosiglitazone and pioglitazone raise HDL-C and LDL-C and increase the size of LDL, with pioglitazone increasing HDL-C up to 15%, in one study, almost twice that achieved by rosiglitazone; pioglitazone, but not rosiglitazone, lowers triglyceride and apo C-III *(69)*.

Based on these considerations and using the more stringent ADA criteria for elevated triglyceride and reduced HDL-C, about 60% of subjects will require treatment for these abnormalities, whereas the corresponding number for the NCEP criteria is about 40%. The focus of the NCEP on non-HDL-C as the secondary treatment target tends to place further emphasis on statins and ezetemibe, because of their effectiveness in lowering non-HDL-C. Statins are the most effective agents for the lowering of non-HDL-C levels, because in addition to lowering LDL-C, they also reduce VLDL-C and IDL-C, probably by enhancing their removal rates through the LDL receptor. It has been suggested that at high doses, statins may reduce VLDL secretion as well *(70)*. Therefore, even if LDL-C are at target levels on statin therapy, increasing the dose of statin or switching to a more potent statin would achieve greater non-HDL-C and triglyceride lowering and help to achieve secondary lipid-lowering goals. Furthermore, if significant triglyceride lowering is achieved with high-dose statins, there is evidence that an increase in LDL particle size may be achieved *(71)*. In addition, treatment with statins also results in a greater reduction of the total number of LDL particles and apo B concentration than other agents. In this regard, it has been argued that apo B may be a better marker of dyslipidemia than non-HDL-C (as discussed in the last section). In comparison fibrates, niacin and high-dose fish oil have a rather modest non-HDL-C-lowering effect (10 mg/dl reduction of non-HDL-C for every 50 mg/dl triglyceride lowering) except in more severe hypertriglyceridemia, where the effect may be significant. By contrast, the ADA has had HDL-C raising as its secondary target. Niacin is by far the most efficacious agent for raising of HDL-C, as neither statins nor fibrates consistently produce >10% HDL-C raising, whereas as little as 1000 mg Niaspan was shown in a year-long clinical trial to produce a 21% increase in HDL-C, with little effect on non-HDL-C *(72)*.

Thus, the two sets of guidelines tend to favor somewhat different second-line pharmacotherapeutic approaches. In part, these disparities result from a lack of clearcut additional evidence for benefit resulting from the lowering of non-HDL-C or raising of HDL-C. Each strategy is supported by circumstantial evidence. In the case of non-HDL-C lowering, there are good data to indicate that non-HDL-C is a better predictor of CHD than LDL-C *(73)*, as well as studies to show that each of the lipoprotein components of non-HDL-C are atherogenic. However, there is as yet no data to show that lowering non-HDL-C with LDL-C held steady at its target has any additional benefit for CHD outcomes. Similarly, there is extensive data demonstrating that HDL-C is a powerful inverse predictor of CHD together with studies indicating that HDL is antiatherogenic through its mediation of reverse cholesterol transport, as well as through anti-inflammatory and antioxidant properties. The only evidence that raising HDL-C is beneficial using traditional lipid-modifying pharmacotherapy in a setting where the LDL-C is at target and kept constant was reported in the recently published Arterial Biology for the Investigation of the Treatment Effects of Reducing Cholesterol (ARBITER 2) study. In this study, 167 subjects with CHD on statin therapy and HDL-C levels <45 mg/dl were randomized either to extended release niacin 1000 mg daily or placebo for a year, and carotid wall intimal medial thickness (IMT) as a surrogate of CHD progression was measured *(72)*. Subjects receiving niacin had no significant progression of carotid IMT as compared with those in the placebo group which progressed significantly. HDL-C levels increased by 21%, and LDL-C levels were unchanged (range of means before and after in placebo and niacin groups was 85–91 mg/dl). However, triglyceride levels fell significantly by 30 mg/dl, so that even in this study, the beneficial effects cannot be attributed to HDL-C raising alone. There is also evidence from the Veterans Administration HDL Intervention Trial (VA HIT) in which gemfibrozil treatment in statin-free men with CHD and a mean LDL-C of 111 mg/dl was associated with a significant reduction in non-fatal MI and CHD death and that about 20% of the beneficial effect could be ascribed to the modest net 6% increase in HDL-C accompanying this treatment *(74)*. Gemfibrozil treatment was also associated with a 25% reduction in triglyceride levels, but this did not correlate with event reduction. The absence of data that triglyceride lowering per se is associated with CVD event reduction suggests that assigning a triglyceride target has little practical value, and the ADA cutpoint of <150 mg/dl for triglyceride probably serves best to identify increased CVD risk rather than a target for treatment. Aside from these two studies, there is also evidence that infusion of nascent HDL as synthetic apo A-I-Milano/phospholipid vesicles is associated with rather rapid angiographic evidence of regression *(75)*. Thus, although there is some evidence supporting both the NCEP and the ADA second-line therapeutic recommendations, clearly more work is needed to substantiate the validity of these strategies.

From a more practical standpoint, the question of what to do beyond LDL-C lowering is limited by the available pharmacotherapeutic agents. These consist of fibrates, niacin, and high-dose omega-3 fatty acids. Combinations of statin + fibrate, statin + niacin, and statin + fish oil have all demonstrated short-term effectiveness in achieving treatment goals in type 2 diabetes or in subjects with combined hyperlipidemia *(64–66)*. Whether these combinations provide additive benefit beyond that achievable with statins is more debatable. Evidence that gemfibrozil which like other fibrates has little effect on LDL-C, but does lower triglyceride and increases HDL-C and LDL particle size, reduced CVD events in the Helsinki Heart Study *(76)* and in the VA HIT *(77)* provided support for the concept that fibrates prevent CVD in a different manner to statins and would therefore likely have an additive vasculoprotective effect when added to statin therapy. Furthermore, in the VA HIT, gemfibrozil appeared to be effective only in subjects with diabetes or insulin resistance *(78)*. However, the Bezafibrate Infarction Prevention and the recently reported Fenofibrate Intervention and Event Lowering in Diabetes (FIELD) trials did not demonstrate a significant effect of these agents on their primary endpoints *(79,80)*. The results of the FIELD study are particularly disappointing, because it was conducted only in type 2 diabetes, most of whom did not have CVD, and it was hoped that this would finally provide the "hard event-" based evidence in type 2 diabetes for fibrate therapy that the earlier, smaller, and positive placebo-controlled angiographic Diabetes Atherosclerosis Intervention Study (DAIS) using fenofibrate had hinted at *(81)*. In FIELD, the primary endpoint—non-fatal MI plus CHD death—was reduced by a non-significant 11% combined; separately, CHD death was increased by 19% (non-significant), and non-fatal MI was reduced significantly by 24%. It is difficult to understand why the results of the VA HIT and FIELD studies differed so significantly, except that participants in the VA HIT trial all had CHD and were not taking statins, whereas, as mentioned, most of those in FIELD did not have CHD, and there was a significant statin "drop-in" rate. Given these results, it is suggested that until further data are available (Action to Control Cardiovascular Risk in Diabetes—ACCORD in 2010), combination treatment with a statin and a fibrate should be used with caution, as the risk of myopathy is increased, particularly in individuals with predisposing conditions like renal failure *(82)*. Myopathy and rhabdomyolysis have been reported with simvastatin, cerivastatin, lovastatin, and atorvastatin in combination with gemfibrozil *(83–85)*. However, several short-term to medium-term studies (*n* = 81–420 subjects) evaluating the efficacy and safety of different statin–fibrate combinations in patients with combined hyperlipidemia have shown a very low incidence of clinically significant myopathy and no cases of rhabdomyolysis *(86–89)*. Additionally, gemfibrozil and fenofibrate differ in their effects on statin pharmacokinetics. Gemfibrozil has been shown to significantly inhibit the glucuronidation of statins, an important but previously unrecognized metabolic pathway of statin catabolism, whereas fenofibrate has little effect *(90,91)*. This probably explains why plasma statin levels are significantly increased with gemfibrozil treatment and not with fenofibrate. In addition, analysis of national databases in the USA found fewer case of rhabdomyolysis associated with fenofibrate compared with gemfibrozil therapy in combination with statin treatment *(92)*. Prior to the results of the FIELD study, fenofibrate has been preferred to gemfibrozil for use in combination therapy with statins but not in the presence of renal insufficiency *(93)*. It is now more difficult to justify this preference in light of the new data.

The addition of niacin to statin therapy has significant lipid-modifying benefit as niacin lowers triglycerides by 20–50%, reduces LDL-C by 5–25%, raises HDL-C by 15–35%, and lowers non-HDL-C and lipoprotein (a) moderately *(94,95)*. Treatment with niacin also results in a shift in LDL and HDL particle density from small dense to larger, more buoyant particles *(96)*. The only study that has evaluated the effect of niacin monotherapy on cardiovascular events is the Coronary Drug Project (CDP), published in 1975 *(97)*. In this study, 1119 men with a history of MI were allocated to treatment with niacin 1–3 g/day, and 2789 participants received placebo. The mean baseline total cholesterol and triglyceride values were 250 mg/dl and 177 mg/dl, respectively. Despite a lack of benefit on total mortality, the risk of recurrent non-fatal MI was reduced by 27% with niacin. A recent re-analysis showed that the benefit of niacin treatment on recurrent MI was similar in patients at all levels of blood glucose, including those with fasting blood glucose >126 mg/dl *(98)*. Evidence for a beneficial effect arising from the addition of niacin therapy to statin treatment was suggested by the HDL Atherosclerosis Treatment Study (HATS) *(99)*. In this trial, the effect of combination therapy with simvastatin and niacin compared with placebo on angiographic end points was evaluated in 160 individuals with prior CHD and low HDL-C levels of whom 16% had diabetes. Simvastatin plus niacin resulted in a significant angiographic benefit with actual regression of lesions, an effect that has not clearly been documented with statin therapy alone. Furthermore, despite the small sample size, treatment with niacin plus simvastatin was associated with a significant 60% reduction in cardiovascular events (CHD death, non-fatal MI, stroke, or revascularization for worsening ischemia), which is a numerically greater effect than has been demonstrated in monotherapy trials. Unfortunately, this study did not have a statin-alone treatment arm, so the conclusions that niacin had an additive effect on simvastatin therapy remain somewhat conjectural, although the ARBITER 2 results discussed above in this section *(72)* strengthen this position. A 5-year clinical trial comparing simvastatin alone versus simvastatin plus extended-release niacin on recurrent events in subjects with established CVD and which includes subjects with type 2 diabetes has just been launched (AIM HIGH) and should answer this question definitively.

However, niacin has significant adverse effects. Hepatotoxicity is the most important of these particularly with "long-acting" or "sustained release" niacin preparations using doses >2000 mg daily. The extended release once-a-day preparation of niacin (Niaspan) has been found to be effective and safe with a low incidence of hepatotoxicity. Myopathy has been reported with the combined use of niacin and lovastatin but has not been described in studies of Niaspan and lovastatin in a single tablet formulation. The incidence of myopathy associated with the combination of niacin and statins appears to be significantly lower than with statins and gemfibrozil *(100)*. Past use of niacin in diabetic patients was limited because of concerns that this agent may lead to deterioration in glucose control. Recent studies have shown only modest increases in HbA1c values in most fairly well-controlled diabetic patients receiving up to 3000 mg of immediate-release niacin *(101)* and up to 1500 mg of Niaspan *(102)*. Nevertheless, care should be exercised when using this agent in diabetic subjects, and it is probably unwise to increase the niacin dose above 1000 mg daily if the HbA1c level is >8.0%. In addition to these safety concerns, niacin may not be well-tolerated by a significant proportion of patients, particularly at higher doses, and it should be remembered that a history of gout, not uncommon in diabetic subjects, is a relative contraindication. However, doses as low as 1000 mg/day may have moderate HDL-C-raising effects (72).

The use of high-dose omega-3 fatty acids (3–8 gm/day) is another intervention that has shown to lower triglyceride levels by 15–30% in diabetic subjects in short-term studies without adverse effects on HbA1c or HDL-C and only a slight increase in LDL-C values, and the availability of high-dose omega-3 concentrates improves the tolerability of this treatment (103,104). Recently the Japan EPA Lipid Intervention Study in a large long-term randomized clinical trial demonstrated that 1.8 gm of esicoapentaneoic acid (EPA) added to pravastatin therapy reduced CHD events by 19%, providing evidence that addition of high dose EPA to statin therapy yielded further benefit. There is in addition clinical trial evidence to show that low-dose omega-3 fat (0.3–1.0 g/day) reduces CVD mortality in populations with CVD, although there are no specific data in diabetes (105).

In summary, the evidence in support of CVD benefit from niacin therapy is somewhat more consistent than the results of fibrate therapy, there is preliminary evidence for an additive effect of niacin when added to a statin, and the case for HDL raising is growing stronger. Limitation of niacin use because of side effects or the presence of more severe hypertriglyceridemia might favor addition of fibrates, and even though statin–fenofibrate combinations may be slightly safer than statin–gemfibrozil combinations, the clinical trial data are more convincing with genfibrozil. High-dose omega-3 fatty acids constitute a potentially safe hypotriglyceridemic agent for use in combination therapy, particularly since it has been demonstrated to reduce coronary events.

IS IT TIME TO INCLUDE NEWER LIPOPROTEIN MEASURES IN THE ASSESSMENT AND MANAGEMENT OF DIABETIC DYSLIPIDEMIA?

A range of technologies have become available for large-scale measurement of lipoprotein subfractions and apoproteins. These have been designated as novel CHD risk factors by NCEP indicating that they may have added value in predicting risk but have not yet acquired the abundance of evidence to warrant being added to the standard lipid profile for risk assessment or management decisions (6). These novel risk factors include apo B, apo E, apo C-III, lipoprotein (a), lipoprotein particle size, especially LDL particle size, and HDL subfractions. The decision to add a new measure to the standard lipid profile would require that the method be widely available, that it demonstrate sufficient precision to be reliable over a wide range of conditions, that it have independent risk-predictive value, that it adds to therapeutic decision-making beyond what is currently available, and that the added cost be justified by the clinical benefit it provides. From among these, measurement of total serum apo B comes closest to meeting most of the above conditions; it is readily available, and modern methods are sufficiently precise and inexpensive for large-scale use (106). It has been argued that it is a more precise predictor of outcomes (particularly when combined as a ratio with apo A-I) than LDL-C or the LDL-C/HDL-C ratio (107,108), and although it correlates strongly with non-HDL-C, it is not as strongly concordant (109), and several studies have now shown it to be a better predictor of CHD than non-HDL-C (110,111). This has been ascribed to the fact that apo B is a better measure of the number of apo B-containing atherogenic particles than is non-HDL-C, and as it has become clear that diabetic subjects tend to have smaller, denser LDL particles (as well as HDL particles) and larger, lighter VLDL particles (112) and that apo B gives a better measure of the number of particles than does non-HDL-C (113). This assumes that the number of atherogenic particles is the most powerful positive lipid predictor of CHD, but this remains to be proven. Certainly, in diabetic subjects, it has been shown that in those with normal non-HDL-C levels, apo B values may be frequently elevated (113). There is also evidence that apo B may predict the response to statin and even fibrate therapy better than does LDL-C (114). The Canadian Lipid Working Group has considered these data and has adopted an apo B target of <0.90 g/l as an alternative to the LDL-C target of <2.5 mmol/l (<100 mg/dl) in its guidelines (115), especially in statin-treated subjects.

Although it has been difficult to prove consistently that LDL particle-size measurements are more powerful predictors of CVD events than LDL-C or non-HDL-C (116), the idea that LDL particle number may be a better predictor than LDL-C, non-HDL-C or even apo B of CVD events, has been proposed by the developers of the nuclear magnetic resonance spectroscopic method that measures lipoprotein particle sizes and then calculates particle concentrations (117). Although this method does not produce the same particle-size measurements as does the more traditional method of gel electrophoresis of LDL, they do correlate well (118) although there is no available method with which to assess and compare the particle concentration results. In a recent analysis of the utility of measuring LDL particle number in the Framingham Heart Study, although LDL particle number identified the metabolic syndrome with high sensitivity, a higher small LDL particle number was not associated with greater CVD event rates in people with the metabolic syndrome (119). In the final analysis, the application of each of these new methodologies is limited by what we know from therapeutic intervention trials. It is difficult to know what further could be done in a diabetic subject with an LDL-C of 65 mg/dl, a non-HDL-C of 100 mg/dl, and an HDL-C of 44 mg/dl on a combination of high-dose statin, ezetemibe, and extended-release niacin, who is shown to have increased numbers of small LDL particles. Too often what is lost in this debate is the benefit that would accrue to the patients we treat if we were simply to adhere efficiently and rigorously to the NCEP and ADA guidelines.

REFERENCES

1. Kannel WB, McGee DL. Diabetes and cardiovascular disease. The Framingham Study. *JAMA* 1979; 241: 2035–2038.
2. Turner RC, Millns H, Neil HA, Stratton IM, Manley SE, Matthews DR, Holman RR. Risk factors for coronary artery disease in non-insulin dependent diabetes mellitus: United Kingdom Prospective Diabetes Study (UKPDS: 23). *BMJ* 1998; 316: 823–828.
3. Solano MP, Goldberg RB. Management of diabetic dyslipidemia. *Endocrinol Metab Clin North Am* 2005; 34: 1–25.
4. Saydah SH, Fradkin J, Cowie CC. Poor control of risk factors for vascular disease among adults with previously diagnosed diabetes. *J Am Med Assoc* 2004; 291: 335–342.
5. Gu K, Cowie CC, Harris MI. Diabetes and decline in heart disease mortality in US adults. *JAMA* 1999; 281: 1291–1297
6. Expert Panel on Detection, Evaluation, and Treatment of High Blood Cholesterol in Adults. Executive summary of the third report of the National Cholesterol Education Program (NCEP) Expert Panel on detection, evaluation, and treatment of high blood cholesterol in adults (Adult Treatment Panel III), *JAMA* 2001; 285: 2486–2497.
7. Haffner SM, Lehto S, Rönnemaa T, et al. Mortality from coronary heart disease in subjects with type 2 diabetes and in nondiabetic subjects with and without prior myocardial infarction. *N Engl J Med* 1998; 339: 229–234.
8. Malmberg K, Yusuf S, Gerstein HC, Brown J, Zhao F, Hunt D, Piegas L, Calvin J, Keltai M, Budaj A. Impact of diabetes on long-term prognosis in patients with unstable angina and non-Q-wave myocardial infarction: results of the OASIS (Organization to Assess Strategies for Ischemic Syndromes) Registry. *Circulation* 2000; 102: 1014–1019.
9. Simons LA, Simons JS. Diabetes and coronary heart disease. *N Engl J Med* 1998; 339: 1714–1716.
10. Hu FB, Stampfer MJ, Solomon CG, et al. The impact of diabetes mellitus on mortality from all causes and coronary heart disease in women: 20 years of follow-up. *Arch Intern Med* 2001; 161: 1717–1723.
11. Lotufo PA, Gaziano M, Chae CU, et al. Diabetes and all-cause and coronary heart disease mortality among US male physicians. *Arch Intern Med* 2001; 161: 242–247.
12. Cho E, Rimm EB, Stampfer MJ, et al. The impact of diabetes mellitus and prior myocardial infarction on mortality from all causes and from coronary heart disease in men. *J Am Coll Cardiol* 2002; 40: 954–960.
13. Lee CD, Folsom AR, Pankow JS, Brancati FL; Atherosclerosis Risk in Communities (ARIC) Study Investigators. Cardiovascular events in diabetic and nondiabetic adults with or without history of myocardial infarction. *Circulation* 2004; 109: 855–860.
14. Hillier TA, Pedula KL. Complications in young adults with early-onset type 2 diabetes: losing the relative protection of youth. *Diabetes Care* 2003; 26: 2999–3005.

15. Krolewski AS, Kosinski EJ, Warram JH, Leland OS, Busick EJ, Asmal AC, Rand LI, Christlieb AR, Bradley RF, Kahn CR. Magnitude and determinants of coronary artery disease in juvenile-onset, insulin-dependent diabetes mellitus. *Am J Cardiol* 1987; 59: 750–755.

16. Centers for Disease Control and Prevention (CDC). *Data & Trends*. Available at http://www.cdc.gov/diabetes/statistics/age/source.htm.

17. Chaturvedi N, Jarrett J, Morrish N, Keen H, Fuller JH. Differences in mortality and morbidity in African Caribbean and European people with non-insulin-dependent diabetes mellitus: result of 20-year follow-up of a London cohort of a multinational study. *BMJ* 1996; 313: 848–852.

18. Dijkstra, M. Klok, D. Hoogenhuyze van, HP Sauerwein, A. Berghout. Ischaemic heart disease in Turkish migrants with type 2 diabetes mellitus in the Netherlands: wait for the next generation? *Neth J Med* 2002; 60: 21–24.

19. Weijers RNM, Goldschmidt HMJ, Silberbusch J. Vascular complications in relation to ethnicity in non-insulin-dependent diabetes mellitus. *Eur J Clin Invest* 1997, 27: 182–188.

20. Hunt KJ, Williams K, Resendez RG, Hazuda HP, Haffner SM, Stern MP. All-cause and cardiovascular mortality among diabetic participants in the San Antonio Heart Study: evidence against the "Hispanic Paradox." *Diabetes Care* 2002; 25: 1557–63.

21. Kittner SJ, White LR, Losonczy KG, Wolf PA, Hebel JR. Black-white differences in stroke incidence in a national sample. The contribution of hypertension and diabetes mellitus. *JAMA* 1990; 264: 1267–1270.

22. Stamler J, Vaccaro O, Neaton J, Wentworth D; Multiple Risk Factor Intervention Trial Research Group. Diabetes, other risk factors and 12 year cardiovascular mortality for men screened in the Multiple Risk Factors Intervention Trial. *Diabetes Care* 1993; 16: 434–444.

23. Adler AI, Stratton IM, Neil HA, Yudkin JS, Matthews DR, Cull CA, Wright AD, Turner RC, Holman RR. Association of systolic blood pressure with macrovascular and microvascular complications of type 2 diabetes (UKPDS 36): prospective observational study. *BMJ* 2000; 12; 412–419.

24. Pavkov ME, Bennett PH, Sievers ML, Krakoff J, Williams DE, Knowler WC, Nelson RG. Predominant effect of kidney disease on mortality in Pima Indians with or without type 2 diabetes. *Kidney Int* 2005; 68: 1267–1274.

25. Dinneen SF, Gerstein HC. The association of microalbuminuria and mortality in non-insulin-dependent diabetes mellitus: a systematic overview of the literature. *Arch Intern Med* 1997; 15: 1413–8.

26. Knowler WC, Barrett-Connor E, Fowler SE, Hamman RF, Lachin JM, Walker EA, Nathan DM; Diabetes Prevention Program Research Group. Reduction in the incidence of type 2 diabetes with lifestyle intervention or metformin. *N Engl J Med* 2002; 346; 393–403.

27. Samaha FF, Iqbal N, Seshadri P, Chicano KL, Daily DA, McGrory J, Williams T, Williams M, Gracely EJ, Stern L. A low-carbohydrate as compared with a low-fat diet in severe obesity. *N Engl J Med* 2003; 348: 2074–2081.

28. Klein S, Sheard NF, Pi-Sunyer X, Daly A, Wylie-Rosett J, Kulkarni K, Clark NG. Weight management through lifestyle modification for the prevention and management of type 2 diabetes: rationale and strategies: a statement of the American Diabetes Association, the North American Association for the Study of Obesity, and the American Society for Clinical Nutrition. *Diabetes Care* 2004; 27: 2067–2073.

29. US Department of Health and Human Services. *Physical Activity and Health: A Report of the Surgeon General: Centers for Disease Control and Prevention and National Center for Chronic Disease Prevention and Health Promotion*. Washington, DC: US Government Printing Office, 1996.

30. American Diabetes Association. Evidence-based nutrition principles and recommendations for the treatment and prevention of diabetes and related complications. *Diabetes Care* 2003; 26: S51–S61

31. Yu-Poth S, Zhao G, Etherton T, Naglak M, Jonnalagadda S, Kris-Etherton PM. Effects of the National Cholesterol Education Program's step I and II dietary intervention program on cardiovascular disease risk factors: a meta-analysis. *Am J Clin Nutr* 1999; 69: 632–646.

32. Temme EH, Van Hoydonck PG, Schouten EG, Kesteloot H. Effects of a plant sterol-enriched spread on serum lipids and lipoproteins in mildly hypercholesterolemic subjects. *Acta Cardiol* 2002; 57: 111–115.

33. Gylling H, Miettinen TA. Serum cholesterol and cholesterol and lipoprotein metabolism in hypercholesterolemic NIDDM patients before and during sitostanol ester-margarine treatment. *Diabetologia* 1994; 37: 773–780.

34. Chandalia M, Garg A, Lutjohann D, von Bergmann K, Grundy SM, Brinkley LJ. Beneficial effects of high dietary fiber intake in patients with type 2 diabetes mellitus. *N Eng J Med* 2000; 342: 1392–1398.

35. Anderson JW, Allgood LD, Turner J, Oeltgen PR, Daggy BP. Effects of Psyllium on glucose and serum lipid responses in men with type 2 diabetes and hypercholesterolemia. *Am J Clin Nutr* 1999; 70: 466–473.

36. Turley ML, Skeaff CM, Mann JI, Cox B. The effect of a low-fat, high-carbohydrate diet on serum high density lipoprotein cholesterol and triglyceride. *Eur J Clin Nutr* 1998; 52: 728–732.

37. Garg A. High-monounsaturated-fat diets for patients with diabetes mellitus: a meta-analysis. *Am J Clin Nutr* 1998; 67: 577S–582S.

38. Bravata DM, Sanders L, Huang J, Krumholz HM, Olkin I, Gardner CD, Bravata DM. Efficacy and safety of low-carbohydrate diets. A systematic review. JAMA 2003; 289: 1837–1850.

39. Vettor R, Serra R, Fabris R, Pagano C, Federspil G. Effect of sibutramine on weight management and metabolic control in type 2 diabetes: a meta-analysis of clinical studies. *Diabetes Care* 2005; 28: 942–949.

40. O'Meara S, Riemsma R, Shirran L, Mather L, ter Riet G. A systematic review of the clinical effectiveness of orlistat used for the management of obesity. *Obes Rev* 2004; 5: 51–68.

41. Pinkney J, Kerrigan D. Current status of bariatric surgery in the treatment of type 2 diabetes. *Obes Rev* 2004; 5: 69–78.

42. Goldberg RB, Capuzzi D. Lipid disorders in type 1 and type 2 diabetes. *Clin Lab Med* 2001; 1: 147–172.

43. Turner RC, Millns H, Neil HA, Stratton IM, Manley SE, Matthews DR, Holman RR. Risk factors for coronary artery disease in non-insulin dependent diabetes mellitus: United Kingdom Prospective Diabetes Study (UKPDS: 23). *BMJ* 1998; 316: 823–828.

44. Heart Protection Study Collaborative Group. MCR/BHF Heart Protection Study of cholesterol lowering with simvastatin in 20,536 high-risk individuals: a randomized placebo-controlled trial. *Lancet* 2002; 360: 7–22.

45. Colhoun HM, Betteridge DJ, Durrington PN, et al. Primary prevention of cardiovascular disease with atorvastatin in type 2 diabetes in the Collaborative Atorvastatin Diabetes Study (CARDS): multicentre randomized placebo-controlled trial. *Lancet* 2004; 364: 685–696.

46. Cannon CP, Braunwald E, McCabe CH, et al. Intensive versus moderate lipid lowering with statins after acute coronary syndromes. *N Engl J Med* 2004; 350: 1495–1504

47. Grundy SM, Cleeman JI, Merz CN, Brewer HB Jr, Clark LT, Hunninghake DB, Pasternak RC, Smith SC Jr, Stone NJ; Coordinating Committee of the National Cholesterol Education Program; Coordinating Committee of the National Cholesterol Education Program: National Heart, Lung, and Blood Institute; American College of Cardiology Foundation; American Heart association. Implications of recent clinical trials for the National Cholesterol Education Program Adult Treatment Panel III guidelines. *Circulation* 2004; 110: 227–239.

48. LaRosa JC, Grundy SM, Waters DD, Shear C, Barter P, Fruchart JC, Gotto AM, Greten H, Kastelein JJ, Shepherd J, Wenger NK; Treating to New Targets (TNT) Investigators. Intensive lipid lowering with atorvastatin in patients with stable coronary disease. *N Engl J Med* 2005; 352: 1425–1435.

49. Shepherd J, Barter P, Carmena R, Deedwania P, Fruchart JC, Haffner S, Hsia J, Breazna A, LaRosa J, Grundy S, Waters D. Effect of lowering LDL cholesterol substantially below currently recommended levels in patients with coronary heart disease and diabetes: the Treating to New Targets (TNT) study. *Diabetes Care.* 2006; 29: 1220–1226.

50. Ballantyne CM, Houri J, Notarbartolo A, Melani L, Lipka LJ, Suresh R, Sun S, LeBeaut AP, Sager PT, Veltri EP; Ezetimibe Study Group. Effect of ezetimibe coadministered with atorvastatin in 628 patients with primary hypercholesterolemia: a prospective, randomized, double-blind trial. *Circulation* 2003; 107: 2409–2415.

51. American Diabetes Association. Standards of medical care in diabetes. *Diabetes Care* 2006; 29(Suppl 1); S4–S42.

52. Gracia PJ. Pleiotropic effects of statins: moving beyond cholesterol control. *Curr Atheroscler Rep* 2005; 7: 34–39.

53. Schwartz GG, Olsson AG, Ezekowitz MD, Ganz P, Oliver MF, Waters D, Zeiher A, Chaitman BR, Leslie S, Stern T; Myocardial Ischemia Reduction with Aggressive Cholesterol Lowering (MIRACL) Study Investigators. Effects of atorvastatin on early recurrent ischemic events in acute coronary syndromes. The MIRACL study a randomized controlled trial. *JAMA* 2001; 285: 1711–1718.

54. Ridker PM, Rifai N, Clearfield M, et al. Measurement of C-reactive protein for the targeting of statin therapy in the primary prevention of acute coronary events. *N Engl J Med* 2001; 344: 1959–1965.

55. Ridker PM, Cannon CP, Morrow D, Rifai N, Rose LM, McCabe CH, Pfeffer MA, Braunwald E; Pravastatin or Atorvastatin Evaluation and Infection Therapy-Thrombolysis in Myocardial Infarction 22 (PROVE IT-TIMI 22) Investigators. C-reactive protein levels and outcomes after statin therapy. *N Engl J Med* 2005; 352(1): 20–28.

56. Ridker PM; JUPITER Study Group. Rosuvastatin in the primary prevention of cardiovascular disease among patients with low levels of low-density lipoprotein cholesterol and elevated high-sensitivity C-reactive protein: rationale and design of the JUPITER trial. *Circulation* 2003; 108: 2292–2297.

57. Ford E. Body mass index, diabetes, and C-reactive protein among U.S. adults. *Diabetes Care* 1999; 22: 1971–1977.

58. Moreno PR, Fuster V. New aspects in the pathogenesis of diabetic atherothrombosis. *J Am Coll Cardiol* 2004; 44: 2293–2300.

59. Alexander CM, Landsman PB, Teutsch SM, Haffner SM; Third National Health and Nutrition Examination Survey (NHANES III); National Cholesterol Education Program (NCEP). NCEP-defined metabolic syndrome, diabetes, and prevalence of coronary heart disease among NHANES III participants age 50 years and older. *Diabetes* 2003; 52: 1210-1214.

60. Cowie CC, Harris ML. *Physical and Metabolic Characteristics of Persons with Diabetes. Diabetes in America.* 2nd ed. National Institutes of Health, Bethesda, MD, USA 1995: 117–164.

61. Manley SE, Frighi V, Stratton E, et al. U.K. Prospective Diabetes Study 27. Plasma lipids and lipoproteins at diagnosis of NIDDM by age and sex. *Diabetes Care* 1997; 20: 1683–1687.

62. Feingold KR, Grunfeld C, Pang M, et al. LDL subclass phenotypes and triglyceride metabolism in non-insulin dependent diabetes. *Arterioscler Thromb Vasc Biol* 1992; 12: 1496–1502.

63. The Diabetes Prevention Program Research Group. Lipid, lipoproteins, C-reactive protein and hemostatic factors at baseline in the Diabetes Prevention Program. *Diabetes Care* 2005; 28: 2472–2479.

64. Capuzzi DM, Morgan JM, Weiss RJ, Chitra RR, Hutchinson HG, Cressman MD. Beneficial effects of rosuvastatin alone and in combination with extended-release niacin in patients with a combined hyperlipidemia and low high-density lipoprotein cholesterol levels. *Am J Cardiol* 2003; 91: 1304–1310.

65. Athyros VG, Papageorgiou AA, Athyrou VV, Demitriadis DS, Kontopoulos AG. Atorvastatin and micronized fenofibrate alone and in combination in type 2 diabetes with combined hyperlipidemia. *Diabetes Care* 2002; 1198–1202.

66. Chan DC, Watts GF, Barrett PH, Beilin LJ, Redgrave TG, Mori TA. Regulatory effects of HMG CoA reductase inhibitor and fish oils on apolipoprotein B-100 kinetics in insulin-resistant obese male subjects with dyslipidemia. *Diabetes* 2002; 51: 2377–2386

67. Emanuele N, Azad N, Abraira C, Henderson W, Colwell J, Levin S, Nuttall F, Comstock J, Sawin C, Silbert C, Marcovina S, Lee HS. Effect of intensive glycemic control on fibrinogen, lipids, and lipoproteins: Veterans Affairs Cooperative Study in type II diabetes mellitus. *Arch Intern Med* 1998; 18: 2485–2490.

68. Palumbo PJ. Metformin: effects on cardiovascular risk factors in patients with non-insulin-dependent diabetes mellitus. *J Diabetes Complications* 1998; 12: 110–119.

69. Goldberg RB, Kendall DM, Deeg MA, Buse JB, Zagar AJ, Pinaire JA, Tan MH, Khan MA, Perez AT, Jacober SJ; GLAI Study Investigators. A comparison of lipid and glycemic effects of pioglitazone and rosiglitazone in patients with type 2 diabetes and dyslipidemia. *Diabetes Care* 2005; 28: 1547–1554.

70. Scharnagl H, Schinker R, Gierens H, Nauck M, Wieland H, Marz W. Effect of atorvastatin, simvastatin, and lovastatin on the metabolism of cholesterol and triacylglycerides in HepG2 cells. *Biochem Pharmacol* 2001; 62: 1545–1555.

71. Pontrelli L, Parris W, Adeli K, Cheung RC. Atorvastatin treatment beneficially alters the lipoprotein profile and increases low-density lipoprotein particle diameter in patients with combined dyslipidemia and impaired fasting glucose/type 2 diabetes. *Metabolism* 2002; 51: 334–342.

72. Taylor AJ, Sullenberger LE, Lee HJ, Lee JK, Grace KA. Arterial Biology for the Investigation of the Treatment Effects of Reducing Cholesterol (ARBITER) 2: a double-blind, placebo-controlled study of extended-release niacin on atherosclerosis progression in secondary prevention patients treated with statins. *Circulation* 2004; 110: 3512–3517.

73. Liu J, Sempos C, Donahue RP, Dorn J, Trevisan M, Grundy SM. Joint distribution of non-HDL and LDL cholesterol and coronary heart disease risk prediction among individuals with and without diabetes. *Diabetes Care* 2005; 28: 1916–1921.

74. Robins SJ. Cardiovascular disease with diabetes or the metabolic syndrome: should statins or fibrates be first line lipid therapy? *Curr Opin Lipidol* 2003; 14: 575–583.

75. Nissen SE, Tsunoda T, Tuzcu EM, Schoenhagen P, Cooper CJ, Yasin M, Eaton GM, Lauer MA, Sheldon WS, Grines CL, Halpern S, Crowe T, Blankenship JC, Kerensky R. Effect of recombinant ApoA-I Milano on coronary atherosclerosis in patients with acute coronary syndromes: a randomized controlled trial. *JAMA* 2003; 290: 2292–2300.

76. Koskinen P, Manttari M, Manninen V, Huttunen JK, Heinonen OP, Frick MH. coronary heart disease incidence in NIDDM patients in the Helsinki Heart Study. *Diabetes Care* 1992; 15: 820–825.

77. Rubins HB, Robins SJ, Collins D, Fye CL, Anderson JW, Elam MB, Faas FH, Linares E, Schaefer EJ, Schectman G, Wilt TJ, Wittes J. Gemfibrozil for the secondary prevention of coronary heart disease in men with low levels of high-density lipoprotein cholesterol. *N Engl J Med* 1999; 341: 410–418.

78. Rubins HB, Robins SJ, Collins D, Nelson DB, Elam MB, Schaefer EJ, Faas FH, Anderson JW. Diabetes, plasma insulin, and cardiovascular disease. Subgroup analysis from the Department of Veterans Affairs High-Density Lipoprotein Intervention Trial (VA-HIT). *Arch Intern Med* 2002; 162: 2597–2604

79. The BIP Study Group. Secondary prevention by raising HDL cholesterol and reducing triglycerides in patients with coronary artery disease. The Bezafibrate Infarction Prevention (BIP) Study. *Circulation* 2000; 102: 21–27.

80. The FIELD Study Investigators. Effects of long-term fenofibrate therapy on cardiovascular events in 9795 people with type 2 diabetes mellitus (the FIELD study): randomised controlled trial. *Lancet* 2005; 366: 1849–1861

81. Diabetes Atherosclerosis Intervention Study Investigators. Effect of fenofibrate on progression of coronary-artery disease in type 2 diabetes: the Diabetes Atherosclerosis Intervention Study, a randomized study. *Lancet* 2001; 357: 905–910.

82. Pierce LR, Wysowski DK, Gross TP. Myopathy and rhabdomyolysis associated with lovastatin-gemfibrozil combination therapy. *JAMA* 1990; 264: 71–75.

83. Tal A, Rajeshawari M, Isley W. Rhabdomyolysis associated with simvastatin-gemfibrozil therapy. *South Med J* 1997; 90: 546–547.

84. Pogson G, Kindred L, Carper B. Rhabdomyolysis and renal failure associated with cerivastatin-gemfibrozil combination therapy. *Am J Cardiol* 1999; 83: 1146.

85. Duell PB, Connor WE, Illingworth DR. Rhabdomyolysis after taking atorvastatin with gemfibrozil. *Am J Cardiol* 1998; 81: 368–369.

86. Ellen RL, McPherson R. Long term efficacy and safety of fenofibrate and a statin in the treatment of combined hyperlipidemia. *Am J Cardiol* 1998; 81: 60B–65B.

87. Iliadis EA, Rosenson RS. Long-term safety of pravastatin-gemfibrozil therapy in mixed hyperlipidemia. *Clin Cardiol* 1999; 22: 25–28.

88. Murdock DK, Murdock AK, Murdock RW. Long-term safety and efficacy of combination gemfibrozil and HMG-CoA reductase inhibitors for the treatment of mixed lipid disorders. *Am Heart J* 1999; 138: 151–155

89. Vega GL, Ma PT, Cater NB, Filipchuk N, Meguro S, Garcia-Garcia AB, Grundy SM. Effects of adding fenofibrate (200mg/day) to simvastatin (10mg/day) in patients with combined hyperlipidemia and metabolic syndrome. *Am J Cardiol* 2003; 91: 956–960.

90. Prueksaritanont T, Zhao JJ, Ma B, Roadcap BA, Tang C, Qiu Y, Liu L, Lin JH Pearson PG, Baillie TA. Mechanistic studies on metabolic interactions between gemfibrozil and statins. *Pharmacol Exp Ther* 2002; 301: 1042–1051.

91. Prueksaritanont T, Tang C, Qiu Y, Mu L, Subramanian R, Lin JH. Effects of fibrates on metabolism of statins in human hepatocytes. *Drug Metab Dispos* 2002; 30: 1280–1287.

92. Jones PH, Davidson MH. Reporting rate of rhabdomyolysis with fenofibrate + statin versus gemfibrozil + any statin. *Am J Cardiol* 2005; 95: 120–122.

93. K/DOQI clinical practice guidelines for management of dyslipidemias in patients with kidney disease. *Am J Kidney Dis* 2003; 41: 1–91.

94. Shepherd J, Betteridge J, Van Gaal L; European Consensus Panel. Nicotinic acid in the management of dyslipidaemia associated with diabetes and metabolic syndrome: a position paper developed by a European Consensus Panel. *Curr Med Res Opin* 2005; 21: 665–682

95. Carlson LA, Hamsten A, Asplaund A. Pronounced lowering of serum levels of lipoprotein Lp(a) in hyperlipidemic subjects treated with nicotinic acid. *J Intern Med* 1989; 226: 271–276.

96. Superko HR, Krauss RM. Differential effects of nicotinic acid in subjects with different LDL subclass patterns. *Atherosclerosis* 1992; 95: 69–76.

97. The Coronary Drug Project Research Group. Clofibrate and niacin in coronary heart disease. *JAMA* 1975; 231: 360–381.

98. Canner PL, Furberg CD, Terrin ML, McGovern ME. Benefits of niacin by glycemic status in patients with healed myocardial infarction (from the Coronary Drug Project). *Am J Cardiol* 2005; 95: 254–257.

99. Brown BG, Zhao XQ, Chait A, Fisher LD, Cheung MC, Morse JS, Dowdy AA, Marino EK, Bolson EL, Alaupovic P, Frohlich J, Albers JJ. Simvastatin and niacin, antioxidant vitamins, or the combination for prevent of coronary disease. *N Eng J Med* 2001; 345: 1583–1592.

100. Omar MA, Wilson JP, Cox TS: Rhabdomyolysis and HMG-CoA reductase inhibitors. *Ann Pharmacother* 2001; 35: 1096–1107.

101. Elam MB, Hunninghake DB, Davis KB, Garg R, Johnson C, Egan D, Kostis JB, Sheps DS, Brinton EA. Effect of niacin on lipid and lipoprotein levels and glycemic control in patients with diabetes and peripheral arterial disease: the ADMIT study. A randomized trial. *JAMA* 2000; 284: 1263–1270.

102. Grundy SM, Vega GL, McGovern ME, Tulloch BR, Kendall DM, Fitz-Patrick D, Ganda OP, Rosenson RS, Buse JB, Robertson DD, Sheehan JP; Diabetes Multicenter Research Group. Efficacy, safety, and tolerability of once-daily niacin for the treatment of dyslipidemia associated with type 2 diabetes. *Arch Intern Med* 2002; 162: 1568–1576.

103. Friedberg CE, Janssen MJ, Heine RJ, Grobbee DE. Fish oil and glycemic control in diabetes. A meta-analysis. *Diabetes Care* 1998; 21: 494–500.

104. Woodman RJ, Mori TA, Burke V, Puddey IB, Barden A, Watts GF, Beilin LJ. Effects of purified eicosapentaenoic and docosahexaenoic acids on glycemic control, blood pressure, and serum lipids in type 2 diabetic patients with treated hypertension. *Am J Clin Nutr* 2002; 76: 1007–1015.

105. Yokoyama M, Origasa H, Matsuzaki M, Matsuzawa Y, Saito Y, Ishikawa Y, Oikawa S, Sasaki J, Hishida H, Itakura H, Kita T, Kitabatake A, Nakaya N, Sakata T, Shimada K, Shirato K. Japan EPA lipid intervention study (JELIS) Investigators. Effects of eicosapentaenoic acid on major coronary events in hypercholesterolaemic patients (JELIS): a randomised open-label, blinded endpoint analysis. *Lancet.* 2007; 369:1090–1098.

106. Kris-Etherton PM, Harris WS, Appel LJ; AHA Nutrition Committee; American Heart Association. Fish consumption, fish oil, omega-3 fatty acids, and cardiovascular disease. *Circulation* 2002; 106(21): 2747–2757.

107. Grundy SM. Low-density lipoprotein, non-high-density lipoprotein, and apolipoprotein b as targets of lipid-lowering therapy. *Circulation* 2002; 106: 2526–2529.

108. Sniderman AD, Furberg CD, Keech A, Roeters van Lennep JE, Frohlich J, Jungner I, Walldius G. Apolipoproteins versus lipids as indices of coronary risk and as targets for statin treatment. *Lancet* 2003; 361: 777–780.

109. Williams K, Sniderman AD, Sattar N, et al. Comparison of the associations of apolipoprotein B and low-density lipoprotein cholesterol with other cardiovascular risk factors in the Insulin Resistance Atherosclerosis Study (IRAS). *Circulation* 2003; 108: 2312–2316.

110. Sniderman AD, St Pierre AC, Cantin B, et al. Concordance/discordance between plasma apolipoprotein B levels and the cholesterol indexes of atherosclerotic risk. *Am J Cardiol* 2003; 91: 1173–1177.

111. Ridker PM, Rifai N, Cook NR, Bradwin G, Buring JE. Non-HDL cholesterol, apolipoproteins A-I and B100, standard lipid measures, lipid ratios, and CRP as risk factors for cardiovascular disease in women. *JAMA* 2005; 294: 326–333

112. Pischon T, Girman CJ, Sacks FM, Rifai N, Stampfer MJ, Rimm EB. Non-high-density lipoprotein cholesterol and apolipoprotein B in the prediction of coronary heart disease in men. *Circulation* 2005; 112: 3375–3383.

113. Garvey WT, Kwon S, Zheng D, Shaughnessy S, Wallace P, Hutto A, Pugh K, Jenkins AJ, Klein RL, Liao Y. Effects of insulin resistance and type 2 diabetes on lipoprotein subclass particle size and concentration determined by nuclear magnetic resonance. *Diabetes* 2003; 52: 453–462.

114. Wägner AM, Pérez A, Zapico E, Ordóñez-Llanos J. Non-HDL cholesterol and apolipoprotein B in the dyslipidemic classification of type 2 diabetic patients. *Diabetes Care* 2003; 26: 2048–2051.

115. van Lennep JE, Westerveld HT, van Lennep HW, et al. Apolipoprotein concentrations during treatment and recurrent coronary artery disease events. *Arterioscler Thromb Vasc Biol* 2000; 20: 2408–2413.

116. Genest J, Frohlich J, Fodor G, McPherson R; Working Group on Hypercholesterolemia and Other Dyslipidemias. Recommendations for the management of dyslipidemia and the prevention of cardiovascular disease: summary of the 2003 update. *CMAJ* 2003; 169: 921–924.

117. Lada AT, Rudel LL. Associations of low density lipoprotein particle composition with atherogenicity. *Curr Opin Lipidol* 2004; 15: 19–24.

118. Cromwell WC, Otvos JD. Low-density lipoprotein particle number and risk for cardiovascular disease. *Curr Atheroscler Rep* 2004; 6: 381–387.

119. Blake GJ, Otvos JD, Rifai N, Ridker PM. LDL particle concentration and size as determined by NMR spectroscopy as predictors of cardiovascular disease in women. *Circulation* 2002; 106: 1930–1937.

120. Kathiresan S, Otvos JD, Sullivan LM, Keyes MJ, Schaefer EJ, Wilson PW, D'Agostino RB, Vasan RS, Robins SJ. Increased small low-density lipoprotein particle number: a prominent feature of the metabolic syndrome in the Framingham Heart Study. *Circulation* 2006; 113: 20–29.

16 Polypills for Treatment of Type 2 Diabetes

Is the Concept of Polypharmacy Correct?

Werner Waldhäusl, MD

CONTENTS

SUMMARY

Type 2 diabetes mellitus (T2DM) is a common disease frequently showing complex multimorbidity in its late phase. Early stages lack clinical symptoms and easily escape diagnosis. Once diagnosed, all treatments of T2DM are based on adopting a healthy lifestyle and attempt to interfere with appetite, body weight, glycemia, insulin sensitivity, blood pressure, and platelet aggregation. But treatment regimens differ with the disease stage. Recently polypharmacy—condensed in a polypill—has been proposed as a tool of primary and secondary prevention of cardiovascular disease and potentially for primary and secondary prevention of T2DM. However, any antidiabetic polypill would need to be tailored to one of the various stages of T2DM, which differ considerably because metabolic and clinical defects evolve as the disease progresses. Although a daily fixed-dose treatment might be helpful from some of its aspects, any such polypill will encounter major obstacles. These are not only due to the size and weight of its formulation but also to the loss of therapeutic flexibility, which is mandatory to overcome acute

From: *Contemporary Endocrinology: Controversies in Treating Diabetes:*
Clinical and Research Aspects
Edited by: D. LeRoith and A. I. Vinik © Humana Press, Totowa, NJ

metabolic derangements and to cope with intermittent increases in blood pressure. Against such a background future, antidiabetic polypills will require thorough testing not only as to their side effects but also as to their metabolic efficacy and effect on normalization of body weight and life expectancy to prove that they are superior to available treatment for the prevention and treatment of T2DM.

Key Words: Polypharmacy, antidiabetic polypill, Type 2 diabetes mellitus, antihyperglycemic agents, depression, psychoneurohormones

INTRODUCTION

For decades, polypharmacy has been a reality for patients suffering from fatefully progressing disorders. These include chronic cardiovascular disease (CVD: requiring diuretics, beta-blockers, ACE-inhibitors, and aspirin), renal disease (requiring diuretics, antihypertensives, resins, and if carrying a renal transplant, immune suppressives), severe "malign" hypertension (requiring multiple antihypertensives), or rheumatoid arthritis (requiring non-steroidal analgetics, steroids, and immunosuppressives). Likewise in the early stages of type 2 diabetes mellitus (T2DM), when obesity and/or hyperglycemia prevail and treatment frequently resorts prematurely to biguanide, α-glucosidase inhibitors, and/or appetite suppressants instead of physical exercise, restriction of calorie intake, and reduction of body weight. This is embarassing as life-style interventions have been shown to prevent and delay T2DM manifestation in those prone to develop this disease (1,2).

Even more drugs are given in the late stages of T2DM when the microan-giopathic sequelae of chronic hyperglycemia can result in diabetic retinopathy, nephropathy, and neuropathy. During these stages, patients with T2DM frequently require antihypertensives and lipid-lowering drugs, aspirin and analgetics, in addition to antihyperglycemic agents.

Complete adherence to prescribed drugs can be as low as 20% (3). With 14% of prescriptions never taken up and 13% of prescribed drugs obtained never ingested (4), it is no surprise that antihypertensive treatment regimens frequently combine a diuretic and an ACE-inhibitor in a single pill to guarantee better patient compliance. Such combipills benefit the patient as long as parallel increases in dose do not cause any undesired side effects by overdosing one of its components.

Wald and Law (5) conceived the idea of a "polypill" to more effectively combat CVD and better protect all those at risk, that is, the entire population above 55 years of age. The recommended contents were a statin, folic acid, aspirin, and three antihypertensive agents each at half standard dose. Wald and Law estimated that by this treatment, ischemic heart disease (IHD) could be reduced by 88% and stroke by 80%, a superb deal if proven correct. In addition, one third of people taking the "polypill" would gain on average about 11 years of life free from events of IHD and stroke. The proposal of a polypill to prevent and delay CVD in people above 55 years of age has provoked a considerable debate *(6,7)*.

The concept of combination pharmacotherapy has been extended beyond CVD *(5)* to metabolic disorders and T2DM *(8,9)*. Before embarking on any project to design an antidiabetic "polypill," (i) the characteristics of T2DM, whose picture changes considerably during its natural course, and (ii) the available treatment forms need to be considered. Only then can we answer the question of whether an antidiabetic polypill might be superior to other forms of intervention.

CHARACTERISTICS OF T2DM

Endocrinology textbooks *(10)* describe T2DM as a disease with a polygenic disposition that is unveiled in response to interference by environmental factors promoting overweight and obesity. Major players in that context include physical inactivity, food intake in excess of energy expenditure, and a long-term positive energy balance resulting in metabolic obesity with increased volume of visceral fat, a predictor of T2DM *(11)*. The prevalence of T2DM, which accounts for 90% of all diabetes worldwide, has almost quintupled during the second half of the twentieth century in the industrialized world—up in Germany from only 0.7–1.0% shortly after World War II, at a time when food supply was short and the burden of manual labor still considerable. Diabetes is now the eighth leading disease in the calculated economic burden of disease in high-income countries *(12)*. This rising trend is set to continue with the life-time risk of people born in the USA in the year 2000 developing T2DM estimated to reach 32.8% for men and 38.5% for women *(13)*. The incidence and prevalence of T2DM depends, however, also on racial background, as best exemplified in non-Hispanic blacks and Mexican Americans, who have a 1.6-fold and 1.9-fold greater prevalence than non-Hispanic whites *(14)*.

In the long term, the burden of T2DM includes the sequelae of diabetic microangiopathy, peripheral and autonomic neuropathy, and accelerated macroangiopathy. These defects can result in manifest diabetic retinopathy and premature cataracts, diabetic foot, and chronic renal failure, all of which surface earlier in elderly than in young diabetic patients. Such secondary "late" diabetic complications, which can become irreversible in the long run, require thorough and specific care although they could largely be prevented by proper and early treatment of T2DM *(15,16,17)*. To be successful, treatment has to rest on a thorough knowledge of the pathophysiology of T2DM and to be specific for each given state of the disease.

PATHOPHYSIOLOGY OF T2DM

Apart from hyperglycemia, key characteristics of T2DM include increased hepatic glucose production, impaired glucose-stimulated insulin release, and reduced insulin sensitivity of target tissues of insulin action (18), all of which can already be seen years before the onset of the disease. These metabolic dysregulations are aggravated in the elderly by age-associated impairments of insulin secretion and insulin sensitivity, decreased physical activity, and co-morbidities of all sorts as well as—in part—by the drugs needed for their treatment. In addition, the aging process impairs "glucose effectiveness," that is, reduced insulin-independent glucose uptake.

Such impaired insulin action also referred to as "insulin resistance" not only affects carbohydrate metabolism but also extends among others to insulin's ability to enhance blood flow, which is markedly impaired in obese insulin insensitive elderly patients with T2DM (19).

Insulin resistance can precede overt hyperglycemia by decades in those prone to later develop T2DM (20) but also associates with physical inactivity, hypertension, and dyslipidemia including severe hypertriglyceridemia, ischemic cardiovascular disease (21), and polycystic ovarian syndrome (22).

Any such loss of insulin sensitivity reduces insulin-stimulated glucose disposal, which is accompanied by hyperinsulinemia in the obese (23) and by impaired glucose transport/phosphorylation and glycogen synthesis in T2DM (24) and obesity (25).

Among the factors detrimentally affecting skeletal muscle insulin sensitivity, lipotoxicity of free fatty acids (FFA) is of considerable importance. FFA inhibit insulin-stimulated glucose uptake at plasma concentrations within the physiological range (26,27) and thereby promote the development of T2DM. This is consistent with the improvement of muscle glucose disposal observed in response to lowering plasma FFA concentration (28).

Glucose-stimulated insulin release, which depends both on glucose entry into the beta cell and on its phosphorylation, seems in parallel to be impaired by the same mechanism, particularly in response to long-term exposure to elevated plasma FFA concentrations (29). Such ubiquitous reduction by FFAs of glucose transport/phosphorylation possibly explains the inseparable coexistence of insulin insensitivity and abnormal insulin secretion in T2DM. Against that background it would appear that chronic lipotoxicity begets hyperglycemia and thus facilitates secondary glucotoxicity (Fig. 1) (30).

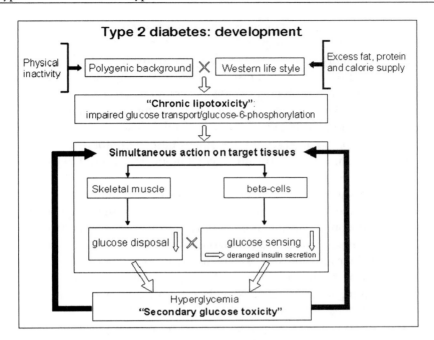

Fig. 1. Scheme of type 2 diabetes mellitus (T2DM) development. Based on excess supply of fatty acids provided by both high fat/high calorie food intake and nocturnal lipolysis reduces glucose transport/phosphorylation in skeletal muscle and potentially simultaneously in beta cells. Such lipotoxicity impairs simultaneously glucose disposal, glucose sensing, and insulin secretion. The resulting hyperglycemia (T2DM) is then further aggravated by added secondary glucotoxicity. Reproduced with permission from *(30)*.

RISK MANAGEMENT AND TREATMENT OF T2DM

Early/premature manifestation of T2DM in those prone to develop the disease therefore largely depends on a positive energy balance due to food intake in excess of energy expenditure resulting in obesity. Proper risk management and prevention of T2DM thus wherever possible have to overcome obesity by restricting food/energy intake and muscle inactivity/atrophy through increasing physical activity. The clinical importance of such change in life-style cannot be exaggerated, and its dominant role in primary and secondary prevention of T2DM has been confirmed in several major randomized clinical studies *(1,2,31)* in people at high risk for developing T2DM. Of note, reduction of body weight and promotion of physical exercise reduced the cumulative incidence of T2DM by 50% over 3.2 years. Not surprisingly, normalization of body weight and regular physical exercise thus are the standard approach in the treatment of T2DM in its early stages.

As T2DM progresses, treatment becomes more complex, because in addition to insulin resistance and impaired glucose-stimulated insulin release, the disease can gradually result in a decline in basal insulin secretion and insiduously approach a state of overall insulin deficiency. Drugs have been approved to tackle the resulting problems (Table 1) including different stages and risk factors of T2DM. These drugs are aimed at reducing body weight (metformin, rimonabont, orlistat; DPP IV inhibitors), insulin resistance (metformin and glitazones), postprandial glycemia (α-glucosidase inhibitors), and increasing endogenous insulin release (insulin secretagogues: sulfonylureas, glinides; GLP-1 mimetics, and DPP IV inhibitors).

Of note, among oral antidiabetic agents unresolved major risks have been attributed – besides hypoglycemia in response to insulin secretagogues – to the use of glitazones causing both removal from the market (troglitazone, Rezulin R) and black boxing (rosiglitazone, Avandia R) of some of their group (Table 1). The incriminated side effects included severe hepatotoxicity, cardiac insufficiency and heart attacks as well as potential premature osteoporosis potentially relating to accelerated osteoclast differentiation and bone resorption in a receptor dependent manner as shown in mice *(32,33)*.

The overall goal of any drug treatment is to improve glycemia and reduce HbA1c, ideally to $\leq 6.5\%$, thereby avoiding or delaying indirectly the development of diabetes-associated microvascular complications *(34)*. To this end, self-monitored blood glucose values have been set as low as 70–135 mg/dl by the joint European cardiovascular prevention guidelines to account also for the close dependence of endothelial function on blood glucose concentration *(35)*.

The goals of treatment of T2DM, however, have to extend beyond the control of hyperglycemia, which is critical for the prevention of microvascular lesions *(34)*. Both dyslipidemia and hypertension have to be tackled as well to prevent or delay macrovascular defects in the late stages of the disease *(15)*. The sequential use of antihyperglycemic drugs follows the natural course of T2DM, whose phenotype is initially dominated by hyperglycemia due to insulin resistance, overweight and obesity, and later, when weight loss occurs spontaneously, by more markedly impaired insulin release. Rational treatment of T2DM accommodates that pattern in its many guidelines with attempts to reduce weight by physical exercise and cutting down food intake. It then continues with metformin in diabetic patients still overweight, followed by insulin secretagogues and glitazones before insulin therapy is instituted (Fig. 2) *(36)*.

In this context, one has to be aware that none of the drugs used for blood glucose control directly treats established diabetes-associated eye and kidney disease or any partial—peripheral or autonomous—breakdown of the nervous system or accelerated macroangiopathy. All these secondary defects of T2DM may require additional and specific treatment particularly by antihypertensive

Table 1

Antidiabetic Drugs for the Treatment of T2DM not to be Substituted for Insulin with Indirect (i) and Direct (d) Antihyperglycemic Action

Goal	Drug	Side effects
Weight reduction	Orlistat (i) (120 mg t.i.d.)	Fecal fat loss (soiling) Loss of fat-soluble vitamins
	Rimonabant (i) (20 mg/day; appetite suppressant) (cannabinoid receptor-1-inhibitor)	Weight loss (approximately 5 kg more than placebo)
Absorption inhibitors	α-Glucosidase inhibitors (d) (100 mg t.i.d.)	Flatulence Weight loss (0–10 kg/year)
Insulin sensitizer	Metformin (d) [500–2550 mg/day)	Abdominal discomfort Nausea (lactic acidosis) Weight loss (0–6 kg/yr)
	Glitazones (i) (4–45 mg/day)	Weight gain (+1–13 kg/year) Edema Anemia (Hepatotoxicity)
	Troglitazone[a]	Hepatotoxicity
	Rosiglitazone[b]	Heart attacks, bone fractures
Insulin secretagogues		
Oral	Sulfonylurea (d) (2nd generation 1–15 mg/day)	Hypoglycemia Weight gain (1–3 kg/year)
	Meglitinides (d) (0.5–120 mg before meals)	Hypoglycemia Weight gain (1–3 kg/year)
	DPP-IV inhibitors (i)[c] (LAF 237 50 mg/day)	Nausea
S.c. injection	GLP-1 mimetics (i) (exenatide 5–10 μg b.i.d.)	Nausea (recovery of beta-cell mass?) Weight loss

[a] Admitted 1997, removed 2000.
[b] Black boxed 2007.
[c] As yet not approved.

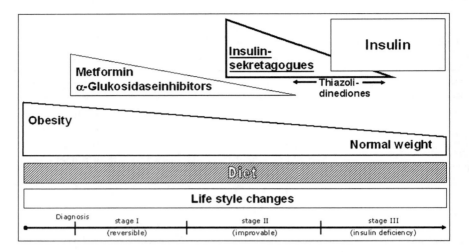

Fig. 2. Rational treatment of type 2 diabetes mellitus (T2DM) accounting for the stages of the disease, the need of lifestyle changes (diet and physical exercise), and the available options of pharmacotherapy (metformin in those overweight, followed by insulin secretagogues and glitazones in stage II and early stage III before insulin therapy is instituted).

and antihyperlipidemic drugs but also local treatment once neuropathic ulcers and proliferative diabetic retinopathy develop.

An analysis of the goals achieved controlling hyperglycemia, hyperlipidemia, and hypertension, however, gives a bleak picture. According to NHANES III *(37)*, 18% of all patients with diabetes surveyed had HbA1c values above 9.5%, 34% had blood pressure greater than 140/90 mm Hg, and 58% had LDL-cholesterol above 130 mg/dl. Other data even show that only 2% of all patients with diabetes had achieved all goals of therapy as recommended by the American Diabetes Association *(38)*.

Major obstacles to achieving the goals of proper diabetes care include among others

1. partial or complete non-compliance by the patient for economic reasons, that is, an inadequate health care system
2. non-compliance because of unrealistic polypharmacy in multimorbid patients, that is, drugs are bought but not consumed
3. lack of patient motivation toward self-management
4. non-professionalism and/or lack of expertise on the side of the healthcare personnel
5. environmental factors favoring obesity by promotion of excess food intake ("junk food") and avoidance of physical exercise (cars and television).

Some, but not all of these obstacles may be tackled by a "polypill" that would reduce the number of pills to be swallowed by a given patient requiring complex treatment. Before proceeding with a polypill, one has, however, to remember that in those prone to develop T2DM removal of detrimental environmental factors, that is, of high energy food intake and physical inactivity, could avoid manifestation of up to 80% of all T2DM, without any pharmacotherapy (1,2,31). In the early stages of the disease, such an approach can even transiently reverse hyperglycemia into a normoglycemic state. So why develop an antidiabetic polypill?

THE ANTIDIABETIC POLYPILL

The concept of a pill to be taken once daily for the prevention, delay, and/or alleviation of chronic disease originates from the desire to lower cardiovascular risk in the population at large and in those over 55 years of age in particular (5). The proposed cardiovascular "polypill" with its six components (three antihypertensives, a statin, aspirin, and folic acid) would serve to reduce blood pressure, plasma LDL-cholesterol, platelet aggregation, and plasma homocystein. Wald and Law estimate the years of life gained by taking the polypill from age 55 years onward would be 11–24 for women and 12–21 for men. By adding omega-3-fatty acids, cardiac rehabilitation, and diet to the polypill, patients with coronary heart disease, post-myocardial infarction, or stroke are projected to respond to such polyportfolio by experiencing a reduction in clinical events of 84, 91, and 77%, respectively (39).

Designing an antidiabetic polyportfolio might help to overcome the difficulty of convincing people at high risk for developing T2DM that a healthy lifestyle can reduce the incidence of the disease (1,2) and in convincing patients that adequate clinical care including proper self-management can minimize the risk of manifest diabetes-associated late complications due to microangiopathy (15,16,17,34). The unwillingness of the public at large and of patients already suffering from T2DM in particular to benefit from available knowledge might even be outwitted. Some obstacles, however, confront that simplistic attitude. Primary and secondary prevention of T2DM require a more complex approach than Wald and Law's polypill (5) if fixed combinations of antidiabetic drugs are to be used atop of necessary changes in lifestyle.

Major problems to be dealt with arise from (i) the need to adequately address the patient's actual metabolic and clinical state, which requires targeted intervention but no polypill and (ii) the change in phenotype with progression of T2DM. These stages of the disease could for the sake of the argument be categorized besides prediabetes (stage 0) as reversible (stage I), improvable (stage II), and insulin deficient (stage III) (Fig. 2).

Table 2

The Antidiabetic "Polypill": Goals and Requirements of Treatment for Different Stages of T2DM (for Definition of Stages, see Fig. 2)

Stage*	Goals	Polypill components	n
	Prevention		
Stage 0	Normalization of body		2
(2)	weight		
	–Appetite control	Rimonabant	
	–Stimulation of physical activity	? (Lifestyle intervention)	
	–Energy wasting	Orlistat	
	Treatment		2
Stage I	Normalization of body		2
(2)	weight		
	–Appetite control	Rimonabant	
	–Stimulation of physical activity	? (Lifestyle intervention)	
	–Energy wasting	Orlistat and α-glucosidase inhibitor	
	Lowering of blood glucose	Metformin	
Stage II	Normalization of body	As in stage 1	2
(6)	weight		
	Lowering of blood glucose		2
	–Insulin secretagogues	Sulfonylurea	
	–Insulin sensitizer	Metformin (if obese) Glitazone (if non-obese)	
	Normalization of blood pressure	ACE-inhibitor	1
	Normalization/reduction of LDL-cholesterol	Statin	1
Stage III	Lowering of blood glucose		
(6)	–Insulin secretagogues	Sulfonylurea or glinide	1
	–Insulin sensitizer	Glitazone, metformin	2
	–Insulin	–	
	Normalization of blood pressure	ACE-inhibitor	1
	Normalization/reduction of LDL-Cholesterol	Statin	1
	Platelet aggregation inhibition	Aspirin	1

* total number of components, *n*.

Polypills of different content would be required to adequately deal with the specifics of a given stage. This would lead to at least four different polypills each embedded in a polyportfolio providing for appropriate changes in lifestyle (Table 2) if the goals to be met are defined as prevention of T2DM and as successful treatment of its different stages.

In this context, polypill I would have to be for the prevention of T2DM in those at high risk of developing the disease. It would need to tame appetite long term (e.g., by rimonabant) and provide for a negative energy balance (e.g., using orlistat). Wishfully, I would like to add to the mix the as yet non-existent drug stimulating the frequently lost natural desire for physical exercise.

Polypill II should then serve for treatment of T2DM in its early phase (stage I). It would contain metformin (maximum dose 2550 mg/day) in addition to the contents of polypill I to overcome insulin resistance and to lower blood glucose.

Polypill III would have to cope with T2DM stage 2. Its task would be to restore insulin availability and action by added sulfonylurea and glitazone compounds, respectively, and to protect with an added statin against the sequelae of hypercholesterinemia. Possibly a DP-IV inhibitor should be added—once available—to stimulate insulin release, delay gastric emptying, and reduce body weight *(40)*.

Polypill IV would most likely omit metformin, as in stage III patients frequently approach normal body weight. In addition, it would complement the other ingredients of polypill III with an ACE-inhibitor to protect against hypertension and a premature decline in renal function and aspirin to inhibit platelet aggregation in the case of cardiovascular disease.

As the concept of the polypill rests on ingestion of a single daily pill *(5)* any design of an antidiabetic polypill will encounter major obstacles due to size and weight (up to 3 g) of its formulation and due to loss of adequate dosing intervals (e.g., t.i.d. for orlistat and metformin and before meals for meglitinide and α-glucosidase inhibitors). Furthermore, the possibility of overdosing single components has to be taken into account, particularly when a polypill is erroneously taken more frequently than once daily.

Thus, antidiabetic polypills would need to be thoroughly tested to prove their superiority over available, more flexible treatments of T2DM. To this end, key evidence-based criteria will have to include metabolic efficacy and normalization of body weight as well as insulin release and, additionally, undisturbed bioavailability of the polypills' single components and absence of any interference with individual drug action.

However, even if an apparently successful antidiabetic polypill could be designed, it remains to be seen how any such formulation can overcome poor regional diabetes care. Such deficiencies could result from an ineffective or individually unaffordable health care system, from inadequate patient motivation for proper self-management, from poor training of those responsible for adequate patient education, or from a mix of them all.

Against such a background, a polymeal could be tastier and an adequate physical exercise program a safer alternative than any antidiabetic polypill. Calculated from the Framingham database, the benefits of a polypill and exercise strategy promise an increase in overall life expectancy of 6.6 years and in life expectancy free from cardiovascular disease of 9.0 years *(41)*. No doubt, such change in life-style would also benefit patients with T2DM at all stages and thus outmaneuver any antidiabetic polypill, particularly if target-oriented incentives were used to motivate patients to reach set therapeutic goals both for their metabolism and body weight *(42)*.

REFERENCES

1. Tuomilehto J, Lindström J, Eriksson JG, Valle TT, Hamalainen H, Ilanne-Parikka P, Keinanen-Kiukaanniemi S, Laakso M, Louheranta A, Rastas M, Salminen V, Uusitupa M. Finnish Diabetes Prevention Study Group: prevention of type 2 diabetes mellitus by changes in lifestyle among subjects with impaired glucose tolerance. N Engl J Med 344: 1343–1350, 2001.
2. Pan XR, Li GW, Hu YH, Wang JX, Yang WY, An ZX, Hu ZX, Lin J, Xiao JZ, Cao HB, Liu PA, Jiang XG, Jiang YY, Wang JP, Zheng H, Zhang H, Bennett PH, Howard BV. Effects of diet and exercise in preventing NIDDM in people with impaired glucose tolerance. The Da Quing IGT and Diabetes Study. Diabetes Care 20: 537–544, 1997.
3. Monane M, Bohn RL, Gurwitz JH, Glynn RJ, Levin R, Avorn J. The effects of initial drug choice and co-morbidity on antihypertensive therapy compliance: results from a population based study in the elderly. Am J Hypertens 10: 697–704, 1997.
4. Berg JS, Dischler J, Wagner DJ, Raia JJ, Polmer-Shevlin N. Medication compliance: a health care problem. Ann Pharmacother 27: S1–S54, 1993.
5. Wald NJ, Law MR. A strategy to reduce cardiovascular disease by more than 80%. BMJ 326: 1419–1424, 2003.
6. Robinson JG, Maheshwari N. A 'poly-portfolio' for secondary prevention: a strategy to reduce subsequent events by up to 97% over five years. Am J Cardiol 95: 373–378, 2005.
7. Franco OH, Steyerberg EW, de Laet C. The polypill: at what price would it become cost effective? J Epidemiol Community Health 60: 213–217, 2006.
8. Scheen AJ. Management of the metabolic syndrome. Minerva Endocrinol 29: 31–45, 2004.
9. Gale E. The polypill and type 2 diabetes. Diabet Med 21: 8–10, 2004.
10. Buse JB, Polonsky KS, Burant CF. Type 2 diabetes mellitus. In: Larsen PR, Kronenberg HM, Melmed S, Polonsky KS (eds) Williams Textbook of Endocrinology. Saunders, PA, 2003, pp 1427–1483.
11. Bennett PH, Bogardus C, Tuomilehto J, Zimmet P. Epidemiology and natural history of NIDDM: non-obese and obese. In: Alberti KGMM, Zimmet P, DeFronzo RA, Keen H (eds) Chichester International Textbook of Diabetes Mellitus, 2nd ed. London: John Wiley & Sons Ltd., 1987, pp. 147–176.

12. Lopez AD, Mathers CD, Ezzati M, Jamison DT, Murray CJL. Global and regional burden of disease and risk factors, 2001: systematic analysis of population health data. Lancet 367: 1747–1757, 2006.

13. Narayan KM, Boyle JP, Thompson TJ, Sorensen SW, Williamson DF. Lifetime risk for diabetes mellitus in the United States. JAMA 290: 1884–1890, 2003.

14. Harris MI, Flegol KM, Cowie CC, Eberhardt MS, Goldstein DE, Little RR, Wiedmeyer H-M, Byrd-Holt DD. Prevalence of diabetes, impaired fasting glucose, and impaired glucose tolerance in US adults. The 3rd National Health and Nutrition Examination Survey, 1988–1994. Diabetes Care 21: 518–524, 1998.

15. UK Prospective Diabetes Study (UKPDS) Group. Intensive blood glucose control with sulfonylureas or insulin compared with conventional treatment and risk of complications in patients with type 2 diabetes (UKPDS 33). Lancet 352: 837–853, 1998.

16. UK Prospective Diabetes Study (UKPDS) Group. Effect of intensive blood glucose control with metformin on complications in overweight patients with type 2 diabetes (UKPDS 34). Lancet 352: 854–865, 1998.

17. Gaede P, Vedel P, Larsen N, Jensen GV, Parving HH, Pedersen O. Multifactorial intervention and cardiovascular disease in patients with type 2 diabetes. N Engl J Med 348: 383–393, 2003.

18. DeFronzo R. The triumvirate β-cell, muscle, liver. A collusion responsible for NIDDM. Diabetes 37: 667–687, 1988.

19. Meneilly GS, Elliot T. Metabolic alterations in middle-aged and elderly obese patients with type 2 diabetes. Diabetes Care 19: 544–546, 1996.

20. Beck-Nielsen H, Groop LC. Metabolic and genetic characterization of prediabetic states. J Clin Invest 93: 1714–1721, 1994.

21. Reaven GM. Role of insulin resistance in human disease. Diabetes 37: 1595–1607, 1988.

22. Moller DE, Fliers JS. Insulin resistance: mechanisms, syndromes and implications. N Engl J Med 325: 938–948, 1992.

23. Haffner SM, Stern MP, Mitchel BD, Hazuda HP, Patterson JK. Incidence of type II diabetes in Mexican Americans predicted by fasting insulin and glucose levels, obesity, and body-fat distribution. Diabetes 39: 283–288, 1990.

24. Cline GW, Petersen KF, Krssak M, Shen J, Hundal RS, Trajanoski Z, Inzucchi S, Dresner A, Rothman DL, Shulman GI. Impaired glucose transport as a cause of decreased insulin-stimulated muscle glycogen synthesis in type 2 diabetes. N Engl J Med 341: 240–246, 1999.

25. Petersen KF, Hendler R, Price T, Perseghin G, Rothman DL, Held N, Amatruda JM, Shulman GI. 13C/31P NMR studies on the mechanism of insulin resistance in obesity. Diabetes 47: 381–386, 1998.

26. Boden G, Chen X, Ruiz J, White JV, Rossetti L. Mechanisms of fatty acid-induced inhibition of glucose uptake. J Clin Invest 93: 2438–2446, 1994.

27. Roden M, Krssak M, Stingl H, Gruber S, Hofer A, Fürnsinn C, Moser E, Waldhäusl W. Rapid impairment of skeletal muscle glucose transport/ phosphorylation by free fatty acids in humans. Diabetes 48: 358–364, 1999.

28. Piatti PM, Monti LD, Davis SN, Conti M, Brown MD, Pozza G, Alberti KG. Effects of an acute decrease in non-esterified fatty acid levels on muscle glucose utilization and forearm indirect calorimetry in lean NIDDM patients. Diabetologia 39: 103–112, 1996.

29. Carpentier A, Mittelman SD, Lamarche B, Bergman RN, Giacca A, Lewis GF. Acute enhancement of insulin secretion by FFA in humans is lost with prolonged FFA elevation. Am J Physiol 276: E1055–E1066, 1999.

30. Waldhäusl WK, Roden M. The effects of free fatty acids on glucose transport and phosphorylation in human skeletal muscle. Curr Opinion Endocrinol Diabetes Obes 7: 211–216, 2000.
31. Knowler WC, Barrett-Connor E, Fowler SE, Hamman RF, Lachin JM, Walker EA, Nathan DM; Diabetes Prevention Program Research Group. Reduction in the incidence of type 2 diabetes with lifestyle intervention or metformin. N Engl J Med 346: 393–403, 2002.
32. Couzin J. Heart attack risk overshadows a popular diabetes therapy. Science 316: 1550–51, 2007.
33. Wan Y, Chong LW, and Evans RM. PPARgamma regulates osteoclastogenesis in mice. Nature Medicine 13: 1496–1503, 2007.
34. The Diabetes Control and Complications Trial Research Group. The effect of intensive treatment of diabetes on the development and progression of long-term complications in insulin-dependent diabetes mellitus. N Engl J Med 329: 977–986, 1993.
35. Pyorala K, Lehto S, De Bacquer D, De Sutter J, Sans S, Keil U, Wood D, De Backer G, EUROASPIRE I Group; EUROASPIRE II Group. Risk factor management in diabetic and non-diabetic patients with coronary heart disease. Findings from the EUROASPIRE I AND II surveys. Diabetologia 47: 1257–1265, 2004.
36. Waldhäusl W. Rational treatment of NIDDM. Does it exist? Diabetes Nutr Metab Rev 4: 259–265, 1990.
37. Saadine J, Engelgau M, Beckles G, Gregg E, Thompson T, Narayan KM. A diabetes report card fort the United States: quality of care in the 1990s. Ann Intern Med 136: 565–574, 2004.
38. Beckles GL, Engelgau MM, Narayan KM, Herman WH, Aubert RE, Williamson DF. Population-based assessment of the level of care among adults with diabetes in the U.S. Diabetes Care 21: 1432–1438, 1998.
39. Robinson JG, Maheshwari N. A 'poly-portfolio' for secondary prevention: a strategy to reduce subsequent events by up to 97% over five years. Am J Cardiol 95: 373–378, 2005.
40. Drucker DJ. Enhancing incretin action for the treatment of type 2 diabetes. Diabetes Care 26: 2929–2940, 2003.
41. Franco OH, Bonneux L, de Laet C, Peeters A, Steyerberg EW, Mackenbach JP. The polymeal: a more natural, safer, and probably tastier (than the polypill) strategy to reduce cardiovascular disease by more than 75%. BMJ 329: 1447–1450, 2004.
42. Waldhäusl W. The metabolic syndrome and type 2 diabetes: what has gone wrong in type 2 diabetes care? Current Diabetes Reports 4: 395–396, 2004.

17 Comorbid Depression and Diabetes

Natural History and Clinical Aspects

Richard R. Rubin, *PhD*

SUMMARY

Depression, the leading cause of disability in the world, is more common in patients with diabetes, and it is associated with negative outcomes in these patients. These negative outcomes include less adherence to treatment recommendations, higher blood glucose levels, higher rates of microvascular and macrovascular complications, lower rates of productivity at work, higher health care costs, and higher mortality rates.

This chapter addresses two key issues concerning comorbid depression and type 2 diabetes: 1) why depression is more common in patients with type 2 diabetes, and 2) whether relieving depression in patients with diabetes improves clinical and other outcomes. It appears that depression is a risk factor for developing type 2 diabetes, while having type 2 diabetes does

From: *Contemporary Endocrinology: Controversies in Treating Diabetes:*
Clinical and Research Aspects
Edited by: D. LeRoith and A. I. Vinik © Humana Press, Totowa, NJ

not seem to increase the risk of becoming depressed. Depression may increase diabetes risk via behavioral and/or psychoneurolhormonal pathways. Depression treatment is effective in relieving depression in patients with diabetes, and it can improve glycemic control in those whose control is poor. This treatment can also improve work productivity and reduce health care costs.

Key Words: Depression, type 2 diabetes, depression treatment

INTRODUCTION

Depression is the leading cause of disability in the world and the third most common reason for seeing a primary care physician. Most studies find an increased risk of depression in patients with diabetes. In a nationally representative sample of adults with diabetes, the 12-month prevalence of major depressive disorder (MDD) was about 50% greater than the rate in the general population: 9.3–6.0% (1,2). A meta-analysis of 20 controlled studies also found higher rates of clinically significant depression symptoms among patients with diabetes (20.5%) compared with those without diabetes (11.4%) (3). Among people with diabetes, depression is associated with a host of negative outcomes, including less adherence to diet, exercise, medication recommendations (4–7), higher blood glucose levels (7), higher rates of microvascular and macrovascular complications (4,8–12), lower rates of productivity at work (13), higher mortality rates (9,14,15), and higher health care costs (4,16).

The human and economic toll of comorbid depression and diabetes has sparked interest in two important questions:

1. Why is depression more common in people who have diabetes?
2. Does relieving depression improve clinical outcomes?

WHY IS DEPRESSION MORE COMMON AMONG PEOPLE WITH DIABETES?

Depression could be more common in patients with diabetes for a variety of reasons. For example, the daily demands of living with diabetes or the challenges created by diabetes complications could increase a person's risk for becoming depressed. Or depression could increase a person's risk for developing diabetes. Behavioral or hormonal effects of depression could have that effect, especially in the case of type 2 diabetes. Finally, some other process, such as aging or an as yet undetermined genetic factor, might increase a person's risk for both diabetes and depression.

Could Being Depressed Increase One's Risk of Developing Diabetes?

In 1674, Thomas Willis, the British physician who identified glycosuria as a sign of diabetes, was the first to address the natural history of comorbid depression and diabetes when he stated that diabetes was caused by "sadness or long sorrow and other depressions and disorders" *(17)*. No one pursued Willis provocative hypothesis for almost 300 years; then interest in the comorbidity of diabetes and depression was renewed with a few studies published in the 1930s through the 1960s. These researchers pursued Willis' general thinking, searching for the "diabetic personality" in people with type 1 diabetes *(18,19)*. This search proved fruitless, and researchers turned from looking for emotional *causes* of diabetes to looking for emotional *consequences* of the disease. The fact that diabetes can be demanding in countless ways large and small led many to assume that diabetes increased a person's risk for depression, not the opposite. There were a few longitudinal studies of psychological adjustment in young people with type 1 diabetes *(20,21)*, but until about 10 years ago, we had essentially no data to help us understand the natural history of depression and type 2 diabetes.

Recent Evidence Suggests it Could

In 1996, Eaton and colleagues *(22)* published an interesting study, suggesting Willis might have been right after all, at least when it came to a person's risk for developing *type 2* diabetes. This study was followed in 1999 by one in Japan conducted by Kawakami and colleagues *(23)* that came to similar conclusions. These studies sparked others, and between 2003 and 2005, eight more papers were published addressing the same question. These studies varied in important respects, including how researchers determined whether a person had diabetes at the beginning of the study, how depression was assessed, the study populations, and the length of follow-up. Despite these differences, the results of all but one of these studies lent at least some support for Willis' hypothesis, even when known risk factors for developing diabetes (demographic, behavioral, and metabolic) were controlled. These studies are discussed below and described in Table 1.

The pioneering study of Eaton et al. *(22)* was the only one to assess depression using a diagnostic interview rather than a self-report questionnaire; the former is considered a more valid method and generally yields lower estimated depression rates. This study followed 1715 people who said they did not have type 2 diabetes when they entered the study. After 13 years, the people who had been depressed at baseline were about twice as likely to have developed type 2 diabetes as those who had not been depressed, controlling for demographic, behavioral, and metabolic risk factors. Because of the small number of people who developed diabetes during

Table 1

Effect of Depression on Subsequent Risk of Developing Type 2 Diabetes

Study	Number of Subjects	Diagnostic method	Duration of follow-up	Findings	Comments
East Baltimore Site of the Epidemiologic Cachment Area Survey (Eaton et al., 1996)	1718 men and women	Diagnostic interview (DIS)	13 years	RR = 2.23, 95% CI = 0.90–5.55	$p = 0.08$
Kawakami et al., 1999	2764 male employees	Zung Depression Screener	8 years	HR = 2.31, 95% CI = 1.03–5.20	$p < 0.05$
Study of Women's Health Across the Nation (SWAN) (Everson-Rose et al., 2003)	2254 premenopausal, middle-aged women	CES-D Depression Screener	2 years	OR = 2.28, 95% CI = 1.2–6.4 for African Americans	$p < 0.30$; too few cases in other ethnic groups for reliable assessment
National Health and Nutrition Examination Epidemiologic Survey Follow-Up Survey (NHEFS) (Carnethon et al., 2003)	6190 men and women	General Well-Being Screener	>15 years	RR = 3.0, 95% CI = 2.0–4.7 for subjects with <HS education	RR is NSD for subjects with ≥ HS education

Study	Sample	Measure	Follow-up	Result	Additional result
NHEFS (Sadyah et al 2003)	8870 men and women	CES-D Depression Screener	9 years	RH = 1.11, 95% CI = 0.79–1.56	RH = 1.27 (95% CI = 0.93–1.73) not adjusting for BMI and physical activity
Nurses' Health Study (Arroyo, 2004)	72,178 female nurses	Mental Health Index Screener	4 years	RR = 1.2, 95% CI = 1.0–1.5	$p = .05$
Atherosclerosis Risks in Communities (ARIC) Study (Golden et al., 2004)	11,615 men and women	Vital Exhaustion Screener	6 years	Highest quartile versus lowest RH = 1.38, 95% CI: 1.10-1.73	
Rancho Bernardo Study (Palinkas et al., 2004)	971 men and women	Beck Depression Screener	8 years	OR = 2.50, 95% CI = 1.29–4.87	Type 2 diabetes at baseline not associated with later depression
Whitehall II Study (Kumari et al., 2004)	10,308 civil servants	General Health Questionnaire Depression Screener	12 years	OR (men) = 1.17, 95% CI = 0.8-1.7; OR (women) = 1.08, 95% CI = 0.6–1.9	OR for diabetes or IGT significant for both genders
Brown et al., 2005	1622 men and women with diabetes; 2279 without diabetes	Population-based, case-controlled administrative database	History of depression in previous 3 years	OR = 1.23, 95% CI = 1.10–1.37 for those 20–50 years of age	OR = 0.92, 95% CI = 0.84–1.00 for those ≥51 years of age

the study, this difference in diabetes rates between depressed and non-depressed subjects was not statistically significant. Kawakami et al. *(23)* published a study several years later on 2764 Japanese men whose diabetes status at baseline was determined by self-report and medical records and reported findings similar to those of Eaton et al. After 8 years, study participants who had been moderately or severely depressed at baseline according to a validated self-report screener were significantly more likely to have developed diabetes, controlling for other risk factors. Those who had been identified as only mildly depressed at baseline did not have an increased risk of developing diabetes during the study. In a result similar to that of Kawakami et al., Golden et al. *(24)* found an increased risk of developing diabetes over 6 years only among those in the highest quartile of vital exhaustion, a proxy for depression symptoms. The study population was 11,615 adults participating in the Atherosclerosis Risk in Communities (ARIC) study.

Other researchers have reported that the effects of depression on diabetes risk vary by demographic factors, including education, age, and race/ethnicity. Carnethon assessed depression symptoms in 6190 adults who participated in the National Health and Nutrition Examination Epidemiologic Follow-Up Study and found a significant association with the risk of developing type 2 diabetes after a 15 year follow-up only in those with less than a high-school education *(25)*. In a retrospective database study, Brown et al. compared earlier depression markers (diagnosis of depression or antidepressant medication use) in a group of patients recently diagnosed with type 2 diabetes and a matched sample that had not been diagnosed with diabetes. Among patients 20–50 years old, prior depression markers were more common in those recently diagnosed with diabetes, but this was not true for those over the age of 50 *(26)*. Everson-Rose et al. *(28)*, following 2662 women in the Study of Women's Health Across the Nation (SWAN) study, reported that depression screener scores were significantly associated with 3-year risk of developing type 2 diabetes in African-American participants but not in Whites *(27)*.

The findings of Arroyo et al. *(28)* were consistent with Willis' hypothesis: among 72,178 participants in the Nurses Health Study, those who had higher depression screener scores were significantly more likely to develop type 2 diabetes over 4 years than participants with lower MHI-5 scores. Kumari et al. *(29)* reported that depression was associated with higher blood glucose levels in people who have normal glucose tolerance (NGT), leading to an increase in the number of people developing impaired glucose tolerance (IGT). In this report on 10,308 civil servants participating in the Whitehall II study, scores on a depression screener predicted a composite measure of type 2 diabetes + new IGT 12 years later, but these scores did not predict developing type 2 diabetes alone.

In a study that included some patients who already had diabetes, Palinkas et al. *(30)* demonstrated not only that depression symptoms at baseline predicted diabetes risk but also that study participants who had type 2 diabetes at baseline were no more likely to be depressed at follow-up than those who did not have diabetes when they entered the study. This is the only study that directly assessed both causal possibilities.

Only Saydah et al. reported findings that provided no support for the hypothesis that depression increases a person's risk for developing type 2 diabetes *(31)*. In this study of 8870 adults who completed a depression screener as part of the National Health and Nutrition Examination Epidemiologic Follow-Up Study, there was no statistically increased incidence of diabetes at 9-year follow-up for those with high or moderate baseline depression screener scores compared with those with no depression symptoms. In this study, reported depression rates were very high (15.9%), and diabetes status at baseline was determined solely by self-report, which might account for the lack of positive findings.

Overall, these studies suggest that depression could well be a risk factor for developing type 2 diabetes, though this effect may vary according to characteristics of the population (i.e., by. age, education, or race/ethnicity), and it might not be present for patients with low levels of depression symptoms. The possibility that depression could increase a person's risk for developing type 2 diabetes appears more likely if one considers risk factors such as BMI and physical activity as *mediators* of depression's effect on diabetes risk (i.e. as mechanisms by which depression affects diabetes risk) rather than considering these risk factors as *confounders* of depression's effect (i.e., as factors to be eliminated in an effort to generate the most accurate estimate of depression's true effect on diabetes risk). If we consider BMI and physical activity to be mechanisms by which depression exerts its effect on diabetes risk, published estimates that control for those factors underestimate depression's true effect.

If depression does increase a person's risk for developing type 2 diabetes, the mechanism for this effect could be behavioral, psychoneurohormonal, or both.

HOW DEPRESSION COULD INCREASE ONE'S RISK
OF DEVELOPING TYPE 2 DIABETES

Behavioral Mechanisms

Depression is associated with behaviors that increase a person's risk of developing type 2 diabetes. For example, depression is associated with physical inactivity *(32–35)* and higher BMI *(36–40)*, and in the Women's Health Study (WHS), BMI and physical inactivity were each independent risk factors for developing diabetes during the 7-year study *(41)*. Physical inactivity can increase diabetes risk indirectly by contributing to weight gain and directly by decreasing insulin sensitivity and impairing glucose metabolism through insulin receptor down-regulation in muscle and inhibited glucose delivery to muscle. Several large randomized controlled trials (RCT) including the Da Qing IGT and Diabetes Study, the Finnish Diabetes Study and the Diabetes Prevention Program, have shown that decreasing BMI and increasing physical activity can reduce the risk of developing type 2 diabetes in those at high risk for the disease *(42–44)*.

Depression is associated with increased smoking, and smoking appears to be associated with an increased risk of developing type 2 diabetes. Most researchers have found higher levels of depression among smokers *(45–48)*. In a 40-year study, the association between smoking and depression was assessed in 1952, 1970, and 1992. In 1992, a smoker was three times more likely to be depressed than a non-smoker *(45)*. Smoking at baseline in this study did not predict the onset of depression, but subjects who became depressed during the 40-year study were more likely to start smoking and less likely to quit than those who had never been depressed. Several studies have found an association between smoking and the risk of developing type 2 diabetes *(49–52)*. In one of the strongest studies that included standardized measures of glucose tolerance to determine incident diabetes, current smokers in the Insulin Resistance Atherosclerosis Study (IRAS) were almost three times as likely to develop type 2 diabetes over 5 years as participants who had never smoked (after multivariate adjustment for other diabetes risk factors) *(49)*. For some reason, this finding did not apply to subjects who entered the study with IGT. Mechanisms by which smoking could increase diabetes risk include inducing hyperglycemia and hyperinsulinemia *(53)*, impaired insulin sensitivity through impaired endothelial function *(54)*, and the effects of cadmium on glucose metabolism *(55)*.

Depression is also associated with sleep disturbances *(56–59)*, but it is unclear whether sleep disturbances are a risk factor for type 2 diabetes. Three studies found that those who slept less (fewer than 5 or 6 h) or more (longer than 9 h) than average (seven or eight hours) had an increased risk of later developing diabetes *(60–62)*; in one of these studies *(61)*, the association remained significant only for long sleep durations after adjustment for BMI and a variety of confounders and was no longer significant for short sleep durations. Other researchers *(63)*, found no association between sleep duration or sleep complaints and diabetes risk in a 32-year follow-up of 1077 women. IGT during sleep deprivation has been demonstrated *(64)*; this could be the mechanism by which sleep problems increase a person's risk for developing diabetes, if these problems have that effect.

PSYCHONEUROHORMONAL MECHANISMS

Depression could also increase a person's risk for developing diabetes through psychoneurohormonal mechanisms. Depression has been called "a stress response gone awry." Stress triggers the release of catecholamines, growth hormone, and glucagon, all of which affect blood glucose levels. In depression, this release is abnormally prolonged. People suffering from depression also experience prolonged elevations in cortisol levels; chronically elevated cortisol levels can contribute to hyperglycemia through a variety of mechanisms, including synergy with other counter-regulatory hormones to stimulate glycogenolysis, gluconeogenesis, lipolysis, and inhibition of peripheral glucose transport and utilization (65). Michelson et al. established that cortisol hypersecretion has clinical consequences when they demonstrated that women who were depressed developed premature osteoporosis, a recognized side effect of elevated cortisol (66). Chronic hypersecretion of cortisol and counter-regulatory hormones could contribute to insulin resistance in patients with major depression (67–70). Winokur et al. (71) demonstrated that during oral glucose tolerance test (OGTT), depressed patients without any diabetes risk factors had a greater increase in plasma glucose levels and a greater decrease in plasma glucagon concentrations than non-depressed individuals.

It is interesting to note that depression is also associated with hypersecretion of proinflammatatory cytokines, including IL-1, IL-6, and tumor necrosis factor-alpha (72), and with the expression of adhesion molecules. Elevated proinflammatory cytokine levels in patients with diabetes are due to increased production by adipose tissue (73) and to age-related increased secretion by monocytes and macrophages (74,75). Cytokine hypersecretion may not only interfere with insulin action and increase diabetes risk but also contribute to increased risk for cardiovascular disease, the leading cause of death in patients with type 2 diabetes.

Conclusions Regarding the Natural History of Depression and Type 2 Diabetes

The current literature provides substantial evidence for the hypothesis that depression increases the risk of developing type 2 diabetes and some evidence for behavioral and psychoneurohormonal mechanisms that might account for this effect. On the other hand, there is evidence that type 2 diabetes does not increase the risk of becoming depressed (30) and that the initial onset of MDD typically precedes the diagnosis of type 2 diabetes by many years (30,76). This does not preclude the possibility that diabetes-related distress contributes to the increased prevalence of depression among people with diabetes (77).

Diabetes-related distress could partially explain the higher recurrence rates and longer duration of MDD and depressive symptoms among those with diabetes *(78)*.

It is possible that the effects of depression on risk for diabetes are appreciable only for those who are already at high risk for diabetes. Depression may worsen glycemic control only among those who already have impairments in glucose tolerance. Or depression may worsen glycemic control in everyone, but this decrement might lead to overt diabetes only in those whose blood glucose levels are already close to the level required for a diagnosis of diabetes.

DOES TREATING DEPRESSION IMPROVE CLINICAL OUTCOMES?

If treating depression could reduce the human and economic toll of comorbid depression and diabetes, this treatment would be a tremendous boon. As noted, depression in patients with diabetes is associated with a broad range of macrovascular and microvascular complications *(79)*. Some studies suggest that depression is not simply associated with complications but may contribute to the development and progression of at least some of them. For example, longitudinal studies have shown that depression is a risk factor for developing retinopathy among children with type 1 diabetes *(80)* and for hospitalization or death over a 3-year period in a study of older adults *(81)*. Others found that depression increased risk for coronary artery disease five-fold among women with diabetes who were followed for 10 years *(11)*. Work problems *(82)* and health care costs are also much higher when a patient with diabetes is depressed *(16)*, and depression is associated with significantly higher rates of death in people with diabetes *(14,15,83)*.

Because we are only beginning to understand the magnitude of depression's impact on clinical outcomes in patients with diabetes, no one seriously considered the possibility of treating depression to improve those outcomes until recently. In fact, until recently we had no evidence from RCT that antidepressant treatment even relieved depression in patients with diabetes because no such studies had been done. The results of these studies are described below and shown in Table 2.

Beginning in 1997, investigators at Washington University School of Medicine (St. Louis, Missouri) conducted three separate, short-term (8–10 weeks), controlled clinical trials to assess the efficacy of tricyclic antidepressants (nortriptyline) *(84)*, selective serotonin reuptake inhibitors (SSRIs) (fluoxetine) *(85)*, and psychotherapy (cognitive behavior therapy or CBT) *(86)* for major depression in people with diabetes.

Table 2
Effect of Depression Treatment on Clinical Outcomes

Study	Subjects (n)	Treatment	Effect on depression	Effect on clinical outcomes
Lustman et al., 1997	Type 1 (14); type 2 (14)	Nortripyline versus placebo (8 weeks)	n > p: reduction in depression screener scores, proportion with depression remission	A1c levels increased in n > p
Lustman et al., 2000	Type 1 (26); type 2 (34)	Fluoxetine versus placebo (8 weeks)	F > p: reduction in depression screener scores, proportion with significant improvement	Trend (p = 0.13): A1c levels decreased in F > p
Lustman et al., 1998	Type 2 (51)	CBT[a] + DE[b] versus DE alone (10 weeks)	CBT + DE > DE alone: proportion with depression remission	A1c levels decreased in CBT + DE > DE alone
Katon et al., 2004	Type 2 (315); type 1(14)	DCM[c] versus UC[d](12 months)	DCM > UC: reduction in depression severity	NSD A1c levels DCM versus UC
Williams et al., 2004	Type not specified (417)	DCM[c] versus UC[d](12 months)	DCM > UC: reduction in depression severity	NSD A1c levels DCM versus UC

[a] Cognitive behavioral therapy.
[b] Diabetes education.
[c] Depression case management.
[d] Usual care.

CBT is designed to help patients identify mistaken and maladaptive thoughts and to replace these thoughts with more accurate and adaptive ones. CBT is also designed to increase patients' engagement in enjoyable activities, and it has been shown to improve depression in the general population (87–89). In the cognitive therapy study (86), the control treatment was an educational intervention combined with supportive counseling, provided by nurses and diabetes educators. The actively treated group received both the CBT and the education/support intervention; the control group received only the latter.

In each study, patients receiving depression treatment (nortripyline, fluoxetine, or CBT) had a significantly higher rate of depression remission compared with the control group (nortriptyline, 57% vs. 35%; fluoxetine, 62% vs. 31%; and cognitive therapy, 85% vs. 27%).

Effects of depression treatment on A1C were mixed in these studies. Nortritpyline had a hyperglycemic effect; fluoxetine use was associated with a trend toward lower A1c levels; and CBT was associated with significantly lower A1C levels compared with control treatments. Nortriptyline improved depression, but A1c levels rose during the 8-week study in the nortriptyline group while they remained stable in the control patients. Path analysis that included all subjects revealed a substantial (0.8–1.2%) reduction in A1C level attributable to depression remission that was offset by an increase of similar magnitude in A1C attributable to nortriptyline treatment. In the fluoxetine study there was a trend (p = .13) toward greater A1C reduction among actively treated patients compared with controls. In the CBT + DE study those in the active treatment arm had a greater reduction in A1C levels compared with controls 6 months after the intervention ended (–0.9 vs +0.7%; p = 0.04).

Although these studies were well controlled, the number of patients involved was small, so statistical power was limited. Very recently, other researchers have studied the benefits of depression treatment in RCT that included more patients with diabetes; their findings confirm the effectiveness of depression treatment while providing little support for the hypothesis that this treatment lowers A1C levels. In the Pathways Study, 329 patients with diabetes and depression were randomized to a depression case management intervention or to usual care (90). The case management intervention was an individualized treatment program run by specially trained nurses who were supervised by psychiatrists and psychologists. Patients began treatment by choosing either short-term counseling with the nurse (following a structured intervention protocol) or antidepressant medication; the treatment was adjusted as needed. Depression symptom and A1C levels were assessed at baseline and 3, 6, and 12 months later. Patients receiving the depression intervention reported less depression severity over time than patients receiving usual care, but both groups had identical reductions in A1C levels during the study (baseline $7.99 \pm 1.55\%$; 6-month assessment $7.58 \pm 1.47\%$; and 12-month assessment $7.64 \pm 1.57\%$).

The Improving Mood-Promoting Access to Collaborative Treatment (IMPACT) Study included 417 people with diabetes and used a design nearly identical to that used in the Pathways Study *(91)*. The results of this study were also very similar—patients assigned to the active intervention had less severe depression at 12-month follow-up than those receiving usual care, but HA1C levels declined to the same small degree in both groups (baseline 7.28 $\pm$ 1.43% and 12-month assessment 7.11 $\pm$ 1.38%).

Only one of the five studies described above found that depression treatment lowered A1C levels. In that study, the only one that used counseling as the exclusive intervention, mean baseline A1C level was 10.2% in the CBT group and 10.4% in the control group, much higher levels than are seen in most patients today. By contrast, the A1C levels of patients in the more recent larger trials were lower (7.3–8.0%) than seen in many settings. Taken together, these studies do not provide much support for the idea that depression treatment, especially medication, will improve A1C levels for most patients, especially those in reasonably good glycemic control.

Although these findings might be considered discouraging, it should be noted that earlier small RCT found that fluoxetine treatment lowered A1C *(92–94)* or increased insulin sensitivity *(95)*. It is also worth noting that in the Pathways study, where A1c levels went down about 0.35% in both groups, about half of the patients in the usual care arm were taking antidepressants as part of their usual care. In addition, 45% of the patients in the intervention group still had significant depression symptoms at 12-month follow-up, so more intensive antidepressant treatment might have yielded additional glycemic benefits. This suggests that study findings might underestimate the true effect of depression treatment. Even if this is true, it is clear in patients with good glucose control that it almost certainly requires enhanced diabetes self-management training as well optimal depression treatment to lower A1C levels.

We should also keep in mind that depression could affect outcomes other than A1C levels. We know, for example, that cardiovascular disease is expressed earlier in the course of diabetes in patients who are also depressed *(96)*; would treating depression protect patients from this process? Studies to address this question would be ambitious undertakings, given the length of time (and the very large number of patients) required to answer questions about long-term cardiovascular outcomes.

Depression treatment might also improve work productivity, another important outcome. Depression has a negative impact on work productivity in people with diabetes *(97)*, and primary care-based depression management incorporating a nurse case manager resulted in an annual improvement in productivity and reduced absenteeism of $2601 in a group of patients not selected for having diabetes *(98)*. The costs of the intervention were not specified, but studies like this one have encouraged a few large health insurance companies to begin paying for depression management programs, including paying primary care physicians additional fees to screen patients for depression and to provide follow-up consultation to patients who are prescribed antidepressant medication or in more severe cases referred to a psychiatrist or psychologist. One large insurer eventually plans to offer this program nationwide *(99)*.

CONCLUSIONS

Depression appears to be a likely risk factor for developing type 2 diabetes, though many important questions about this relationship remain unanswered, including the level of depression symptoms required to increase diabetes risk (some have suggested that mild depression does not have an effect), the magnitude of the depression-related risk (some found only statistically non-significant effects), whether depression elevates diabetes risk only in certain demographic populations (some found depression effects risk only in African Americans, younger patients, or those with less education), and the degree to which behavioral and psychoneurohormonal factors mediate the relationship between depression and diabetes risk.

Studies designed to answer these questions should include a population sufficiently large and diverse to allow assessment of demographic variation in depression-related diabetes risk. Participants ought to have an oral glucose tolerance test to objectively determine their precise metabolic status at baseline and during follow-up (a procedure not used in some previous studies). In addition, the severity of depressive symptoms should be assessed, by means of diagnostic interview if possible. Depression has cognitive, emotional, and vegetative symptoms. Future research should determine whether each type of symptom has the same association with diabetes risk.

Studies should also assess mechanisms that might explain the relationship between diabetes and depression, should one be observed. For example, one could test the theory that chronic mild cortisol excess causes the deterioration of glucose tolerance leading to type 2 diabetes. At least in the early stages of progressive glucose intolerance, agents that block cortisol secretion or cortisol action should ameliorate glucose metabolism in some depressed patients. In patients with abnormal cortisol function, blocking cortisol should improve glucose tolerance; in patients with normal cortisol function it should have no effect on glucose tolerance. This approach could help determine whether cortisol hypersecretion causes both depression and glucose intolerance or depression leads to cortisol hypersecretion, which leads to glucose intolerance (and perhaps worsened depression as well) Answering these questions could lead to new treatments for preventing type 2 diabetes.

Depression in patients with diabetes can be treated effectively with medication or counseling (84–85,90–91). To date most randomized clinical trials found that depression treatment was not associated with a greater reduction in A1C levels than usual care (84–85,90–91), though the populations in recent large trials had rather low A1C levels at baseline, and many patients in the usual care groups received depression treatment. Future studies should address important unanswered questions, including the effect of depression treatment on outcomes other than A1C level (e.g., level of functioning, complications, health care utilization, and mortality), the effects of treatment rather than treatment arm (to deal with the fact that in RCT many usual care patients receive treatment), the efficacy of therapy rather than its effectiveness (to deal with the fact that treatment in treatment arms of studies is often suboptimal), and the effects of combined antidepressant treatment and diabetes self-management training on clinical outcomes.

This review has clinical implications. It indicates the potential benefits of depression screening in those at high risk for developing type 2 diabetes, because in this case, depression may well represent an additional diabetes risk factor. Depression treatment should always be provided to patients who need it, and it could prevent or delay the development of diabetes in some individuals. Recognizing depression as an additional diabetes risk factor should also heighten the clinician's attention to reducing other risk factors.

The association between depression and bad outcomes in those who already have diabetes means clinicians should regularly screen patients for depression. The clinician can identify patients likely to be depressed by asking two questions about mood and anhedonia (the diagnostic and statistical manual (DSM) -IV cardinal diagnostic criteria): "During the past 2 weeks, have you felt down, depressed, or hopeless?" and "During the past 2 weeks, have you felt little interest or pleasure in doing things?" Positive responses to one or both questions should trigger questions about the remaining seven DSM-IV symptoms, verifying the severity, frequency, and duration of any symptoms that are present. Screening questionnaires may also be used before seeing the patient to guide the discussion or determine whether the issue needs discussion or after seeing the patient to confirm or document impressions.

Clinicians can choose from a variety of validated self-report questionnaires for depression screening. Most patients can complete one of these questionnaires in <5 min; scoring takes <2 minutes, so results are available to discuss at the same visit. One of the most widely used of these, especially in recent years, is the Patient Health Questionnaire-9 (PHQ-9) *(100)*, which has questions that match the DSM-IV diagnostic criteria for depression.

Patients identified as depressed should be treated or referred for treatment. In 1994, 60% of patients being treated for depression received antidepressant medication; 10 years later, the figure was over 80%. All commonly prescribed antidepressant agents seem to be similarly effective when it comes to relieving depression, so prescription decisions should be based on the patient's prior experience with these agents, cost, and likely side-effects. Tricyclic antidepressants and similar agents are more likely to contribute to sleepiness and weight gain, and more likely to be associated with cardiac toxicity than bupropion or the SSRIs and related agents (SSNRI and SSRIB), though some of the latter agents also cause weight gain. Some SSRI and related agents have also been associated with sexual problems in both men and women *(101,102)*. Effective treatment is more likely when (i) the dose is titrated (patients are often exquisitely sensitive to side-effects and may stop treatment as a result); (ii) patients understand that side-effects will diminish (and that full therapeutic effect will not be felt for a few weeks); and (iii) insomnia is treated proactively (begin a sleep normalizing agent along with the antidepressant). As noted, counseling, especially CBT, is also a proven treatment for depression in patients with diabetes *(86)*.

In summary, depression appears to be a risk factor for diabetes, depression can be treated effectively in people with diabetes, and this treatment could help reduce the great and growing human and economic toll of comorbid depression and diabetes.

REFERENCES

1. Egede LE, Zheng D. Independent factors associated with major depressive disorder in a national sample. *Diabetes Care* 2003, 26:104–111.
2. Kessler RC, Berglund P, Demler O, Demler O, Jin R, Koretz D, Merikangas KR, Rush AJ, Walters EE, Wang PS. The epidemiology of major depressive disorder: results from the National Comorbidity Replication (NCS–R). *JAMA* 2003, 289:3095–3105.
3. Anderson RJ, Freedland KE, Clouse RE, Lustman PJ. The prevalence of comorbid depression in adults with diabetes. *Diabetes Care* 2001, 24:1069–1078.
4. Ciechanowski PS, Katon WJ, Russo JE. Depression and diabetes: impact of depressive symptoms on adherence, function, and costs. *Arch Intern Med* 2000, 160:3278–3285.
5. Ciechanowski PS, Katon WJ, Russo JE, Hirsch IB. The relationship of depressive symptoms to symptom reporting, self-care and glucose control in diabetes. *Gen Hosp Psychiatry* 2003, 25:246–252.
6. Kilbourne AM, Reynolds CF, Good CB, Sereika SM, Justice AC, Fine MJ. How does depression influence diabetes medication adherence in older patients? *Am J Geriatr Psychiatry* 2005, 13:202–210.

7. Lustman PJ, Anderson RJ, Freedland KE, De Groot M, Carney RM, Clouse RE. Depression and poor glycemic control: a meta-analytic review of the literature. *Diabetes Care* 2000, 23:934–942.

8. de Groot M, Anderson R, Freedland KE, Clouse RE, Lustman PJ. Association of depression and diabetes complications: a meta-analysis. *Psychosom Med* 2001, 63: 619–630.

9. Black SA, Markides KS, Ray LA. Depression predicts increased incidence of adverse health outcomes in older Mexican Americans with type 2 diabetes. *Diabetes Care* 2005, 28:2822–2828.

10. Rosenthal MJ, Fajardo M, Gilmore S, Morley JE, Naliboff BD: Hospitalization and mortality of diabetes in older adults. A 3-year prospective study. *Diabetes Care* 1998, 21:231–235.

11. Clouse RE, Lustman PJ, Freedland KE, Griffith LS, McGill JB, Carney RM. Depression and coronary heart disease in women with diabetes. *Psychosom Med* 2003, 65:376–383.

12. Wingard DL, Barrett-Connor E: Heart disease and diabetes. In: Harris MI, Editor, 2nd Ed., *Diabetes in America*, Bethesda, MD: National Institutes of Health. 1995, p. 429–48.

13. Tuncell K, Bradley CK, Nerenz D, Williams LK, Pladevall M, LaFata JE. The impact of diabetes on employment and work productivity. *Diabetes Care* 2005, 28:2662–2667.

14. Zhang X, Norris SL, Gregg EW, Cheng YJ, Beckles G, Kahn HS. Depressive symptoms and mortality among persons with and without diabetes. *Am J Epidemiol* 2005, 161: 652–660.

15. Katon WJ, Rutter C, Simon G, Lin EHB, Ludman E, Chiechanowski P, Kinder L, Young B, Von Korff M. The association of comorbid depression with mortality in patients with type 2 diabetes. *Diabetes Care* 2005, 28:2668–2672.

16. Egede LE, Zheng D, Simpson K: Comorbid depression is associated with increased health care use and expenditures in individuals with diabetes. *Diabetes Care* 2002, 25:464–470.

17. Willis T. *Diabetes*: A Medical *Odyssey*, New York: Tuckahoe. 1971.

18. Menninger WC. Psychologic factors in the etiology of diabetes. *J Nerv Ment Dis* 1935, 81:1–13.

19. Slawson DF, Flynn WR, Kollar EJ. Psychologic factors associated with the onset of diabetes mellitus. *JAMA* 1963, 185:166–170.

20. Kovacs M, Obrosky DS, Goldston D, Drash A. Major depressive disorder in youths with IDDM: a controlled prospective study of course and outcome. *Diabetes Care* 1997, 2045–2051.

21. Jacobson AM, Hauser ST, Wertlieb D, Wolfsdorf JI, Orleans J, Vieyra M. Psychological adjustment of children with recently diagnosed diabetes mellitus. *Diabetes Care* 1986, 9:323–329.

22. Eaton WE, Armenian H, Gallo J, Pratt L, Ford DE. Depression and risk of onset of type II diabetes: a prospective population-based study. *Diabetes Care* 1996, 19:1097–1102.

23. Kawakami N, Takatsuka N, Shimizu H, Ishibashi H. Depressive symptoms and the occurrence of type 2 diabetes among Japanese men. *Diabetes Care* 1999, 22:1071–1076.

24. Golden SH, Williams JE, Ford DE, Yeh H, Sanford CP, Nieto FJ, Brancatti, FL. Depressive symptoms and the risk of type 2 diabetes: the Atherosclerosis Risk in Communities study. *Diabetes Care* 2004, 27:429–435.

25. Carnethon MR, Kinder LS, Fair JM, Stafford RS, Fortmann SP. Symptoms of depression as a risk factor for incident diabetes: findings from the National Health and Nutrition Examination Epidemiologic Follow-Up Study, 1971–1992. *Am J Epidemiol* 2003, 158:416–423.

26. Brown LC, Majumdar SR, Newman SC, Johnson JA. History of depression increases risk of type 2 diabetes in younger adults. *Diabetes Care* 2005, 28:1063–1067.

27. Everson-Rose SA, Meyer PM, Powell LH, Pandey D, Torrens JI, Kravitz HM, Bromberger JT, Matthews KA. Depressive symptoms, insulin resistance, and risk of diabetes in women in midlife. *Diabetes Care* 2003, 26:2856–2862.

28. Arroyo C, Hu FB, Ryan LM, Kawachi I, Colditz GA, Speizer FE, Manson J. Depressive symptoms and risk of type 2 diabetes in women. *Diabetes Care* 2004, 27:129–133.

29. Kumari M, Head J, Marmot M. Prospective study of social and other risk factors for incidence of type 2 diabetes in the Whitehall II Study. *Arch Intern Med* 2004, 164:1873–1880.

30. Palinkas LA, Lee PP, Barrett-Connor E. A prospective study of type 2 diabetes and depressive symptoms in the elderly: the Rancho Bernardo Study. *Diabet Med* 2004, 11:1185–1191.

31. Saydah SH, Brancatti FL, Golden SH, Fradkin J, Harris MI. Depressive symptoms and the risk of type 2 diabetes mellitus in a US sample. *Diabetes Metab Res Rev* 2003, 19:202–208.

32. Yancey AK, Wold CM, McCarthy WJ, Weber MD, Lee B, Simon PA, Fielding JE. Physical inactivity and overweight among Los Angeles County adults. *Am J Prev Med* 2004, 27:183–184.

33. Garrett NA, Brasure M, Schmitz KH, Schultz MM, Huber MR. Physical inactivity: direct cost to plan. *Am J Prev Med* 2004, 27:304–309.

34. Wang G, Brown DR. Impact of physical activity on medical expenditures among adults downhearted and blue. *Am J Health Behav* 2004, 3:208–217.

35. Fukukawa Y, Nakashima C, Tsuboi S, Kozakai R, Doyo W, Niino N, Ando F, Shimokata H. Age differences in the effect of physical activity on depressive symptoms. *Psychol Aging* 2004, 19:346–351.

36. McElroy SL, Kotwal R, Malhotra S, Nelson EB, Keck PE, Nemeroff CB. Are mood disorders and obesity related? A review for mental health professionals. *J Clin Psychiatry* 2004, 65:634–651.

37. Johnston E, Johnson S, McLeod P, Johnston M. The relation of body mass index to depressive symptoms. *Can J Public Health* 2004, 95:179–183.

38. Dong C, Sanchez LE, Price RA. Relationship of obesity to depression: a family-based study. *Int J Obes Relat Metab Disord* 2004, 28:790–795.

39. Roberts RE, Deleger S, Strawbridge WJ, Kaplan GA. Prospective association between obesity and depression: evidence from the Alameda County Study. *Int J Obes Relat Metab Disord* 2004, 28:514–521.

40. Stunkard AJ, Faith MS, Allison KC. Depression and obesity. *Biol Psychiatry* 2003, 54:330–337.

41. Weinstein AR, Sesso HD, Lee IM, Cook NR, Manson JE, Buring JE, Gaziano JM. Relationship of physical activity vs body mass index with type 2 diabetes in women. *JAMA* 2004, 292:1188–1194.

42. Pan XR, Li GW, Hu YH, Wang JX, Yang WY, An ZX, Hu ZX, Lin J, Xiao JZ, Cao HB, Liu PA, Jiang XG, Jiang YY, Wang JP, Zheng H, Zhang H, Bennett PH, Howard BV. Effects of diet and exercise in preventing NIDDM in people with impaired glucose tolerance. The Da Qing IGT and diabetes study. *Diabetes Care* 1997, 20:537–44.

43. Tuomiletho J, Lindstorm J, Riksson JG, Valle TT, Hamalainein H, Ilanne-Parikka P, Keinanen-Kiukaaniemi S, Laakso M, Louheranta A, Rastas M, Salminen V, Uusitupa M. Prevention of type 2 diabetes mellitus by changes in lifestyle among subjects with impaired glucose tolerance. *N Engl J Med* 2001, 344:1343–1350.

44. Knowler WC, Barrett-Connor E, Fowler SE, Hamman RH, Lachin JM, Walker EA, Nathan D for the Diabetes Prevention Program Research group. Reduction in the incidence

of type 2 diabetes with lifestyle intervention or metformin. *N Engl J Med* 2002, 346: 393–403.

45. Murphy JM, Horton NJ, Monson RR, Laird NM, Sobol AM, Leighton AH. Cigarette smoking in relation to depression: historical trends from the Sterling County Study. *Am J Psychiatry* 2003, 160:1663–1669.

46. La Rosa E, Consoli SM, Clesiau H, Soufi K, Lagrue G. Psychosocial distress and stressful life antecedents associated with smoking: a survey of subjects consulting a preventive health center (article in French). *Presse Med* 2004, 33:919–926.

47. Benjet C, Wagner FA, Borges GG, Medina-Mora ME. The relationship of tobacco smoking with depressive symptomatology in the Third Mexican National Addictions Survey. *Psychol Med* 2004, 34:881–888.

48. Haas AL, Eng C, Dowling G, Schmitt E, Hall SM. The relationship between smoking history and current functioning in disabled community-living older adults. *Ann Behav Med* 2005, 29:166–173.

49. Foy CG, Bell RA, Farmer DF, Goff DC, Wagenknecht LE. Smoking and incidence of diabetes among US adults: findings from the Insulin Resistance Atherosclerosis Study. *Diabetes Care* 2005, 28:2501–2507.

50. Manson JE, Ajani UA, Liu S, Nathan DM, Hennekens CH. A prospective study of cigarette smoking and the incidence of diabetes mellitus among US male physicians. *Am J Med* 2000, 109:538–542.

51. Wannamethee SG, Shaper AG, Perry IJ. Smoking as a modifiable risk factor for type 2 diabetes in middle-aged men. *Diabetes Care* 2001, 28:1590–1595.

52. Rimm EB, Chan J, Stamfer MJ, Colditz GA, Willett WC. Prospective study of smoking, alcohol use, and the risk of diabetes in men. *BMJ* 1995, 310:555–559.

53. Fratti AC, Iniestra F, Ariza CR. Acute effect of cigarette smoking on glucose tolerance and other cardiovascular risk factors. *Diabetes Care* 1996, 19:112–118.

54. Celermajer DS, Sorensen KE, Georgakopoulous D, Bull C, Thonas O, Robinson J, Deanfield JE. Cigarette smoking is associated with dose-related and potentially reversible impairment of endothelium-dependent dilation in healthy young adults. *Circulation* 1993, 88:2149–2155.

55. Schwartz GG, Il'yasova D, Ivanova A. Urinary cadmium, impaired fasting glucose, and diabetes in the NHANES III. *Diabetes Care* 2003, 26:468–470.

56. Quan SF, Katz R, Olson J, Bonekat W, Enright PL, Young T, Newman A. Factors associated with incidence and persistence of symptoms of disturbed sleep in an elderly cohort: the Cardiovascular Health Study. *Am J Med Sci* 2005, 329:163–172.

57. Spoormaker VI, van den Bout J. Depression and anxiety complaints: relations with sleep disturbances. *Eur Psychiatry* 2005, 20:243–245.

58. Foley D, Ancoli-Israel S, Britz P, Walsh J. Sleep disturbances and chronic disease in older adults: results of the 2003 National Sleep Foundation Sleep in America Survey. *Psychosom Res* 2004, 56:497–502.

59. Buyesse DJ. Insomnia and depression in aging: assessing sleep in older adults. *Geriatrics* 2004, 59:47–51.

60. Gottlieb DJ, Punjabi NM, Newman AB, REsnick HE, Redline S, Baldwin CM, Nieto FJ. Association of sleep time with diabetes mellitus and impaired glucose tolerance. *Arch Intern Med* 2005, 165:863–867.

61. Ayas NT, White DP, Al-Delaimy WK, Manson JE, Stampfer MJ, Speizer FE, Patel S, Hu FB. A prospective study of self-reported sleep duration and incident diabetes in women. *Diabetes Care* 2003, 26:380–384.

62. Nilsson PM, Roost M, Engstrom G, Hedblad B, Berglund G. Incidence of diabetes in middle-aged men is related to sleep disturbances. *Diabetes Care* 2004, 27:2464–2469.

63. Bjorkelund C, Bondyr-Carlsson D, Lapidus L, Lissner L, Mansson J, Skoog I, Bengtsson C. *Diabetes Care* 2005, 28:2739–2744.

64. Spiegel K, Leproult R, Van Cauter E. Impact of sleep debt on metabolic and endocrine function. *Lancet* 1999, 23:1435–1439.

65. Musselman DL, Betan E, Larsen H, Phillips LS. Relationship of depression to diabetes types 1 and 2: epidemiology, biology, and treatment. *Biol Psychiatry* 2003, 54:317–329.

66. Michelson D, Startakis C, Hill L, Reynolds J, Galliven E, Chrousos G, Gold P. Bone mineral density in women with depression. *N Engl J Med* 1996, 335:1176–1181.

67. DeFronzo R, Sherwin RS, Felig P. Synergistic interactions of counterregulatory hormones: a mechanism for stress hyperglycemia. *Acta Chir Scand* 1980, 498 (supplement):33–42.

68. Brindley DN, Rolland Y. Possible connections between stress, diabetes, obesity, hypertension and altered lipoprotein metabolism that may result in atherosclerosis. *Clin Sci* 1989, 77:453–461.

69. Weinstein SP, Paquin T, Pritsker A, Haber RA. Glucocorticoid-induced insulin resistance: dexamethsone inhibits the activation of glucose transport in rat skeletal muscle by both insulin- and non-insulin-related stimuli. *Diabetes* 1995, 44:441–445.

70. Dimitriadis G, Leighton B, Parry-Billings M, Sasson S, Young M, Krause U, Bevan S, Piva T, Wegener G, Newsholme EA. Effects of glucocorticoid excess on the sensitivity of glucose transport and metabolism to insulin in skeletal muscle. *Biochem J* 1997, 321:707–712.

71. Winokur A, Maislin G, Phillips JL, Amsterdam JD. Insulin resistance after oral glucose tolerance testing in patients with major depression. *Am J Psychiatry* 1988, 145:325–330.

72. Ross R. Atherosclerosis: an inflammatory disease.*N Engl J Med* 1999, 340:115–126.

73. Fried SK, Bunkin DA, Greenburg AS. Omental and subcutaneous adipose tissue of obese subjects release interleukin-6: depot differences and regulation by glucocorticoid. *J Clin Endocrinol Metab* 1998, 83:847–850.

74. Fernandez-Real JM, Vayreda M, Richart C, Gutierrez C, Broch M, Vendrell J, Ricart W. Circulating interleukin-6 levels, blood pressure, and insulin sensitivity in apparently healthy men and women. *J Clin Endocrinol Metab* 2001, 86:1154–1159.

75. Paolisso G, Rizzo MR, Mazziotti G, Tagliamonte MR, Gambardella A, Rotondi M, Carella C, Giugliano D, Varricchio M, D'Onofrio F. Advancing age and insulin resistance: role of tumor necrosis factor alpha. *Am J Physiol* 1998, 275:E294–E299.

76. Talbot F, Nouwen A. A review of the relationship between depression and diabetes in adults: is there a link? *Diabetes Care* 2000, 23:1556–1562.

77. Engum A, Mykletun A, Midthjell K, Holen A, Dahl AA. Depression and diabetes: a large population-based study of sociodemographic, lifestyle, and clinical factors associated with depression in type 1 and type 2 diabetes. *Diabetes Care* 2005, 28:1904–1909.

78. Rubin RR, Ciechanowski P, Egede LE, Lin EHB, Lustman PJ. Recognizing and treating depression in patients with diabetes. *Curr Diab Rep* 2004, 4:119–125.

79. de Groot M, Anderson R, Freedland KE, Clouse RE, Lustman PJ. Association of depression and diabetes complications: a meta-analysis. *Psychosom Med* 2001, 63: 619–630.

80. Kovacs M, Mukerji P, Drash A, Iyengar S: Biomedical and psychiatric risk factors for retinopathy among children with IDDM. *Diabetes Care* 1995, 18:1592–1599.

81. Rosenthal MJ, Fajardo M, Gilmore S, Morley JE, Naliboff BD. Hospitalization and mortality of diabetes in older adults. A 3-year prospective study. *Diabetes Care* 1998, 21:231–235.

82. Von Korff M, Katon W, Linn EHB, Simon G, Ciechanowski P, Ludman E, Oliver M, Rutter C, Young B. Work disability among individuals with diabetes. *Diabetes Care* 2005, 28:2464–2469.

83. Egede LE, Nietert PJ, Zheng D. Depression and all-cause mortality and coronary heart disease mortality among adults with and without diabetes. *Diabetes Care* 2005, 28: 1339–1345.

84. Lustman PJ, Griffith LS, Clouse RE, Freedland KE, Eisen SA, Rubin EH, Carney RM, McGill JB. Effects of nortriptyline on depression and glycemic control in diabetes: results of a double-blind, placebo-controlled trial. *Psychosom Med* 1997, 59:241–250.

85. Lustman PJ, Freedland KE, Griffith LS, Clouse RE. Fluoxetine for depression in diabetes: a randomized, double-blind, placebo-controlled trial. *Diabetes Care* 2000, 23: 618–623.

86. Lustman PJ, Griffith LS, Freedland KE, Kissel SS, Clouse RE. Cognitive behavior therapy for depression in type 2 diabetes mellitus: a randomized, controlled trial. *Ann Intern Med* 1998, 129:613 –621.

87. Toner BB, Segal ZV, Emmott S, Myran D, Ali A, DiGasbarro I, Stuckless N. Cognitive-behavioral group therapy for patients with irritable bowel syndrome. *Int J Group Psychother* 1998, 38:215–243.

88. Turk DC, Meichenbaum D, Genest M. *Pain and Behavioral Medicine: A Cognitive-Behavioral Perspective*, New York: Guilford Press. 1978.

89. Carney RM, Freedland KE, Stein PK, Skala JA, Hoffman P, Jaffe AS. Change in heart rate and heart rate variability during treatment for depression in patients with coronary heart disease. *Psychosom Med* 2000, 62: 639–647.

90. Katon WJ, Von Korff M, Lin EHB, Simon G, Ludman E, Russo J, Ciechanowski P, Walker E, Bush T. The pathways study: a randomized trial of collaborative care in patients with diabetes and depression. *Arch Gen Psychiatry* 2004, 61:1042–1049.

91. Williams JW, Katon W, Lin EHB, Noel PH, Worschel J, Connell J, Harpole L, Fultz BA, Hunkeler E, Mika VS, Unutzer J. The effectiveness of depression care management on diabetes-related outcomes in older patients. *Ann Intern Med* 2004, 140:1015–1024.

92. Gray DS, Fujioka K, Devine W, Bray GA. Fluoxetine treatment of the obese diabetic. *Int J Obesity* 1992, 16:193–198.

93. O'Kane M, Wiles PG, Wales JK. Fluoxetine treatment of obese type 2 diabetic patients. *Diabet Med* 1994, 11:105–110.

94. Connolly VM, Gallagher A, Kesson CM. A study of fluoxetine in obese elderly patients with type 2 diabetes. *Diab Med* 1995, 12:416–418.

95. Maheux P, Ducros F, Bourque J, Garon J, Chiasson JL. Fluoxetine improves insulin sensitivity in obese patients with non-insulin dependent diabetes mellitus independently of weight loss. *Int J Obesity* 1997, 21:97–102.

96. Forrest KYZ, Becker DJ, Kuller LH, Wolfson SK, Orchard TJ. Are predictors of coronary heart disease and lower-extermity arterial disease in type 1 diabetes the same? A prospective study. *Atherosclerosis* 2000, 148:158–169.

97. Von Korff M, Katon W, Lin EHB, Simon G, Ciechanowski P, Ludman E, Oliver M, Rutter C, Young B. Work disability among individuals with diabetes. *Diabetes Care* 2005, 28:1326–1332.

98. Rost K, Smith JL, Dickinson M. The effect of improving primary care depression management on employee absenteeism and productivity: a randomized trial. *Medical Care* 2004, 42:1202–1210.

99. Freudenheim M. Aetna to pay for program to manage depression. *New York Times*, November 2, 2005.

100. Spitzer RL, Kroenke K, Williams JBW, et al. Validation and utility of a self-report version of the PRIME-MD: the PHQ Primary Care Study. *JAMA* 1999, 282:1737–1744.
101. Rosen RC, Lane RM, Menza M. Effects of SSRI on sexual function: a critical review. *J Clin Psychopharmacol* 1999, 21:241–242.
102. Rudkin L, Taylor MJ, Hawton K. Strategies for managing sexual dysfunction induced by antidepressant medication. *Cochran Database Syst Rev* 2004, 18(4):CD003382.

INDEX

Printed in the United States of America.